The Management of Terminal
Malignant Disease

The Management of Terminal Malignant Disease

Cicely Saunders, OM, DBE, FRCP,
Chairman, St Christopher's Hospice, London

and

Nigel Sykes, MA, MRCGP
Consultant Physician, St Christopher's
Hospice, London

Edward Arnold
A member of the Hodder Headline Group
LONDON BOSTON SYDNEY AUCKLAND

Edward Arnold is a division of Hodder Headline PLC
338 Euston Road, London NW1 3BH

© 1993 Edward Arnold

First published in the United Kingdom 1984
Third edition 1993

3 5 7 6 4
95 97 99 98 96

Distributed in the Americas by Little, Brown and Company,
34 Beacon Street, Boston MA 02108

British Library Cataloguing in Publication Data
Management of Terminal Malignant Disease. - 3Rev.ed
I. Saunders, Dame Cicely   II. Sykes, Nigel
362.196994

ISBN 0 340 56354 0

Whilst the advice and information in this book is believed to be true and
accurate at the date of going to press, neither the author nor the publisher
can accept any legal responsibility for any errors or omissions that may
be made. In particular (but without limiting the generality of the
preceding disclaimer) every effort has been made to check drug dosages;
however, it is still possible that errors have been missed. Furthermore,
dosage schedules are constantly being revised and new side effects
recognised. For these reasons the reader is strongly urged to consult the
drug companies' printed instructions before administering any of the
drugs recommended in this book.

Typeset in 10/11 Palatino by Anneset, Weston-super-Mare, Avon
Printed and bound in the United Kingdom by
St Edmundsbury Press Ltd, Bury St Edmunds, Suffolk and
J W Arrowsmith Ltd, Bristol

Preface

The last two editions of this book established themselves as authoritative and inclusive guides for those seeking to provide palliative care. This edition has been almost entirely re-written in order to fulfil the same objectives and to widen its usefulness among the many disciplines whose combined contributions are needed to make good palliation a reality for those with terminal malignant disease.

For this edition, the founding Editor has been joined by Dr. Nigel Sykes who works with her at St. Christopher's Hospice, London. As before, most of the contributors are connected with St. Christopher's, being either past or present members of staff or being known to the hospice for the helpful application of expertise in their own fields to the needs of palliative care. The Editors are very grateful to all the authors for their work and patience.

Although the formation of this book has been centred in a hospice, not all its contributors work in a hospice setting. Much of what is written here is relevant to those working in the community or in general hospitals, whether in a specialist palliative care role or in another specialty. Indeed, it is increasingly recognised that the principles of cancer palliation have relevance to people with a wide range of terminal diseases, and this is the concern of the book's final chapter. We hope that those in many fields of medicine who have in their care patients with incurable progressive diseases may find this volume of use and be able to extrapolate from it to their own practice.

Even since the second edition of this book, palliative care has expanded greatly as a specialist area both in the United Kingdom and throughout the world. New services are being developed in forms that are shaped by the needs of their local community. The number of health care professionals who have become aware of palliative care and who seek to gain relevant knowledge is increasing correspondingly. Both as a consequence of, and a stimulus to, these changes the public expectation of what palliation can achieve is deepening. The Editors hope that this new edition will be a helpful support to those who are participating in these developments and that, through them, it may benefit terminally ill people and their families.

Dame Cicely Saunders and Nigel Sykes
January 1993

Contents

9. Ethical and Legal considerations

10. Wider Applications of Palliative Care *Robert Dunlop*

Contributors

Mary J. Baines, OBE., MRCP.,
Consultant Physician, St. Christopher's Hospice, London

Peter Byrne, BA., B.Phil.,
Senior Lecturer in the Philosophy of Religion, King's College, London

Bruce Cleminson, DRCOG., MRCGP.,
General Practitioner, Scalloway, Shetland Isles

Robert Dunlop, FRACP.,
Medical Director, St. Christopher's Hospice, London

Anne Gibson, Dip. COT.,
Day Centre Manager, St. Christopher's Hospice, London

Carol Haigh, RGN., DPSN., FETC., BSC(Hons.),
Nurse Teacher, Department of Continuing Education, Blackpool Campus,
Lancashire College of Nursing and Health Studies

Louis Heyse-Moore, DObstRCOG., DCH., MRCGP., MRCP.,
Medical Director, St. Joseph's Hospice, London

Josephine Hockley, SRN., MSc.,
Clinical Nurse Specialist (palliative care), Western General Hospital,
Edinburgh

Gail Hodgson, PhD., MRCPsych.,
Consultant Psychiatrist, Coney Hill Hospital, Gloucester

Andrew Hoy, MRCP,. FRCR.,
Medical Director, Princess Alice Hospice, Esher, Surrey

Avril Jackson, B.Ed.,
Information Officer, St. Christopher's Hospice, London

Peter Kaye, MA., MRCP., MRCGP., DRCOG.,
Consultant in Palliative Medicine, Cynthia Spencer House,
Northampton

Wendy Lethem, RGN., BSc(Hons)., Dip N.,
Clinical Nurse Specialist, Greenwich Support Team, London

Leonard Lunn,
Chaplain, St. Christopher's Hospice, London

Alexander McCall Smith,
Department of Scots Law, University of Edinburgh, Scotland

Barbara Monroe, BA., B.Phil., CQSW.,
Director of Social Work, St. Christopher's Hospice, London

Marie Murphy, MRCPI.,
Senior Hospice Physician, St. Ann's Hospice, Worsley, Greater Manchester

Tony O'Brien, MRCPI.,
Consultant Physician in Palliative Medicine, Marymount Hospice, County Cork, Ireland

Betty O'Gorman, MCSP., SRP.,
Superintendent Physiotherapist, St. Christopher's Hospice, London

David Oliviere, MA., CQSW.,
Social Work Director, North London Hospice, London

Cicely Saunders, OM., DBE., FRCP.,
Chairman, St. Christopher's Hospice, London

Frances Sheldon, MA,(cantab), MPhil., CQSW.,
Macmillan Lecturer in Psychosocial Palliative Care, University of Southampton

Anthony Smith, FRCS., Ed.,
Director of Studies, St. Christopher's Hospice, London

Penny Smith, SRN., RM., HV.,
Director of Home Care, St. Christopher's Hospice, London

Nigel Sykes, MA., MRCGP.,
Consultant Physician, St. Christopher's Hospice, London

Tom West, OBE., MB., BS.,
Former Medical Director, St. Christopher's Hospice, London

1

Introduction – 'History and Challenge'

Cicely Saunders

The modern hospice movement, beginning in the 1960s, grew from opportunities to listen to patients and to pay attention both to their needs and to their achievements. From it has grown the now worldwide specialty of palliative care, carried out by a great variety of multidisciplinary teams and interpreted according to differences in culture and resources. National and regional associations are increasing in number and the World Health Organisation brings palliative and cancer care together in the same section and has inspired a number of WHO collaborative centres and reports from expert committees.[1,2]

The breadth of interest and its actual and potential impact on the treatment of people in other fields of medical care will be apparent in this new edition of a textbook first published in 1978.[3] Originally commissioned by Professor Gordon Hamilton Fairley not long before his untimely death, the emphasis of the given title was upon the management of the disease in all its impact upon a patient and his family network. The implication was that if the symptoms of the inexorable advance of an incurable disease were relieved or controlled and communication established, the central characters themselves, given appropriate support, would have greater potential for their own management of its consequences.

Much that follows in this book, which reflects advances both in symptom control and in the understanding of the intense feelings aroused in both patient and family, and, indeed in staff, is also relevant to earlier stages of this progress. The concern here is with 'terminal disease' which may be recognized weeks or even months before death. 'Terminal care' is part of palliative care, often lasting a few days only and its problems are more easily handled where effective support of all kinds has been given at earlier stages. The words 'terminal patient' should rarely, if ever, be used. They give an impersonal and negative impression and the whole message of the hospice movement has been one of the unique and often creative possibilities that occur, even at the ending of life.

History of the movement

In 1935 Alfred Worcester published a small classic *The Care of the Aged, the Dying and the Dead*,[4] three lectures he had been giving to Boston medical students. He was already eighty when they were printed after a lifetime of service as a family doctor with a particular interest in nursing. He acknowledged that much of his knowledge of care at the ending of life came from the Protestant deaconnesses of Kaiserswerth and the Augustine Sisters of Paris.[5] He is rightly regarded as a pioneer in palliative care and this was one of the few writings on the subject to be found when I first began to search the literature as a medical student in the 1950s.

Another seminal work was published by the Marie Curie Memorial Foundation in 1952.[6] The result of a questionnaire sent to District Nurses, it catalogued much physical and social distress among cancer patients at home. This charity has since founded homes, home care nurses, basic research, and an expanding programme of internal and external education.[7]

In 1947, as a recently qualified medical social worker and former nurse, I met in my first ward a Jewish patient aged forty named David Tasma, who had come originally from the Warsaw Ghetto. He received a palliative colostomy for an inoperable and obstructed carcinoma of the rectum. After a few months follow-up in out-patients, he was admitted to another hospital and I visited him frequently, in a well-run but extremely busy surgical ward, until he died two months later. Discussions of a setting that could have helped him find not only symptom relief but also time and space to make his own terms with an apparently unfilfilled and meaningless life, led not only to an initial inspiration but also his own quiet peace. Two key phrases from those long conversations were founding insights for the hospice movement. When he said of a small legacy, 'I'll be a window in your Home' he gave a commitment to openness. Seen first as openness to the world, it grew later to a challenge to be open not only to patients and families but also among ourselves. In another, more personal, exchange he said, 'I only want what is in your mind and in your heart.' Again, later thought led to a commitment to all that could be brought together of continually developing skills, understanding and research, with a readiness for personal concern.

When he died, having made a quiet and personal peace with the God of his forefathers, David Tasma left me with the assurance that he had found his answers and that all our caring must give total freedom to others to make their own way into meaning.

Hospice openness, scientific rigour and personal concern, and freedom for the spirit were built on these foundations and led directly to the ever-widening impetus of the modern movement. Many were Christian foundations, both Catholic and Protestant, but the early challenge to responsibility for openness and respect for differing perceptions of the right way to give the best and most appropriate care for dying patients and their families, has led to various settings and teams coming from very different backgrounds. To suggest that such care could only be based in a separate building, still more only one with some form of religious foundation, would have been to close doors when the commitment from the beginning was to open them and to spread effective care as widely as possible.

After St Christopher's Hospice opened for in-patient care in 1967 and for home care in 1969, pioneers visited from North America on sabbatical leave. Florence Wald, Dean of the Graduate School of Nursing at Yale and the University Hospital Chaplain, Ed Dobihal, were among the founders of the first hospice home care team with no backup beds of its own based in New Haven, Connecticut. Sylvia Lack, from St Joseph's and St Christopher's, joined them as they began caring for patients at home in 1974. Chaplain Carleton Sweetser, from St Luke's Hospital, New York, became Chairman of the Committee that set up the first consulting team within a hospital later that same year, again with no designated beds of its own. Finally, Balfour Mount, now a professor, after a period of clinical experience at St Christopher's, founded the Palliative Care Service of the Royal Victoria Hospital, Montreal, early in 1975. Based in the small Palliative Care Unit it also included home care and a small hospital consulting team. This was the first use of the word 'Palliative' in this field, the older word 'hospice' having come to mean custodial, or less than optimal care, in French-speaking Canada.

These three different patterns for planning palliative care, together with Day Centres first established by St Luke's Hospice in Sheffield, England in 1975, were thus demonstrated by the mid-1970s. Together with the independent hospices (usually developing or working with a home care programme) these formed the impetus which has led to such a proliferation of services, now spreading worldwide. Notable in the United Kingdom has been a series of wide reaching initiatives by the National Society for Cancer Relief, now the Cancer Relief Macmillan Fund.

All these teams developed the principles now set out by the WHO, in that 'palliative care:

- Affirms life and regards dying as a normal process.
- Neither hastens nor postpones death.
- Provides relief from pain and other distressing symptoms.
- Integrates the psychological and spiritual aspects of patient care.
- Offers a support system to help patients live as actively as possible until death.
- Offers a support system to help the family cope during the patient's illness and in their own bereavement.

Radiotherapy, chemotherapy and surgery have a place in palliative care, provided that the symptomatic benefits of treatment clearly outweigh the disadvantages. Investigative procedures are kept to a minimum.'[1]

Decisions to limit treatment to whatever is most appropriate for a particular patient and gives due regard to his own view of what is in his best interests have been made easier by the developments of this now recognized branch of medicine. Making such decisions still remains difficult in many situations, often demands full family and multidisciplinary consultation and a recognition that the relief of suffering is as much a medical commitment as the search for and pursuit of a cure. So often this becomes increasingly illusory and may itself greatly add to suffering. It is fear of what is seen as pointless prolongation of an increasingly painful and depersonalized life that leads to much of the demand for some form of active and deliberate shortening of life.

Earlier history

Although at first there was only sketchy knowledge of hospice history and little conscious connection, today's principles are a modern development of aims comparable to those of the hospices of the early Christian era. Beginning first in the Eastern Mediterranean as Christianity spread as much because of its care for the disadvantaged as from its preaching[8] it reached the Latin world in the second half of the fourth century CE when Fabiola, a Roman matron and disciple of St Jerome, opened a hospice for pilgrims and the sick. From then on many monastic orders set out to obey the commands of the Parable of the Sheep and the Goats (Matthew 25: 35,36) to feed the hungry, give drink to the thirsty, welcome strangers, clothe the naked and visit the sick and prisoners. This, together with the command 'Inasmuch as you did it to the least of these my brethren, you did it to me' (Matthew 25: 40) was the foundation of a service spreading across Europe.[9] They were very different from the Hippocratic tradition which had excluded care for the incurable and dying as contrary to the will of the gods.[10] They also differed in aim from the Roman 'hospitals' established to restore soldiers and gladiators to health and action. The words 'hospes' came to mean both stranger or guest and host and 'hospitium', both the place where they met and the relationship between them, while an equivalent in Hebrew has the same connotation of hospitality. Although many of these centres of service looked above all to the peace of the soul, they did their best for the care of the body, saw their pilgrims as travellers on important journeys and welcomed with honour 'Our Lords the sick'.[11] They were not, however, especially concerned with dying, although no doubt they kept their patients with them to the end.

The first use of the word 'hospice' specifically for dying people came long after many of these services in their often beautiful old buildings were closed after the Reformation. Others were changed and became almshouses for the elderly, while much of their earlier work was taken over by a number of new 'hospitals'. In 1842 Jeanne Garnier, a young widow who had also lost her two children, opened the first of her refuges for the dying in Lyon. It was called both a Hospice and a Calvaire. Several more were opened later by her 'Dames de Calvaire' in other parts of France. Some still remain and at least one of them is becoming involved in today's growth of the Palliative Care Movement in that country. The choice of a different name is due in part to the association with the changes in the medieval institutions noted above. If hospice denotes shelter for the elderly, or largely custodial care, it is not a word easily used for a modern home care or hospital team. Hopefully, however, the main challenge to relationships with the best personal hospitality still remains.

The Irish Sisters of Charity quite independently chose the same name when they founded Our Lady's Hospice for the Dying in Dublin in 1879. Mother Mary Aikenhead's Order, dating from much earlier in the century, had always been concerned with the poor, the sick and the dying but this was their first institution founded specifically for such care. By the time the Order opened St Joseph's Hospice in London's East End in 1905, at least three Protestant homes had opened in the City under other titles, the Friedensheim Home of Rest (later St Columba's) in 1885, the Hostel of God in 1891, and St Luke's Home for the Dying Poor in 1893. The last, founded by Howard Barrett and the Methodist West London Mission, published detailed and vivid Annual Reports which reveal how much of today's respect for personal worth to the end of life was present in this obviously lively institution. When I arrived there as a volunteer Registered Nurse in early 1948, the Matron, Lilian Pipkin, was still giving copies of these reports to new members of staff as embodying the spirit of what was by then called St Luke's Hospital. From the beginning Dr Barrett was telling compelling stories about individual people. He wrote little about symptom control but gave vivid pictures of the courage and indiosyncrasies of his patients and showed a deep concern for the families left at home in dire poverty, unrelieved by any form of social security.

The other main gift of St Luke's to the Hospice Movement and thence to the whole spectrum of palliative medicine was the regime of the regular giving of oral morphine to control the constant pain of much far advanced cancer. Lilian Pipkin dated this from before she had joined the staff in 1935 and believed it was a routine established by the Matron of that time rather than by the team of visiting family doctors. This must have been soon after the Brompton Hospital had put together its Brompton Cocktail of opioids, cocaine and alcohol for patients with advanced tuberculosis. When I arrived in 1948 I had met such a cocktail before but not the regularity nor the careful assessment in balancing the dose to the patient's need. Elsewhere one saw patients, as a medical student later expressed it, 'earning their morphine', with the fear of drug dependence leading to the sadly common phrase 'See if you can hold on a little longer.'

It was the first few years of experience at St Luke's and an awareness of much pain and isolation both in hospital and at home that led me to another step, a medical training, with this area of need in mind. It was Norman Barrett, a thoracic surgeon, who discussed the problem and suggested this. He said, 'Go and read medicine. It's the doctors who desert the dying. There's so much more to be learned about pain. You will only be frustrated if you don't do it properly, and they won't listen to you.'

By 1958 a clinical research fellowship enabled me to begin work in St Joseph's Hospice. Welcomed by the wonderfully caring nuns who had been looking for more medical help, I was able to introduce a regular routine to the drugs they were giving on an 'on demand' basis, introduce medical and nursing records and with taped conversations with patients build up the analysis of the treatment of 1100 who had stayed longer than a few days. The patients of St Joseph's, even more than those of St Luke's, provided the inspiration and evidence for many lectures and papers and thence the funds that founded St Christopher's. This soon proved to be the major catalyst for the modern hospice movement. A series of articles on The Care of the Dying was commissioned by the *Nursing Times*.[12] In the same year the psychologist Herman Feifel published *'The Meaning of Death'*.[13] A fascinating chapter by Carl Jung on 'The Soul and Death' introduced a selection of theory, concept and study.

By this time the Marie Curie Report had been published[6] and Hinton was undertaking his research on 'The Physical and Mental Distress of the Dying'.[14] Home and Hospital distress had been documented before the beginning of the National Health Service and funds were awarded by the DHSS for a research and development project in home care, a controlled clinical comparison of morphine and diamorphine and evaluative studies of the need for and impact of the Hospice on the locality of St Christopher's. The work of Parkes[15] and Twycross[16] is well known and St Christopher's (opened in 1967) became the first of countless hospice and palliative care teams. The need for ever-improving symptom control leading to a research based programme of education, was added to plans for home care, family and bereavement support and an awareness of the need for patient and family choice and control wherever possible.

The majority of patients with far advanced disease, however, will continue to have most, if not all, their care from the professionals working in general wards and oncology units and with the primary care teams. The relevant literature now culminates in major textbooks for the specialist but a primary concern from the beginning of hospice development has been that wherever a patient and his family face mortal illness, they should meet with the attitudes and skills that they need if they are to reach their full potential. This volume is planned for the wider field as well as for those with a focus on palliative care. The first modern units and teams saw themselves as examples of ways of giving appropriate care rather than as models to be copied. They all demonstrated the difference that could be made in the situation of a patient with mortal illness and his family if skilful and continuing symptom control was matched by good communication and family support. A major aim was to define principles that could be interpreted according to various settings.

'Total pain'

In 1986, Wall wrote of the whole field of the research and treatment of pain:

> A second clinical controversy had been created from the his-
> torical development of medicine itself. Up to the nineteenth

century, most medical care related to the amelioration of symptoms while the natural history of the disease took its course toward recovery or death. By 1900, doctors and patients alike had turned to a search for root cause and ultimate cure. In the course of this new direction, symptoms were placed on one side as sign posts along a highway which was being driven toward the intended destination. Therapy directed at the sign posts was denigrated and dismissed as merely symptomatic. By the second half of this century a reaction set in as seen by such remarkable developments as the hospice movement. The immediate origins of misery and suffering need immediate attention while the long-term search for basic cure proceeds. The old methods of care and caring had to be rediscovered and the best of modern medicine had to be turned to the task of new study and therapy specifically directed at pain.[17]

Some fifty years earlier, Leriche had written as his definition, 'Pain is the resultant of a conflict between a stimulus and the whole individual.[18]

Between these two, in 1963, a patient in St Joseph's expressed it in one long answer to the simple question, 'Mrs H., tell me about your pain.' She said, 'Well doctor, it began in my back but now it seems that all of me is wrong . . . I could have cried for the pills and the injections but I knew that I mustn't. It seemed as if all the world was against me and no one understood how I felt. My husband and son were marvellous but they were having to stay off work and lose their money. But it's so wonderful to begin to feel safe again.' She had described 'Total pain', the division of a whole experience into physical, emotional, social and spiritual, which has helped many workers to be aware of the components of such a situation. We try to understand and respond to them and free the patient to find his own path along his final journey and the unexpected gains that are so often found there.

Tackling total pain

The experience of such pain may be overwhelming and, although it may seem somewhat artificial to classify separate components in what for the patient is indivisible, a careful analysis will help towards rational treatment. It is tantamount to making the diagnosis of a new disease, the entity of terminal pain and it can give us a structure for our activities and concerns which we can continually review.

Much knowledge has been acquired through basic and clinical pain research in recent years. Nevertheless, the physical component of such total pain is often inadequately analysed and ineptly treated. Sometimes it is scarcely addressed at all. The majority of these patients can be satisfactorily treated with opioids but in many countries the prescribing of these drugs is severely limited and their 'benefits have clearly not reached all patients . . . Future research may hold great promise for future patients but much greater benefit to existing patients can be gained from the proper application of current knowledge'.[19] Far too many are suffering at this moment.

Nor do we only address pain itself but pay attention to what may be a whole symptom complex. Far advanced cancer may well be a multi-system disease and call for vigorous treatment of nausea, vomiting, breathlessness and the other problems which are addressed in this book. Mrs H., in saying 'all of me is wrong', was referring to more than the pelvic pain of her carcinoma of the cervix.

Her feeling that no one understood how she felt, and that all the world was against her, vividly describes her emotional and mental pain. Elements of anxiety and depression may seem to exist together but as communication opens up it becomes possible to facilitate adjustment to this understandably threatening situation. Isolation enhances any suffering and too many people remain alone with their questions and fears. One unhurried interview can create a new climate and while it may not bring relief, it can open up the way to acceptance which can grow, often in several much shorter exchanges. This may be with different members of a team, especially where they are able to share enough to work constructively together.

This progress may not be either simple or straightforward and the opportunity to express feelings may reveal that there is much understandable anger and bitterness to work through. Not everyone has the time to reach a resolution but people move fast in crisis and unexpected strengths are often revealed and peace found.

This may also be true for the family, thought of from the beginning of the modern movement as the unit of care and often, of course, the main caring team. The history of the disease and its treatment may be full of pain, misunderstandings and unshared threats. Once again, the approach to this stage of illness and its impact is dealt with fully later in this book. The discovery of resources and strengths within the family will ease the pain of bereavement and help the survivors on the path to new ways of living. It is not so much the length of time that can be given, but the way it is planned and used.

The line between emotional and spiritual pain will be drawn differently by each worker, depending to some extent on their own perceptions in this area. As we care for the needs of the body and of the family, however, and turn to our patient's inner life or, as Mrs H. put it, 'the need for safety', we are, I believe, reaching an important centre. We must respect each person's integrity and at times a confirmed wish for privacy, but there may be a surprising readiness to open up discussion and questions to share rather than to answer. We will only do this if we have been competently concerned with the other areas of total pain.

For the body we strive for growing understanding and expertise in symptom control, for due regard to appearance and self-esteem, while maintaining activity and independence and all that keeps going something of a normal life. So far as is practicable, this should be carried out at home. For most people home is the place of choice and where they will most easily maintain their sense of self and self-worth and some control over their situation.

For the family we have to be aware of the whole group and the understanding and support they need if they are to find and use their own resources and strengths. Sometimes we have to help the patient reassert his own place in that group; people may withdraw because of their own fears and the pain of watching someone else's distress, and others begin to behave as if the patient's place were already empty. Somehow there needs to be enough security for communication to open up if sharing is to happen and choices are to be made. The whole question of helping people to face truth is one of the constant challenges in our task of enabling people to be themselves in as honest a way as they can, to find reconciliation, and to make their farewells. All this is not just a salvage operation but the chance for a creative moment. Here the whole team has learned much from the social workers and chaplains who have been involved in this field, especially where there has been joint working with each member of the team contributing as they make their own relationships with the patient and family, both alone and together.

For the essential person we need to concern ourselves with work, interests and accomplishments, for so many people identify themselves with what they do. But there is more to consider than that. What are the inner concerns and values, what has deepest meaning, where is the spirit of this person focused? If someone is able to lay down life with some degree of peace and satisfaction, if it is all to make some sense to him (whether or not he thinks it is the final end) where does he have to look? Is this indeed what we may call the spiritual dimension? And from that, define spiritual pain? This is a challenge posed to us all in the various definitions of palliative care that are put forward, but it tends either to be thought of only as a religious issue or else it is not defined or addressed in any depth. Here, the dictionary gives some clues. *Spirit* is defined as the animating or vital principle in man, the breath of life. *Spiritual* is given as that which 'concerns the spirit or higher moral qualities, especially as regarded in a religious aspect'. Some people we meet have had long links with religious beliefs and practices, held to more or less faithfully. For many they offer support at the deepest level, though for others they may be instead a source of disquiet or guilt. The chaplains among us are constantly involved with these problems and with the various answers of our patients' different religions.

But *spiritual* surely covers much more than that. It is the whole area of thought concerning moral values throughout life. Memories of defections and burdens of guilt may not be seen at all in religious terms and hardly be reachable by the services, sacraments, and symbols that can be so releasing to the 'religious groups'. The realization that life is likely to end soon may well stimulate a desire to put first things first and to reach out to what is seen as true and valuable – and give rise to feelings of being unable or unworthy to do so. There may be bitter and most understandable anger at the unfairness of what is happening, and at much of what has gone on before, and above all a desolating feeling of meaninglessness. Here lies, I believe, the essence of spiritual pain and the greatest challenge to our patients and to the members of the team committed to care for them.

The search for meaning

Most of us have a desire to belong safely to something greater than our insecure and vulnerable selves. The search for meaning in things that includes oneself has recently been shown in nursing research studies[20,21] to be the major concern of a group of hospitalized patients and of a number of nurses.

Many people involved with dying patients and their families have found much help in Viktor Frankl's book *Man's Search for Meaning*. Writing from the extreme situation of a Nazi labour and extermination camp, he says, 'The hopelessness of our situation did not detract from its dignity or meaning.' Not knowing what had happened to his wife, he finds a moment of deep fulfilment in thinking of her – even though he does not know if she is still alive. That love, finding its deepest meaning in his inner self, his spiritual being, is still undefeated. He believes meaning can be found in such love, but also in the memory of accomplishment, and even in the suffering itself. If we are held in suffering, we then have responsibility for the attitude in which we suffer. He believes that no one can tell another what the meaning of his life should be, but that each must not only look back at achievements stored in memory but also seek out the questions that life is asking of him in the present.[22]

Facing meaninglessness

The Old Testament Book of Job presents the classic sufferer, and a recent book by Kahn and Solomon has taken a fresh look at his desperate search for meaning in his own trials and in the whole mystery of unjust suffering. As they point out, it is in the whirlwind that enlightenment comes, the source of the pain itself was the source of revelation. Job 'finds peace and maturation to levels which could only be attained after intense inner suffering'. Because he faces it, he finally comes through.[23]

So how do we help others in their struggle to find a way out of the pain of meaninglessness? We come from such different backgrounds, our stories are radically other, and we do not have mortal illness facing us. Can we build some kind of bridge between us so that we can meet and help their search? We start in concern for the body, with the freedom and space we can give by skills in symptom control and care for role and appearance; we welcome the whole family group and help in their search for their own resources – but what else should hospice or palliative care have to offer? Hospitality to our patients must surely include the readiness to help them as they look at what is most important of all, their inner griefs, guilts, and longings. Discussion will not always be appropriate and hospitality includes the right to privacy.

It is a question of time – and timing – a readiness on the part of all staff to stop and listen at the moment this particular area of pain is expressed and to stay with it. We are not there to take away or explain, or even to understand, but simply to 'Watch with me', as Jesus asked of his disciples in the Garden of Gethsemane. As we have worked so hard and so successfully to relieve physical pain and other symptoms, we may have been tempted to believe that spiritual pain should be tackled and solved in a similar way. Sometimes unrealistic fears can be explained and lead to resolution or a new vision, as came to Job, but sometimes we have to wait beside an apparent failure of resolution. Only as a team becomes more experienced and confident do its members find it easy to allow or even encourage the expression of anger and other negative feelings that may express this inner pain, and the frequent question 'Why?' to which there is no answer.

We have to learn to listen in a way that will help the questioner to find the route to the real trouble and the way to face and handle it. Even to the end, the inner self can still stretch and broaden. This gift of listening to the story may be made by any member of staff but because they are often not concerned with any form of treatment, many social workers, specially trained volunteers and chaplains find they have a place here. But we all have to listen. Not all are as unfortunate as he claims, but in ancient Rome, Seneca complained, 'Who is there in all the world who listens to us? Here I am – this is me in my nakedness, with my wounds, my secret grief, my despair, my betrayal, my pain which I can't express, my terror, my abandonment. Oh, listen to me for a day, an hour, a moment lest I expire in my terrible wilderness, my lonely silence. Oh God, is there no one to listen?' He is not asking for more than a fellow human being to stay there. This is the need of those who are dying and sometimes, even more poignantly, the bereaved.

A short time of true attention can often reach such bitterness and quieten angers and fears. Answers are not really expected and long sessions are not always needed. Old structures and values can emerge almost unbidden to make sense again, and sometimes new discoveries develop from the interchange with a committed person. As a patient said, 'I thought it so strange. Nobody wants to look at me. And then, doctor, I came here and you listened to me. I felt you understood. It seems the pain went with me speaking to you!'

The often simple exchange that arises in such meetings may be felt as a gift. But we are not the only givers. Sooner or later all who work with dying people know they are receiving more than they are giving as they meet endurance, courage and often humour. We need to say so, recognizing, too, the common conviction that there is an enabling grace coming in from beyond us both.

It is hard to remain near pain, least of all an anguish for which we feel we can do nothing. Job's friends are often condemned, but as Kahn points out, they came together to him, they rent their garments in a gesture of solidarity, and they sat down on the ground beside him for a long time in silence. Only after Job himself began to speak did they bring forward their inadequate answers. And it was partly in indignation at them that Job begins to dig deep into his own pain and finally comes face-to-face with a vision of God that leaves him in a new humility that accepts his human condition and all its mystery.

We are not alone in these sometimes very taxing situations. Like Job, our patients may find unexpected resources and new self-awareness and life growing up within themselves once they accept the mystery and the inadequacy of our human sense of justice and desert. Life is not fair, there are no easy answers, but there is a way to acceptance and peace for the last part of the journey and there are many who find it.

Sometimes we will see this happen in terms of our own beliefs but only when asked are we called to share more personally. But unless we are occupied in our own search for meaning we may not create the climate in which patients can be helped to make their own journeys of growth through loss.

Persevere with the practical

But many of us have little or no opportunity for the time these meetings may call for – our patients are too ill and we are sometimes too busy. That, too, we often have to accept, but we can always persevere with the practical. Care for the physical needs, the time taken to elucidate a symptom, the quiet acceptance of a family's angry demands, the way nursing care is given, can carry it all and can reach the most hidden places. This may be all we can offer to inarticulate total pain – it may well be enough as our patients finally face the truth on the other side of death. It may certainly be all that is possible for the member of an overloaded primary health care team, especially where a caring family tries to protect their dying relative from the pain that the knowledge is causing them. Any attempt to reach the patient's inarticulate and by no means, deluded, fears of the future, is hampered. The time needed for opening up communication throughout the family may not be available in a heavy day's work. This may also be true of a busy hospital ward even where the institution of team or primary care nursing gives nurses an increased responsibility to show different authorities the facts of their patient's feelings. The time needed to give the patient freedom to express these may not be given adequate priority among many other more immediate pressures.

Yet very small acts of human courtesy take surprisingly little time compared to the importance they can have. Many patients and families on reaching the more leisurely pace of a specialist unit have referred to help given them in what the staff concerned must have thought were trivial ways.

The Uncomforted

This new edition sets out to answer not only the doctor who says 'There is nothing more I can do' but also the patient who says the same. If we can manage the progress of inexorable disease, even when pressed for time, in such a way that the patient feels affirmed at every step, there is often a surprising amount that he can do, not only in physical ability but in relationships and in a final discovery of worth and meaning.

A few patients, however skilled the symptom control and in spite of concerned listening by experienced staff, do not believe their lives any longer have sense or value. As was pointed out above, appropriate treatment need not include every effort to prolong life regardless of its quality but must recognize that what should be done for a patient with an acute remediable condition may be burdensome and is not necessarily indicated for someone with a chronic and, still more, a terminal condition. An adequately informed patient can decide on his own best interests. Palliative support only may be the choice and may resolve the request, 'Let me die'.

Certain symptoms may demand a constant review of treatment and occasionally medication for their control that may itself lead to a life-threatening condition, such as respiratory depression.Here, too, the patient may be able to discuss and decide on their choice in the matter, while for a patient who is no longer competent the doctor will consider the views of the family and the multidisciplinary team as he decides as best he can how to proceed. 'The proper medical treatment that is administered and that has an incidental effect in determining the exact moment of death is not the cause of death in any sensible use of the term.'[24]

The more definite, and much less common request, 'Kill me' cannot, I believe, be legalized and acted upon without leading to involuntary as well as voluntary euthanasia. The evidence from the Netherlands does not reassure those with any experience in palliative care that this will not be the case.[25]

But the challenge remains from the desperate patient who cannot have his wish without laws which will themselves have dangerous social consequences and put pressure on many of the vulnerable. For such a person, with their understandable, but so far impossible, request we may perhaps go back to the original hospice commission as it may be interpreted today.

To give food can mean to give yourself even briefly to the person hungry for recognition; it can mean give attention, give presence. To give drink can mean to give a moment of refreshment where before was only drought and meaninglessness, where there is hardly a voice strong enough to express thirst. Hospitality, even the giving of a name, or an unspoken understanding, welcomes those unsure of their destination and those made to feel isolated by unshared truth. It means being aware, often without words, of our own inner homelessness and oneness with the 'stranger'. We can clothe or cover exposure and its humiliation with goodwill, we can respect the mystery of the individual by the way we give even momentary privacy. Above all we can come with personal respect. 'I was sick and you visited me', means to call people by name, give courtesy, be ourselves. We are concerned with visiting and opening the prisons of pain, of unrelieved symptoms and of non-communication. These are all gifts of individuals to each other which can be given in brief exchanges but are demanding and draining as well as challenging and often rewarding. Openness and the giving of mind and heart 'in a spirit of freedom'[26] are even more taxing than clinical excellence but match well together.

This book attempts to present what can be offered not only in these extreme circumstances but to all those we meet who are battling with terminal disease and face all their own challenges.

Notes and References

1. World Health Organisation. *Cancer Pain Relief.* Geneva, WHO, 1986.
2. World Health Organisation. *Cancer Pain Relief and Palliative Care.* Report of WHO Expert Committee, Geneva, WHO, 1990.
3. SAUNDERS, C. (ed.). *The Management of Terminal Malignant Disease*, 2nd edn. London, Edward Arnold, 1984.
4. WORCESTER, A. *The Care of the Aged, the Dying and the Dead.* Springfield, Ill., Charles C. Thomas, 1935.
5. KERE, D. 'Alfred Worcester: A pioneer in palliative care,' *American Journal of Hospice and Palliative Care*, May/June, 1992, 13–14 and 36–8.
6. Marie Curie Memorial Foundation. Report on a national survey concerning patients nursed at home. London, Marie Curie Memorial Foundation, 1952.
7. FORD, G. 'A palliative care system – the Marie Curie model,' *The American Journal of Hospice and Palliative Care*, May/June, 1992, 15–17.
8. PHIPPS, W.E. 'The origin of hospices/hospitals,' *Death Studies*, 1988, **12**, 91–9.
9. GOLDIN G. and THOMPSON, J.D. *The Hospital: a Social and Architectural History*, New Haven and London, Yale University Press, 1975, p. 6.
10. WALTON, J. 'Method in medicine,' *The Harveian Oration of 1990.* London, Royal College of Physicians, 1990.
11. STODDARD, S. *The Hospice Movement: A Better Way of Caring for the Dying.* Briarcliff Manor, NY, Stein and Day, 1978.
12. SAUNDERS, C. 'Care of the dying,' *Nursing Times*, September/October, 1959.
13. FEIFEL, H. *The Meaning of Death*, New York, McGraw-Hill, 1959.
14. HINTON, J.M. 'The physical and mental distress of the dying,' *Quarterly Journal of Medicine*, 1963, **32**, 1–21.
15. PARKES, C.M. 'Psychological aspects.' In: *The Management of Terminal Malignant Disease*, 2nd edn, Saunders, C. (ed.), London, Edward Arnold, 1984.
16. TWYCROSS, R. 'Relief of pain.' In: *The Management of Terminal Malignant Disease*, 2nd edn, Saunders, C. (ed.) London, Edward Arnold, 1984.
17. WALL, P.D. 'Editorial – 25 years of pain,' *Pain*, 1986, **25**, 1–4.
18. LERICHE, R. *The Surgery of Pain* (trans. A. Young). London, Ballière, Tindall and Cox, 1939, p. 489.
19. MACRAE, W.A., DAVIES, H.T.O., CROMBIE I.K. 'Editorial – pain: paradigms and treatments,' *Pain*, 1992, **49**, 289–91.
20. SIMSEN, B. 'The spiritual dimension,' *Nursing Times*, November, 1986.
21. WAUGH, L. Spiritual aspects of nursing care: a descriptive study of nurses' perceptions. Unpublished PhD thesis, Edinburgh, 1992.
22. FRANKL, V. *Man's Search for Meaning* (revised and enlarged edition), London, Hodder and Stoughton, 1987.
23. KAHN, J. and SOLOMON, H. Job's Illness: *Loss, Grief and Integration – a Psychological Interpretation*, London, Gaskell, Royal College of Psychiatrists, 1986.
24. DEVLIN, P. *Easing the Passing – the trial of Dr John Bodkin Adams*, London, The Bodley Head, 1985, p. 171.
25. GOMEZ, C.F. *Regulating Death: the Case of the Netherlands*, New York, The Free Press, 1991.
26. WYON, O. *Aim and Basis*, London, St Christopher's Hospice, 1965.

2

Communication

Frances Sheldon

Introduction

Every moment that professionals spend with a person who is dying or their carers is spent in communicating with them. This chapter aims to help professionals from a variety of different backgrounds understand what influences this communication and how to improve what they are doing.

Communication is about dialogue. Each party in the dialogue brings a bundle of assumptions, expectations and behaviour styles with them which influence their interpretation of the dialogue and therefore its outcome. The first part of this chapter is about the expectations and assumptions that might be brought by someone who is dying or their carer, and the values and theoretical framework which underpin the skills that the professional brings. The second part will discuss particular communication problems that often come up in this area of care. The particular issue of communicating with children when someone they love is dying will be covered in Chapter 4.

How individuals communicate is, of course, heavily influenced by their ethnic and cultural background, by their spiritual framework and by the society that they live in. These issues are dealt with in other chapters of this book but they must form the backcloth to any consideration of communicating with patients and families in the crisis of facing death and bereavement. It is important to be aware that much of the research on communication skills and the most commonly used methods of counselling have been developed in Western cultures and neither may apply to those who come from other cultures.

What do patients and their carers bring to the dialogue?

Those living in Western societies in the twentieth century have learnt to expect that the vast majority of children will live to adulthood and that death is reserved for the late middle-aged and elderly and a few unlucky and poignant younger people. They expect that doctors have immense technological resources and considerable power over life and death. They may therefore unrealistically credit doctors with knowledge about the course and length of an illness.

A funeral director discussed his dying wife's illness with her doctor and pressed him for the likely length of her life. This was all the more important to him because he was having an affair with another woman and wished to know how long it might be before he would be free to marry her. The doctor carefully and honestly explained that it was not possible to say. The funeral director left the room with a social worker who had also been present at the interview. He commented to her; 'Of course he *does* know, all doctors do, he's just not saying.'

Conditioned by his society's belief in the foreknowledge of the doctor and impelled by his own particular circumstances, this man could never be convinced that information was not being withheld.

People who come to a professional for help when facing death or bereavement come with life experience and a family history which may have built up beliefs and myths about death and about the illness from which they are suffering. Death is relatively unfamiliar to those in Western societies, because it is much more likely to take place in hospitals or other institutions where it may feel out of the control of relatives and friends and of the dying person too. Carers are less likely to be present at the death in hospital than at home, and bodies are seldom kept at home after death but whisked off to the funeral home. This inexperience can add to the common fear of the unknown which those facing death may feel, and can fuel anxieties about the inevitability of pain and suffering. These may have a basis in fact if a member of an earlier generation did suffer greatly when dying, because modern methods of symptom control were unavailable. It is always important for one member of the professional team to explore with the person who is dying or with the carers what past experience of death may be influencing the way this death is being approached.

There may also be beliefs about the particular illness which are affecting the way the patient and carers feel and behave. Cancer has been especially feared in the second half of the twentieth century. The man who casually said to his doctor 'Of course, my wife and I are sleeping in separate rooms since her cancer was diagnosed' and then revealed that they thought cancer was infectious and that he and their children might catch it, opened up huge anxieties and guilt which needed to be gently explored and challenged with both husband and wife. Today AIDS is another illness which may bring real anxieties, but misconceptions too.

The life experience that patients and their carers bring will influence the way they deal with the situation in a variety of ways.

Mary was fifty-four when she developed bony metastases following a cancer of the breast. The palliative care team were puzzled by her great reluctance to take medication for her pain. When this was explored, she revealed that she saw her cancer as a punishment. She worked in her father's small grocer's shop on Saturdays without payment and used to steal money from the till. Forty years later she felt she was paying the price for this behaviour with her cancer, and that she should not try to avoid her punishment.

The team were able to show her that there were other ways of understanding her pain, and she became more ready to be helped. Barkwell's[1] research showed that 23 per cent of her sample of 100 patients saw their illness as punishment, and 36 per cent as a challenge. Those who saw it as a challenge had less pain and depression than those who saw it as a punishment. Professionals need to explore these beliefs and experiences with patients and their carers to enable them to use the help that is offered.

What should professionals bring to the dialogue?

The values that the professional brings to communication with patients and carers are crucial to the success of that communication. An essential component is a nonjudgemental approach which asserts the unique value of this individual and their experience. Many people may behave in ways which the professional cannot endorse. Limits may need to be set by a team about, for example, the extent to which alcohol can be consumed by a patient in hospital. But unacceptable behaviour should not alter the commitment to value this person. Stedeford[2] comments 'How a person dies depends on at least three factors: the way he has lived, the type of illness, and the quality of care. Staff share grief about the first and second, but only the third is their responsibility.' An associated value is that of self-determination for the patient within the limits set by the legitimate interests of others. Balancing competing interests, for example, between the patient who wishes to stay at home to die and the exhausted wife whose own health is suffering, or between the patient who feels safe in hospital and wishes to stay there and the patient in pain at home who needs admission, requires an open and honest approach with all those involved. The concept of partnership with patients and families builds on this value and has been influenced by improvements in education and easier access to knowledge in the second half of the twentieth century. It requires a sharing of information and joint decision-making with patient and carers about areas which in the past may have been decided by professionals alone. It needs careful negotiation with each new patient as to how far he or she wishes to exercise this right to self-determination. Cultural factors may influence this.

Alongside these values some particular qualities will assist the professional working in this field. The ability to face reality but maintain hope, not the hope of cure, but a sense that life may still offer good things, can be sustaining to both patients and their carers. A positive belief in the potential of individuals for change, even when they face the crisis of death, is an asset. Lichter[3] has reminded us that 'Past coping does not appear to be an accurate indicator of how death will be faced'.

Jane was a single parent with a twelve year-old daughter. She had had many admissions to psychiatric care following suicide attempts at moments of difficulty. When she learnt she was dying many expected that she would repeat this pattern. However she worked hard at making appropriate arrangements for the care of her daughter and then waited with great serenity for her death.

The quality of genuineness is basic in this field of care. Genuineness or self-awareness was defined by Truax and Carkhuff[4] as involving 'the very difficult task of being intimately acquainted with ourselves, and of being able to recognize and accept, as well as respect, ourselves as a whole, containing both good and bad'. Professionals need to understand which situations may be particularly challenging for them as individuals and with which they may need help, and conversely, those situations to which they may be able to make a unique contribution. Professionals, no less than those they wish to help, are formed by their society and their individual experience, and need to understand how this has happened to work sensitively with others. Such self-awareness will help in treading the narrow line between an over-involvement which may destroy the professional and stifle the patient, and the cool detachment which communicates 'I don't care' to patient and carers. This self-awareness needs to operate both at the general level and as part of particular situations. A critical, internal self-monitoring in an interview – 'What exactly made me feel particularly sad at this moment?' 'Why am I finding eye contact difficult now?' – contributes to a full and sensitive evaluation of a situation.

The ability to empathize must go alongside this. Tuson[5] suggests 'the experience of having someone empathize accurately and deeply implies the possibility of change. If someone understands my despair that well, but is not despairing themselves, and is regarding enough to spend time experiencing my despair, then change might be possible.' Such deep empathy may bring pain. Those prepared to offer this must learn to take care of themselves and establish a network of support if they are not to suffer the 'battle fatigue' described by Vachon.[6]

Kübler-Ross stage theory – the right way to die or a defence mechanism for staff?

One of the most widely known 'theories' of the psychological response to the process of dying is that described by Kübler-Ross[7] in her seminal work *On Death and Dying*. She herself did not claim the status of a theory for the work described in that book, but her ideas were rapidly elevated into a prescription for the right way to die which remains extraordinarily powerful. She interviewed 200 dying patients in the USA and identified from these interviews five common experiences which she called 'stages' in the process of dying. These were:

- *Denial* – a refusal to believe that death would be the likely outcome of this illness: 'No, not me.'
- *Anger* – questioning and anger, 'Why me?', 'It's not fair!' 'Someone is to blame'.
- *Bargaining* – An attempt to delay the disaster, often a secret pact with God.
- *Depression* – the two manifestations of this were a reaction to the losses that the illness brought, and preparatory withdrawal at a later stage of the illness.
- *Acceptance* – peaceful resignation.

Kübler-Ross's power as a communicator, her great clinical skills, and her concern for the dying have had great influence in improving care and developing education in this field. Kastenbaum[8] and others who have evaluated her work acknowledge this but suggest that it is important to recognize its limitations. It did not attempt to investigate the influence of age, sex, ethnic background, stage of development or the environment on the reactions of those studied. It was a descriptive study but the findings have been used to imply that all dying people should react in these ways and in a pattern that moves from denial to acceptance. Kastenbaum suggests that it may have been so enthusiastically taken up by professionals because it provided a way of distancing themselves from the suffering of the dying by enabling them to check off feelings against a list, rather than actually listen to the anguish being expressed. So it is important to value Kübler-Ross's insights, but not use them as a straitjacket, and to recognize that, while people who are dying may experience these emotions, they may not experience them all, and that they are just as likely to swing in and out of them.

Jim, a sixty-seven year-old man who had recently learnt that he had inoperable cancer, was referred to a social worker for advice on benefits. His first words to her were 'It's a rotten thing this cancer'. He described his feelings as 'living under the guillotine', knowing that death would come, but not when. At the end of the conversation he said, 'We've just been talking theoretically, you know, it may never happen.'

In this interview he moved through emotions of angry recognition of what was to come and back to denial.

Different approaches to communication

During the 1980s there was increasing awareness that people who are dying have been isolated and their questions and concerns avoided, often because professionals felt anxious about their own emotional survival if they opened up painful issues.[9] There has been an explosion of interest in counselling skills among health care professionals. Maguire in articles with Faulkner,[10] and videotapes with Buckman[11] has developed ways of exploring feelings and establishing key concerns with open questions which allow the person who is dying or their carer to feel a partner in the dialogue and allow doctors or nurses to be open about things they do not know. Moorey and Greer[12] have described the use of cognitive therapy with cancer patients which gives them techniques to manage hitherto overwhelming feelings of anxiety and fear. From this body of work a range of necessary skills has been identified.

What skills do professionals need?

Non-verbal communication

In typical interaction between two people about one-third of what is exchanged is done through words, and two-thirds through non-verbal channels. Professionals anxious about their communication skills usually concentrate on these verbal aspects – 'I don't know what to *say*.' 'How should I *talk* to someone who is dying?' If they are standing in the doorway with their bleep going intermittently, they are unlikely to receive a truthful answer to the question 'How are you feeling about your illness?' however sensitively they ask it. There are some clear guidelines, at their most essential when breaking bad news, but relevant in any communication.

- Make the environment as secure, comfortable and free from distraction as possible. Ask permission to turn off the television (having made sure that this is not the start of a favourite programme). Shut the door or draw the curtain at least part way round the bed.
- Concentrate on the other person, make eye contact comfortably.
- Use touch but tentatively at first until it is clear what this particular person feels comfortable with.

People in distress often initiate conversations in less than ideal circumstances. The relative who pounces on a nurse, rushing with a bedpan to another patient, with the anxious enquiry 'My husband seems much worse today?' still needs the reassurance that the nurse will give her anxieties proper attention at another time. That reassurance is communicated as much by the non-verbal elements of the interchange – stopping for a moment, eye contact, smiling – as by the words used.

Counselling skills

A number of these skills must form part of the basic tool kit of any professional. Attentive listening hears not just the words themselves but their tone, picks up additional clues to the meaning of what is being said from nonverbal behaviour and conveys interest and concern by its concentration which also encourages openness. Reflecting and summarizing build on this listening, checking that the interviewer's perceptions are accurate, focusing on key issues and thus moving discussion forward. Questioning can elicit information using closed questions – 'When did you have your operation?' or attitudes, feelings and opinions by using open questions – 'What do you think the problem is now?' Challenging unclear or distorted statements – 'You say your mother has always hated you, why does that make you a bad person?' 'How will you make sure that you have time for yourself at weekends as well as caring for your sick wife?' – helps the interviewee to reassess situations and develop new strategies for managing them.

However, an important distinction needs to be made between the use of these skills as part of every interaction and the offer of counselling sessions to those who are dying or their carers. This distinction needs to be clear to both client and worker.

Andrew, thirty-two, had cancer of the stomach and was being visited at home by a palliative care nurse. He had a good relationship with her, appreciating her care and concern. He heard that a counsellor had been appointed at a local cancer treatment centre and asked her to arrange an appointment for him with the counsellor. The nurse felt rejected and diminished. She had viewed her intervention as counselling sessions but had not made this clear to Andrew.

Concern to offer a more personal and caring service to those facing their own death and their carers has sometimes lead to the misconception that every patient or carer is looking for, or ought to be offered, formal counselling sessions in this situation and has led professionals to underrate the potential for sensitive use of counselling *skills* while doing a wound dressing or arranging admission for a period of respite care. What the nurse learnt from the experience with Andrew was the importance of being clear about the skills she had, of negotiating openly with her patient the purpose of her visits and of reviewing this regularly. This would have enabled them to consider when and if formal sessions were appropriate and who might offer them. Clarity about the nature and purpose of a professional intervention is all the more necessary in highly charged emotional situations.

Presenting a case and cooperating with others

Not all communication is with patients or their families. Working in the field of terminal disease means working with a wide variety of different professionals, perhaps with volunteers, or with public or charitable organizations whose services or interventions are needed. Here negotiating skills and an ability to be appropriately assertive are a vital part of advocating on behalf of someone more vulnerable. Working in teams is discussed elsewhere in this book. Just as one-to-one communication needs to be underpinned by a value base, so teamwork needs to have a common ethical base and common aims for the overall work of the team even if individuals within it have individual goals for their own work within that. This is only likely to occur if the team takes time to have open discussion about the challenging ethical issues arising in this field separate from such issues arising in practice, and if team aims are regularly reviewed and not just assumed to be shared. Self-awareness and empathy are just as necessary in working with team members as in work with those who are dying and their carers. Wilkinson's research on nurse communication has shown how significant the attitudes of a team leader may be in enabling others to use their skills, or limiting their use.[23]

Particular communication problems

Breaking bad news

Jenny, aged thirty-two, a professional employed in health care, was under investigation for cancer of the breast. She was told she had cancer by a doctor who told her he was in a hurry. On reading her case notes later she found that she had not been told that she had metastases, but that her brother, who was a doctor but not her doctor, had been telephoned and told this.

Breaking bad news poses both ethical and communication challenges. Jenny's doctor did not rise to either. The ethical issue needs to be clarified first, since that will determine what can be communicated. The key decision is who has a right to the information about a particular person's diagnosis and prognosis? A research study by Cartwright[13] carried out in 1969 and repeated in 1987 by Cartwright and Seale[14] demonstrates the changes in attitudes to this issue. In the later study the proportion of those said to know their diagnosis had risen considerably. So it is now more common practice to share this information with the person suffering the disease, though it also should be understood that that person has a right *not* to know the truth, if this is their wish.

The doctor is the team member most likely to take the responsibility for breaking bad news about diagnosis or prognosis, but any member of the team may be drawn into discussion by patient or carer afterwards. Team members need to be clear about what the patient has been told so that any member, be they physiotherapist, chaplain or nurse, may be able to respond appropriately. They may be informed by using a special sheet in the patient's notes or at a multidisciplinary ward meeting.

Maguire and Faulkner[10] suggest that breaking bad news too abruptly may disorganize the patient psychologically and provoke denial. A step-wise approach is the best way to test the pace at which this individual wishes to understand what is happening.

The best moment to start to prepare to break bad news is at the start of the investigative process when the doctor has a suspicion that the outcome is unlikely to be good. This is the moment to discuss with the patient whether information about the disease should be shared with a spouse or a partner or another family member, and in very general terms how much the patient wishes to know of the detail of any results of the investigations. This will begin to give the doctor a 'feel' for the style of communication this individual prefers.

When there is some bad news to discuss the doctor should secure as safe and comfortable an environment as possible, following the guidelines outlined above in the section on non-verbal communication. Acknowledging the well-established research finding that anxiety prevents patients retaining much of what they are told in a consultation, it is now common practice to ask the patient's permission (and carer's, if present) for a nurse or social worker to be present at the interview. This second professional can then remain after the doctor has left and be available for both questions and support. Another method, reported by Hogbin and Fallowfield,[15] is to tape the interview with the patient's permission and offer them the tape to take away. Patients in this study were very positive about using the tape and the majority did so.

One way to start the interview is with a warning: 'We have now had the results of the tests, and I am afraid they are not as good as we hoped. Would you like me to tell you what we found?' This gives the patient the option of asking for the detail or signalling that this is too threatening today by saying, for example: 'I'll leave the detail to you, doctor, just let me know what treatment you are going to give me.'

If the patient asks for the information, a short, clear, jargon-free explanation is needed: 'I am sorry to tell you that we have found some cancer cells in your liver. I'm afraid this may be rather a shock.'

This gives the opportunity for the patient to express what he may be feeling – bewildered, terrified, stunned, resigned. This may be the time to explore past experience of this disease, or particular fears about it. Once feelings and fears have been expressed, the doctor may introduce a discussion on the management of the situation. 'I'd like to discuss with you how we can tackle this problem.'

Even if there are no options for curative treatment, the patient should be reassured that symptoms will be managed, though not given false reassurance that no pain or problems will be experienced, and that this team, or another more appropriate one will continue to be concerned. Ideally after an opportunity has been given for asking any other questions, an appointment should be arranged with the same doctor in a day or two for further discussion. If this is not possible it should be made clear that full information will be passed promptly to a doctor who will be able to give on-going care, such as the general practitioner. This signals the doctor's commitment to the patient's future care. It demonstrates too that breaking and receiving bad news is a process for doctor and patient. A series of short interviews will take no longer and use time more effectively than a heroic session which attempts to tie everything up at once.

Some excellent leaflets are now available on particular illnesses or particular anxieties that may be generated by serious illness. The British organization Cancerlink has produced good ones on sexuality, for example. Such leaflets or suitable books provide a valuable reinforcement and amplification of what has been said.

News about deterioration during the course of an illness can be handled slightly differently. Here the patient has had some experience of the disease and is likely to be having some symptoms. It is then important to find out what they suspect or know about what is happening to them. So starting with an open question: 'How do you think your illness is going?', 'How do you feel at the moment?', or responding to the questions: 'Am I getting worse?', Am I going to die?', by saying: 'Let's discuss that, but tell me what makes you think so?', will help professional and patient start from the same place. Again, a gentle, stepwise procedure can proceed at the patient's pace. Maguire and Faulkner[10] suggest that 'this strategy of moving from acknowledging and exploring the nature and basis of any strong feelings to identifying key concerns is essential if the breaking of bad news is to be managed effectively. It allows the patient to be "lifted" from being overwhelmed to feeling hopeful that something can be done.'

The protective carer

The carer who buttonholes the professional at the front door or in the hospital corridor and firmly says 'He mustn't be told' is not uncommon. If the strategy of discussing with a patient at the start of an investigation how communication should be handled has been followed, the professional should have some idea of the patient's wishes, and can react accordingly. If not, then the ethical issue again comes to the fore. Who has a right to this information? However, even if the professional wishes to assert the primacy of the patient's right to know, a stark statement of this principle is likely to be counter-productive. The fears, anxieties and concern of the carer need to be explored first, and their more intimate knowledge of the person drawn out. Asking: 'What would worry you particularly about him knowing?' gives the opportunity for this, and shows that the listener values the carer's opinions. The majority of carers with such anxieties will then accept a reassurance that the professional will undertake not to initiate any discussion on the outcome of the illness, but that if the dying person raises the issue, the professional will respond truthfully in order to maintain and deserve that person's trust.

Anger

Buckman[16] describes three main types of anger in this situation:

- Anger at the rest of the world who will survive when this person will not.
- Anger at fate/God/destiny.
- Anger at anyone who is trying to help, such as doctors or nurses.

Behind anger are feelings of powerlessness and a desperate search to regain some sort of meaning in a world out of control. Team members themselves may feel some of the second sort of anger from time to time and may be drawn into discussion on this topic with someone who is dying. The chapter on spiritual issues covers this area.

Professionals may be involved in situations where a person who is dying is making life difficult for a carer by their angry behaviour to them. Here the carer may need support and help in understanding why this previously loving person is so awkward now. Carers can be helped to set appropriate boundaries for the dying person. The odd episode of rudeness and rage can be understood and forgiven, but a constant battery will wear out their love, and result in further loss for someone who is losing so much that is important already. Professionals can strengthen carers to ask for proper consideration of their needs without feeling guilty.

Most professionals in this field have experienced being blamed by a dying person or their carer for failing to cure or to alleviate a problem. Defensiveness is never useful. Real shortcomings need to be honestly acknowledged and it always helps to say 'I'm sorry that you feel things went so badly', even if everything possible has been done. Allowing the angry person a chance to talk about their dissatisfaction will often help them to see things in proportion.

A social worker visited by appointment a bereaved husband whose wife had recently died in the local hospice. He was unkempt and unsmiling, and made it clear that he blamed her for encouraging his wife to agree to hospice care. They talked about why he thought this, and he agreed to her visiting again to continue the discussion. On her next visit he was neatly dressed and more friendly. He acknowledged that he had known how ill his wife was and that the admission itself was not the cause of her death.

However, it has sometimes to be accepted that someone will need to hang on to their anger as the only way of dealing with their distress. Teams may then need to be supportive of a team member who is the focus of that anger.

Denial

Denial is a useful protective psychological mechanism in a dangerous situation, provided it does not prevent the person denying from taking action which could protect themselves or others from further harm. So a woman who finds a lump in her breast but denies that it could damage her is denying inappropriately because it prevents her seeking treatment. A woman with well-established and untreatable cancer of the lung, who asserts that she has another twenty years yet and will make that round the world trip, is distancing herself from an unbearable reality. Denial can be uncomfortable for professionals if they prefer to be open with those they work with. The secret is not to collude with the denial by pretending to share it but to understand that individual's need to protect themselves, and to speak to the feelings underneath. To say, 'When things are difficult it helps to think about something pleasant', recognizes the pain of the situation.

Less frequently it is the carer who denies the illness is serious and continues to expect the sick person to carry on as usual. This desperate attempt to maintain normality needs a caring rather than a punitive response from professionals whose first concern may be the effect on their patient.

There are some circumstances in which denial needs to be tackled. If the person who is dying is a single parent with young children who will require care in future, then that parent has to be helped to start the process of planning. Similarly, if there is someone with a learning disability, or a frail elderly person dependent solely on someone who is dying, plans need to be made. Useful mechanisms here are 'What if' and 'planning for the worst and hoping for the best'. Discussing with a single parent what they would like to happen to their children if they were not around, helps to maintain some of the protective distance.

However, if the dying person has a partner who is caring for the children and will continue to be able to do so, then there is no need to breach the denial. Professionals may regret that those who are dying do not take opportunities to speak to those they love about their own death, but each person has to die the death they choose. It will certainly be important for the parent who is going to survive to prepare the children for the death.

Another situation in which denial needs to be tackled is when someone is overtly denying what is happening but is displaying an unusual amount of distress or pain which is not responding to treatment. Again this is best done in a way which avoids direct confrontation. Kearney[17] gives an interesting example of using image work successfully to relieve distress in a young man. Image work can form part of a psychotherapeutic approach and uses imagery to help create a bridge between the conscious and unconscious self. The imaginary material is often visual, but may be auditory or tactile, or from the client's dreams. Kearney comments that 'because the imagery enabled emotional expression in symbolic form it did not challenge the protective shield of Sean's denial, which was allowed to remain intact'.

Depression and depair

Standing alongside another human being in despair at their coming death is a real challenge. The usual methods for dealing with sadness and despair involve reassurance that in the long run things will improve. This is plainly untenable when someone is dying and to a bereaved person seems so unlikely as to be insulting to the person they have lost and to their own fidelity.

Cyril was fifty-six. He had taken early retirement, had a large lump sum in the bank and an ample pension. He had planned to travel and enjoy sun, good food and wine after a lifetime's hard work. Now he was lying in a palliative care bed with cancer of the stomach, unable to eat, his money useless to him. He could not even spend his weekly income.

To jolly him along would have been insensitive. He needed an honest acknowledgement that life can be unfair, and empathy with his misery and sense of loss. Given this understanding, and clear messages from the caring team that they value this despairing individual and have not given up their attempts to make the quality of life as good as possible, some patients may be enabled to recover the coping abilities or even find new ones. Some will never lift, and team members need to help each other not to be drawn down into the pit with the person in despair and thereby become ineffective. If such sadness does spill over into a clinical depression, antidepressant drugs may be considered as an adjunct to the strategies already described.

Fear

The person who shows panic and fear in their final illness can create great unease in the caring team, fellow patients in a ward, and in those who love them. It provides a painful challenge to one of the basic assumptions of palliative care – that it is possible to enable people to have a good quality of life at the end of life. It reminds those who may soon follow of how much is unknown and how tenuous is the control they may have achieved. Like any other emotion fear may be communicated in words or in behaviour. The patient who frequently calls for extra pain relief during the night when that level of medication is effective during the day, may be in reality asking for help with fears in a way that is socially acceptable. The test will be if the patient can be helped to settle without medication if a nurse spends time in gentle exploration of anxieties and stays until the patient is calm.

Common fears are of the manner of death – sudden haemorrhage, being unable to breathe, choking to death, being buried alive – or of what may lie beyond the moment of death. The first essential is not to assume what the fear is, but ask 'You don't seem comfortable, and sometimes you look really scared. One of the team may be able to help. Is there anything that is frightening you particularly?' A discussion of anxieties about the manner of death may lead to concrete reassurance about the way the distressing event can be handled. Patients may see that, for instance, the level of sedation as the end approaches is something that can be negotiated and be more under their control than they had expected. Some fears may be to do with after death.

Peter, aged sixty-eight and knowing he was within a few weeks of death from cancer of the pancreas, seemed to staff to be uneasy and unsettled. A social worker was asked to talk to him on behalf of the team to try to discover what was troubling him. It became clear that he was ruminating for much of the time on what might happen after he died. His wife had died some years before and he now feared that he would not be allowed to join her in heaven because he had been a nominal rather than an active Christian. Together he and the social worker decided on a two-pronged approach. An opportunity would be made for him to talk to the chaplain about these fears, and to help with his constant rumination, he would be supplied with some jigsaws. He had found these a good distraction in the past.

Much has been learnt in recent years about the ways those facing crises can be helped to gain greater control over their fears. The use of cognitive therapy has been mentioned above. Relaxation techniques, incorporating music or guided imagery, can help here. Art therapy can offer a release. Massage and aromatherapy have become much more readily available in health care and can contribute to a sense of peace.

Uncertainty

Common uncertainties faced by those who are dying and their carers are how much hope is there, how long before death comes, what will the intervening period be like and how will death come. For some the uncertainty about the possibility of cure or remission may be with them until the day of death. For others the knowledge that death is coming may be a sort of relief. In their efforts to deal with the tremendous anxiety that living with uncertainty creates, both those who are dying and their carers may press professionals to give them concrete statements on any of these issues.

Studies have shown how unreliable forecasts of prognosis usually are, and that they are likely to be too optimistic. Maguire and Faulkner[10] suggest 'it is better to acknowledge your uncertainty and the difficulties this will cause'. They go on to describe a scheme of responses which checks if the enquirer would like to know what signs may herald further deterioration, encourages positive use of the present time, shows a willingness to monitor the situation regularly and a readiness to respond to any emergency. This gives the security of feeling that someone with more experience recognizes the problem and can be called on if there are particular worries or difficulties.

For some the strategy of 'hoping for the best and planning for the worst' is helpful. When carers come with such questions as, 'Shall I take unpaid leave from my job now or later?', 'Shall I get my daughter over from Australia?', or when some one for whom there is no hope of cure asks, 'Shall I take early retirement?', 'Shall I have more chemotherapy?', this strategy offers a framework for reviewing options. Thinking with patient or carer what the situation would be if the best happened and what they would need to consider if the worst happened, enables them to take a variety of considerations into account without necessarily focusing too heavily on one scenario or the other.

The uncommunicative patient

There is no such thing as an uncommunicative patient, though there may be patients who do not talk as professionals think they should. The issue here is not silence alone. A patient may not talk but by a smile or squeeze of the hand may convey trust or grief. These are the patients who do not talk about their fears and sadness, patients who only converse in monosyllables, patients who shut their eyes when someone asks how they are, and who do this in a way that makes professionals feel uncomfortable and not in control. Some questions need to be asked here.

How has this person dealt with life crises in the past? Can family or friends identify this as a common way of coping? Has every professional in the team in turn tried to start up a deep conversation about feelings and is the patient just plain irritated with intrusive questions? An unfortunate effect of the greater concern for the feelings of those who are dying and the increased openness in discussing them is that there may almost be an expectation that people *should* be ready to talk. They may be pressed to do so, as much to satisfy a professional's view of how people should die, as meet any real need or wish of the patient.

Are the professionals picking up the patient's own feelings of angry hopelessness?

Casement[18] shows how valuable the therapist's own feelings are as a guide to the patient's experience. If this seems the likely explanation it should be tackled with the patient, who needs to be given some responsibility for their own feelings and the effect of them on others. One way might be: 'Mr Jones, recently I [the team] have felt very uncomfortable and helpless when with you, as if nothing I [we] do is any good? Is this how you are feeling?' This may produce an angry outburst that clears the air, or a continuing silence. In the latter case a firm statement about appropriate boundaries may help.

> Mr Jones, I know this is a difficult time for you. I am sorry that we cannot cure you/relieve your pain as we would wish. We do want to go on trying to help but we need to work on it together. I won't press you to talk again unless you show me that you are ready to do so, but until then I won't be able to be as useful as I could be.

Professionals need to be clear about what is properly their responsibility. They cannot be responsible for making everything right, they are responsible for working with the patient to the best of their ability.

Asking for euthanasia

Patients may ask for assistance in ending their lives directly or they may be more indirect. 'You wouldn't let a dog live like this.' The ethical aspects of this issue will be dealt with in Chapter 9 on ethics. The communication approach should be based on principles already outlined in this chapter, a readiness to explore with patient or carer what particular aspects of the situation are most painful, and acknowledgement of and empathy with the emotional pain. Only after this should the professional gently outline the boundaries set by the law and conscience. This needs to be done in a way which does not make the person who has asked feel either ashamed or abandoned. It may well be appropriate to give an assurance that nothing will be done to prolong life. It can be painful to face the reproach or even anger which refusing such a request can bring. This is another situation when the support of team members is vital.

Around the death

There is a particular need for good communication skills in the period around the actual death. The person who is dying communicates increasingly through non-verbal means, but this should not stop professionals talking to them, describing what they are about to do, and treating them as persons with feelings. The carers are likely to be tense and distressed. Good preparation is the key here. If there has been open and honest discussion with the person who is dying and the carers at an earlier stage about possible wishes at the time of death, professionals will feel clearer about how to meet their needs. If someone in the later stages of a life-threatening disease is admitted to a hospital or other institution, carers should be asked on admission about the degree of involvement they wish at the time of death and whether they wish to be called in the night. This should be done even when death is not immediately expected, since it is in practice so hard to predict. Hampe's study of spouses of dying patients in hospital found that only 74 per cent of those who wished to be informed of impending death, and 63 per cent of those who wished to be present at the death achieved this.[19] Lunt et al. showed that relatives of those dying in specialist palliative care settings were twice as likely to be present at the death as those in general wards.[20]

If the death is planned to be at home similar early exploration of all parties' views is needed. In addition carers need to be aware of what actual sources and levels of help there may be. The vague promise 'You'll have all the help you need' may lead to unrealistic expectations of 24-hour care being provided when all that is available is a night sitter once a week.

Once the death is approaching the carers' wishes should be reviewed with them regularly. What they expected they would wish may not turn out in practice to be so, or they may change their view if the death is particularly long drawn out. This is a time when the likely manner of death may be much clearer, and doctor or nurse should explore whether carers would like to be aware in more detail what the event might be like. Special attention needs to be paid to those who may often be excluded at this time – children, those with learning disabilities and the mentally frail elderly. The professionals involved can give a lead in ensuring that they are properly informed and participating appropriately, for example, by including them in family conferences or specifically asking their opinion of how things are going on home visits.

Margaret, aged sixty-five with metastases from breast cancer, was referred to a palliative care home care service. The referral stated that her son Peter, who lived with her and had a learning disability, 'does not know she is dying'. The visiting nurse quickly established that Peter was in fact very well aware of the seriousness of his mother's illness. No one had thought to ask him before. He was keen to continue caring for her. He was very skilled domestically but rather anxious and rigid in his thinking. Margaret did not want to die at home. She felt this would make Peter too anxious, but she remained there until three weeks before her death, lovingly cared for by Peter and still able to give him some emotional support.

There is no 'right' amount of time for carers to spend with the body once the person has died, nor any 'right' way to grieve. Here different cultural practices need to be especially respected. At home carers can be in control. It may be useful to point out to those unused to death at home that there is no need to rush the body out of the house immediately. Farewells can be taken slowly. Grandchildren can come and say goodbye to their grandmother after school in familiar surroundings. In hospital there may be pressure on beds which means unlimited time is not available. If staff know they will soon need that space for another patient they need to give some warning 'In about a quarter of an hour we will need to move your husband elsewhere. You will be able to see him there if you wish or you can finish your goodbyes here in that time.' A frequent source of distress to carers are the procedures for obtaining the death certificate and recovering the patients' belongings from hospital.[21] Making procedures clear and efficient, training staff to carry them out sensitively and providing something more presentable than a black plastic rubbish bag for the belongings communicates a great deal to carers about the degree of concern for them and the value of the person they cared for.

In hospital there are other participants in the death besides the carers and the staff. Other patients will certainly be keen observers and may be more deeply involved if they have known the patient. On the positive side they may learn from seeing how this death has been handled how caringly their own end may be dealt with. On the negative side this death may be a terrifying reminder of their own mortality, especially if the death has not been peaceful. So deaths on the ward should not be ignored. Staff can take the opportunity to say 'Perhaps you saw that Mrs Brown died last night.' This gives permission to ask questions about the death and may lead to some discussion of that patient's own death. If the death was distressing it gives an opportunity to reassure that not all deaths are like that one.

Conclusion

This chapter has attempted to establish some principles for good practice in communication with those who are dying and their carers, and has discussed some particular issues. However there can be no exact blueprint for this work. Egan[22] observes 'helpers tend to over-identify the helping process with the communication skills that serve it. Technique can replace substance. Communication skills are essential of course, but they still must serve the outcomes of the helping process.' Communication is a creative process – herein is its excitement and its danger. It is not possible to be perfectly prepared for whatever comes. So courage is needed with a solid value base and some understanding of basic skills. Most important though is a faith in the potential of the partner in the dialogue, whether that person is dying or bereaved, to change and grow in response to the crisis of loss and death.

Notes and References

1. BARKWELL, D.P. 'Ascribed meaning: a critical factor in coping and pain attenuation in patients with cancer-related pain', *Journal of Palliative Care*, 1991, 7(3), 5–14.
2. STEDEFORD, A. *Facing Death: Patients, Families and Professionals*, Oxford, Heinemann Medical Books, 1984.

3. LICHTER, I. 'Some psychological causes of distress in the terminally ill', *Palliative Medicine*, 1991, **5**, 138–46.
4. TRUAX, C.B. and CARKHUFF, R.R. *Towards Effective Counselling and Psychotherapy*, Chicago, Aldine, 1967.
5. TUSON, G. 'Schindler's Ark: a study in heroism, therapy and change', *Journal of Family Therapy*, 1985, **7**, 161–73.
6. VACHON, M. 'Battle fatigue in hospice/palliative care.' In: Gilmore, A. and Gilmore, S. (eds), *A Safer Death*, New York, Plenum Press, 1988.
7. KÜBLER-ROSS, E. *On Death and Dying*, New York, Macmillan, 1969.
8. KASTENBAUM, R. 'Is death a life crisis?' In: Datan, N. and Ginsberg, L.H. (eds), *Life-span Developmental Psychology: Normative Life Crises*, New York: Academic Press, 1975.
9. MAGUIRE, P. 'Barriers to psychological care of the dying', *British Medical Journal*, 1985, **291**, 1711–3.
10. MAGUIRE, P. and FAULKNER, A. 'How to do it. Communicate with cancer patients: 1. Handling bad news and difficult questions. 2. Handling collusion uncertainty and denial', *British Medical Journal*, 1988, **297**, 907–9, 972–4.
11. MAGUIRE, P. and BUCKMAN, R. *Why Won't They Talk to Me?* Shepperton, Middx: Videotape Linkward Productions, 1985.
12. MOOREY, S. and GREER, S. *Psychological Therapy for Cancer Patients*, Oxford, Heinemann Medical Books, 1989.
13. CARTWRIGHT, A., HOCKEY, L. and ANDERSON, R. *Life Before Death*, London, Routledge and Kegan Paul, 1973.
14. SEALE, C. 'Communication and awareness about death; a study of a random sample of dying people', *Social Science and Medicine*, 1991, **32**(8), 943–52.
15. HOGBIN, B. and FALLOWFIELD, L. 'Getting it taped: the "bad news" consultation with cancer patients', *British Journal of Hospital Medicine*, 1989, **4**(4), 330–33.
16. BUCKMAN, R. *I Don't Know What to Say*, London, Macmillan, 1988.
17. KEARNEY, M. 'Imagework in a case of intractable pain', *Palliative Medicine*, 1992, **6**, 152–57.
18. CASEMENT, P. *On Learning from the Patient*, London, Tavistock, 1985.
19. HAMPE, S.O. 'Needs of the grieving spouse in hospital', *Nursing Research*, 1975, **24**, 113–9.
20. LUNT, B., NEALE, C. and CLIFFORD, C. A comparison of hospice and hospital care for terminally ill cancer patients and their families. Accompanying paper B. Family support in terminal care. Unpublished report of DHSS funded research.
21. WRIGHT, A., COUSINS, J. and UPWARD, J. A study of bereavement support in NHS hospitals in England. Kings Fund Project Paper No. 77. London: King Edward's Hospital fund for London, 1988.
22. EGAN, G. *The Skilled Helper*, Belmont, Brooks Cole, 1990.
23. WILKINSON, S. Factors which influence how nurses communicate with patients. *Journal of Advanced Nursing*, 1991, **16**, 677–688.

3

Symptom Control

Pain

Tony O'Brien

> Despite all the recent advances in knowledge, the management of
> pain in the terminally ill throughout the world remains a disgrace.
> What is needed now is not a stunning new understanding of pain
> pharmacology, but the consistent and rational application of what
> we already know. History will judge us harshly if we continue to
> fail to meet even this modest goal.
>
> Conolly, 1987[1]

For many patients, a diagnosis of cancer equates with the expectation of a
painful and debilitating illness, culminating in a distressing and perhaps
a meaningless death. The process of dying, and in particular concern
regarding uncontrolled pain, are often feared more than death itself. The
prompt and effective relief of pain is a fundamental principle of palliative
care which is enshrined in its very definition.

> The active total care of patients whose disease is not responsive
> to curative treatment, where control of pain, of other symptoms
> and of psychological, social and spiritual problems is paramount,
> and where the goal is the achievement of the best quality of life for
> patients and their families.[2]

By definition therefore, palliative care is concerned with the management
of patients whose disease is 'not responsive to curative treatment'. This
must not be taken to infer that palliative care assumes a role only at a point
when all measures aimed at achieving a cure have been fully exhausted.
The majority of patients with cancer are not cured of their illness, and for
many, this fact is evident from the time of first diagnosis. Kearney (1991)
has highlighted the need for a basic attitudinal change.

> Patients with incurable illness must no longer be viewed as medical
> failures for whom nothing more can be done. They need palliative
> care, which does not mean a hand-holding second-rate soft
> option, but treatment, which most people will need at some

point in their lives, and many from the time of diagnosis, demanding as much skill and commitment as is normally brought into preventing, investigating and curing illness.[3]

Pain occurs in approximately 70 per cent of patients with advanced cancer. In the vast majority of cases, it is amenable to treatment. Indeed, of all the symptoms that occur in advanced cancer, pain is perhaps the one that is most amenable to treatment. Yet, even in developed countries, over half of such patients do not receive an adequate level of analgesia. This tragic and unacceptable situation has developed for a variety of reasons.

- In part, there is a limited understanding of the nature of cancer pain, and specifically there is a failure to appreciate fully that pain is not simply a physical sensation.
- There is also a belief amongst many patients and indeed amongst some doctors and nurses, that pain in cancer is inevitable and untreatable.
- Finally, there is a reluctance to apply well-established principles to the management of cancer pain, arising from inadequate education and compounded by irrational fears concerning the use of opioids.

Experience in hospice and palliative care settings worldwide, has shown that it is possible to achieve good pain control in approximately 95 per cent of all patients. It is important to note that nobody claims to control pain in one-hundred per cent of cases. Statistically, a figure of ninety-five per cent is very encouraging but equally it must be recognized that at any point in time, one patient in twenty will continue to suffer uncontrolled pain. The impact that even this one patient will have on the individuals and on the teams caring for him is quite profound, and far in excess of what would be expected when viewed in pure statistical terms. Such patients must be assured of our continuing efforts to relieve their suffering, even if we cannot fully control their pain. These patients must not be abandoned.

Nature of cancer pain

Despite all the advances in our understanding of pain, we still lack a totally satisfactory definition. Perhaps the most widely accepted definition is that proposed by the International Association for the Study of Pain:

> Pain is an unpleasant sensory and emotional experience associated with actual or potential tissue damage, or described in terms of such damage. Pain is always subjective. Each individual learns the application of the word through experiences related to injury in early life. It is unquestionably a sensation in a part or parts of the body but it is also always unpleasant and therefore an emotional experience.[4]

Melzack and Wall (1988) commend this definition for identifying the association between tissue injury and pain, although this is by no means consistent, and also for highlighting the emotional dimension of the pain experience. However, they are concerned that the word 'unpleasant' is wholly inadequate to describe the 'misery, anguish, desperation and urgency that are part of the pain experience'.[5]

In clinical terms, the above definition has two major strengths. Firstly, it identifies the fact that pain is always subjective. As clinicians, we must at least begin by learning to believe patients when they complain of pain. There is sometimes a temptation to question the validity or reliability of a patient's history when we fail to understand their pain in terms of its pathophysiology or when our best therapeutic efforts are consistently ineffective.

Secondly, it recognizes the importance of emotional factors in the appreciation of pain. Twycross has described pain as being a 'dual phenomenon'. One part of this phenomenon is the perception of the stimulus and the others is the patient's emotional reaction to the stimulus.[6]

It follows therefore, that the potential of any given stimulus to cause distress and suffering will be influenced by the emotional state of the patient at that time. For example, a patient who is feeling frightened, angry, sad or isolated will experience a greater degree of suffering than one who is feeling supported, understood and loved. For although the *pain perception threshold* (the least experience of pain which a subject can recognize) may be relatively constant for all individuals, the *pain tolerance threshold* (the greatest level of pain which a subject is willing to tolerate) is subject to considerable variation. The capacity of emotional factors to influence the pain tolerance threshold must be fully recognized and appreciated.

In trying to understand some of the complexities of pain, it is useful to use the model of *total pain* as described by Dame Cicely Saunders.[7] The pain that a patient describes may be seen as the tip of an iceberg. Underlying this pain, are a whole range of factors – physical, emotional, social and spiritual, each contributing to the total pain experience and each inextricably entwined.

It follows, therefore, that if we focus all our efforts on achieving control of physical pain, without regard to these other factors, it is highly unlikely that we will achieve an optimal level of success. The pain of a patient who is trying to come to terms with the loss of role as a parent and spouse; the pain of a patient readjusting to an altered body image consequent on the effects of surgery or chemotherapy; the pain of someone who struggles in vain to find some meaning in their life and in their suffering; these are pains which do not carry opioid receptors and which are beyond the scope of even the most carefully sited anaesthetist's needle.

Not surprisingly, considerable ingenuity and an openness to explore new approaches to the problem is sometimes required. Kearney has reported on the value of image work in the management of intractable pain, requiring not just the application of the necessary skills involved in using such an approach, but also requiring that a relationship, which is based on trust, be established between the patient and the professional.[8]

Cancer – a chronic pain

One of the major advances in the field of pain has been the recognition that chronic, persistent pain is a distinct medical entity different from acute pain in many respects.[9] Acute pain occurs in response to tissue injury or damage and the expectation is that as healing occurs, so will the pain lessen. The pain may even serve a useful function by forcing the patient to rest the damaged part, thereby enhancing the process of healing.

In contrast, chronic pain occurs in a situation where it is unlikely that further healing will occur. In fact, because cancer is a dynamic disorder, further tissue damage is probable. The chronic pain associated with advancing cancer serves no useful purpose. It is no longer a symptom of tissue disease or injury, but a pain syndrome in its own right. In advanced cancer, the symptoms are the disease.[10]

Measurement of pain

In order to continue to study pain and measures to control pain in a scientific way, it is essential that we have a clear, reliable and accurate way of measuring pain. Many of the methods in common use, are designed to measure the intensity of pain. One such method, the verbal rating score, asks a patient to describe the intensity of his pain as none, mild, moderate or severe. Another method is the visual analogue scale. The patient is presented with a straight line which is 10 cm long. One end represents 'no pain' and the other end represents 'the most severe pain you can imagine'. The patient is asked to mark the line at a point appropriate to the intensity of his pain. This is then measured to get a numerical indication of the intensity of the pain. Both of these methods measure pain in a single dimension – intensity.

In an effort to develop a more comprehensive system of pain measurement, the McGill pain questionnaire was developed.[11] It is now widely recognized as a valid, reliable instrument to measure pain experience. It identifies and measures three major categories of pain experience – sensory, affective and evaluative. One of the principal purposes of this questionnaire is to bridge the gap between the measurement and assessment of pain in the laboratory and the clinical setting.

St Christopher's Hospice, in common with many palliative care centres, has developed and modified its own pain chart. (Figure 3.1) This chart recognizes that patients will commonly have pain at multiple sites. The intensity of each pain is measured by using a verbal rating score, and an attempt is made to assess the impact that the pain is having on a patient's life in terms of mobility and sleep disturbance. Furthermore, the previous use and efficacy of medication and other pain relief procedures is recorded.

The classification of a patient's pain as mild, moderate or severe provides a useful basis on which to select an appropriate drug treatment. Having

PAIN CHART

Indicate each pain numerically on diagram and detail in table below

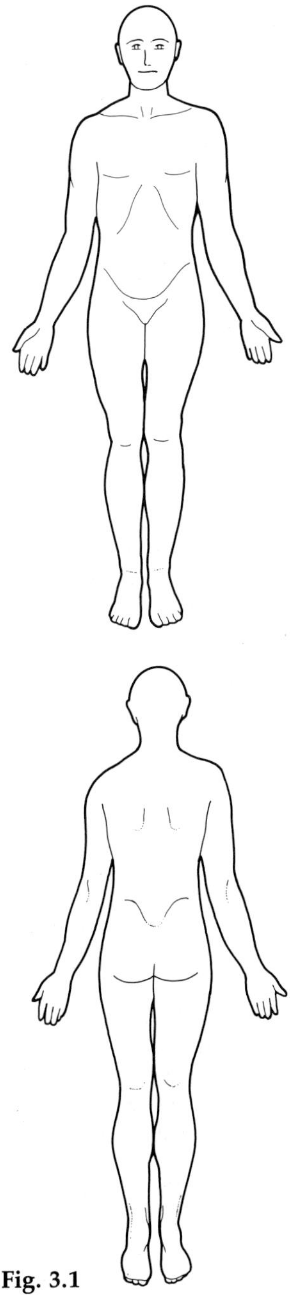

		1	2	3	4
INTENSITY	CONTROLLED				
	MODERATE				
	SEVERE				
	OVERWHELMING				
DURATION	1–2 weeks				
	2–6 weeks				
	6–12 weeks				
	>–12 weeks				
PERIODICITY	CONSTANT				
	INTERMITTENT				
EFFECT ON	SLEEP				
	MOBILITY				

EFFECT OF PRESENT
MEDICATION:

	1	2	3	4
NO DIFFERENCE				
PARTIAL CONTROL				
COMPLETE CONTROL				

OTHER TREATMENT:

	1	2	3	4
nerve block				
radiotherapy				
other				

EFFECT:

	1	2	3	4
NO DIFFERENCE				
PARTIAL CONTROL				
COMPLETE CONTROL				

RELATIVE'S VIEWS:

OTHER INFORMATION:

POSSIBLE CAUSES OF EACH PAIN:

1.
2.
3.
4.

Fig. 3.1

completed the pain chart, the clinician is then asked to record the probable underlying cause of each pain. This is a useful discipline, particularly in the setting of a training institution.

Evaluation of pain

Pain in cancer will usually occur at a number of distinct anatomical sites. Twycross and Fairfield (1982) reported that 34 per cent of patients will have pain at four or more separate sites[12] This is of practical importance in that the underlying cause of each of these pains may well be different, and consequently each may require a separate line of management.

In general the causes of pain in cancer can be classified into four main groups.[13]

- *Pain caused by the cancer*: This is by far the most common cause of pain in cancer, responsible for over two-thirds of all cancer pains. Bone pain, neuropathic pain, visceral pain and soft tissue pain may all be caused by direct involvement of pain sensitive structures by the cancer.
- *Pain caused by the treatment*: Pain may also result as a side effect of cancer treatment, including surgery, chemotherapy and radio-therapy.
- *Pain caused by general weakness/debility*: The aches and stiffness associated with profound weakness and prolonged immobility, may be classified under this heading. In addition, problems such as constipation and pressure sores may also give rise to pain.
- *Pain unrelated to cancer or its treatment*: When a diagnosis of cancer is made, there is a temptation to assume that all subsequent problems are related to the cancer. Osteoarthritis and angina for example, are pains which may occur in patients with cancer, but are clearly unrelated to cancer or its treatment.

Approach to physical pain

Establish the cause

It is essential to establish the cause of each pain, before planning treatment. This will involve taking a careful history and conducting a thorough symptom-focused examination. The site, radiation, quality and severity of each pain will be recorded, and note taken of whether it is intermittent or continuous, and also if there are any aggravating or relieving factors. Record also the extent to which any drugs or other treatments have helped in the past, and if adverse effects have been troublesome.

The information thus gathered, when considered in the context of the known or suspected primary and secondary sites of tumour, and including an assessment of a patient's mental state, will generally be adequate to establish a clinical diagnosis as to the cause of each pain. Uncommonly, it will be necessary to conduct more formal investigations, involving X-rays, scans, etc. Once a reasonably confident diagnosis as to the cause of each pain is established, then rational treatment options may be pursued.

Appropriate treatment

Figure 3.2 summarizes some of the approaches which may be employed as part of the management strategy. Given the nature and complexity of cancer pain, it is unlikely that any single approach will in itself prove entirely effective. More commonly, it is necessary to use a combined approach, using both drug and non-drug measures.

Part of the process of selecting appropriate treatments, will involve offering a clear explanation to the patient regarding the cause of his pain and discussing the relative advantages and disadvantages of the various treatment options. This is a good time to establish what the patient's expectations are of any proposed treatment, and to advise accordingly. It is important at this stage to undertake to continue to work to relieve the pain even if the initial therapeutic efforts are unsuccessful. Equally, it is important not to make false or unrealistic promises, which with the passage of time may only serve to demoralize and further undermine a patient's confidence.

Review

Cancer is a dynamic disorder. Whatever treatment options are started, it is vital to review the care of each patient in a systematic fashion and on a regular basis. The dose of each drug must be individually titrated to match that patient's needs at that point in time. Side effects of treatments must be

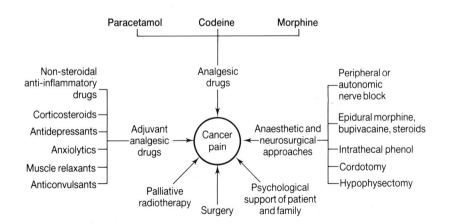

Fig. 3.2 Approach to cancer pain. Reproduced from Baines M. *British Medical Journal* **298**; 36–38, © 1989 British Medical Journal.

anticipated and prevented. Persistent and troublesome side effects must prompt a reassessment to determine the role of alternative approaches.

Analgesic drugs

Analgesic drugs are the mainstay of cancer pain management. The World Health Organization has promoted the concept of the analgesic ladder for cancer pain management. Using this principle, non-opioids such as aspirin and paracetamol are used for mild pain. If they are not adequate to control pain, then a drug of greater potency in the form of a weak opioid is used. Similarly, if drugs of this potency are not sufficient, then an increase to a more potent, strong opioid is recommended. At each stage, it is recognized that it may well be necessary to use adjuvant drugs. Adjuvant drugs are agents, other than those classified as pure analgesics, which when used appropriately will have a useful analgesic effect. The correct use of adjuvant drugs may facilitate a reduction in the opioid dose. The following principles apply to the use of analgesic drugs for cancer pain.

Use oral medication

The oral route is the route of choice for cancer pain management. The only indication to give medication by any other route is for those patients who cannot tolerate drugs by mouth because of severe weakness, dysphagia or vomiting. Severe pain per se, is not necessarily an indication for parenteral therapy.

Give drugs regularly

The frequency with which any drug is given is dictated strictly by the duration of action of that drug. Morphine elixir for example has a duration of action of four hours. MST continus has been specially formulated to have a duration of action of twelve hours. Pethidine is effective for only two to three hours, which makes it unsuitable as the sole analgesic in the management of cancer pain.

The objective is to give the medication at regular intervals, in anticipation of the pain. The exact same principle applies to the use of insulin in the treatment of Diabetes Mellitus. There is no role for PRN medication in the ongoing management of cancer pain.

Use a drug of adequate potency

The essential principle of the analgesic ladder is to match the intensity of the pain with a drug of adequate potency. It follows that if for example

a weak opioid is not sufficiently potent to control pain, then the introduction of a more potent strong opioid is required. The timing of the
introduction of a strong opioid must be based on an assessment of the
nature and severity of the pain, and must not be influenced by any crude
assessment of the likely prognosis.

Non-opioids

Aspirin

Aspirin has analgesic, anti-pyretic and in higher doses anti-inflammatory
properties. In common with other non-steroidal anti-inflammatory drugs,
it appears to exert its effects primarily through inhibition of prostaglandin
synthesis.

The recommended dose of aspirin is 600 mg every four to six
hours. Damage to the gastric mucosa is an important side effect of
aspirin therapy. Other side effects include prolonged bleeding time,
bronchospasm and skin reactions in hypersensitive patients.

Paracetamol

Paracetamol is a synthetic analgesic and anti-pyretic but unlike aspirin
has no anti-inflammatory effects. Surprisingly, its precise mode of action
is ill understood. In therapeutic doses of 1 g four to six hourly, it is generally well tolerated. In overdose, potentially fatal hepatocellular damage
may occur. As little as 10–15 g of paracetamol may be associated with
such damage.

Opioids

An opioid is a general term which describes both naturally occurring
and synthetic drugs which possess opioid like activity and which are
antagonized by naloxone.

The term opiate is a more specific one describing only naturally occurring compounds which are derived from the juice of the opium poppy.

In clinical terms, opioids are classified as weak or strong. These terms
are imprecise, but they serve to highlight one important clinical difference. Weak opioids typically exhibit a ceiling to their analgesic effects.
Further increase in dose, will result in an unacceptable level of side
effects. In contrast, strong opioids have a much wider dose spectrum,
and therefore can be used to relieve more severe pain.

Opioids are also classified in terms of their affinity to bind to specific
receptor sites (Table 3.1). Receptor sites are specialized areas on the
cell membrane which when activated by a specific drug or molecule,

produce the characteristic pharmacological response associated with that drug.

At least four main types of opioid receptor are recognized – *mu, kappa, sigma,* and *delta.* The existence of a fifth receptor type, *epsilon,* has been proposed. In addition, there is now evidence of a further subdivision of *mu* receptors into mu_1 (high affinity) and mu_2 (low affinity) receptors. High affinity mu_1 sites are responsible for mediating anti-nociception, as distinct from low affinity mu_2 sites which mediate the respiratory depressant effects of opioids. Naloxazone is a specific mu_1 antagonist which will reverse analgesia but has no effect on respiratory depression.

The potency of a drug is a measure of its affinity to bind to specific receptor sites – the more potent the drug, the greater the affinity. For example, when comparing two drugs, the more potent drug will produce the same response at a lower dose.

The efficacy of a drug is a measure of the intrinsic activity of that drug. An opioid with low intrinsic activity at individual receptors will not exert a full agonist effect, and is therefore termed a partial agonist.

Table 3.1   Opioid classification by receptor activity

Agonist	A drug which combines with a receptor and activates it, initiating the pharmacological response associated with that drug.	e.g. morphine
Antagonist	A drug which interferes with the action of an agonist: a pure antagonist has minimal or no agonist activity.	e.g. naloxone
Partial agonist	A drug which elicits less than maximal response from interaction with the receptor; if a partial agonist displaces a complete agonist, the result may be a decreased response.	e.g. buprenorphine
Mixed agonist-antagonist	A drug acting simultaneously on the different receptor sub-types, with the potential for both agonist action on one or more types and antagonist action on one or more types; the agonist activity may be partial or complete.	e.g. pentazocine

Source: Reproduced by permission of Churchill Livingstone from Twycross, R.G. and Lack, S.A. *Therapeutics in Terminal Cancer,* 2nd ed, Edinburgh, Churchill Livingstone, 1990.

Opioid receptors are found throughout the brain and spinal cord, particularly in the periaqueductal grey matter, the thalamus and hypothalamus and the substantia gelatinosa of the spinal cord. Opioid receptors have also been demonstrated at sites outside the central nervous system, including the bronchial epithelium and the gut.

Although, our understanding of opioid pharmacology has increased dramatically in recent years, it is as yet incomplete. Galer et al. (1992) highlight the individual variability that may occur in the response to both the analgesic effects and the toxicity profile of different opioid drugs.[14] This phenomenon occurs even with drugs possessing similar pharmacological profiles as for example the *mu* receptor agonists morphine and hydromorphone. The authors recommend a trial of an alternative opioid when dose escalation with morphine or any other opioid, yields intolerable and unmanageable side effects.

Weak opioids

In cancer pain management, weak opioids are used when pain is not adequately controlled by a non-opioid.

Codeine

Codeine is the standard weak opioid. It is closely related to morphine chemically and indeed morphine is one of its metabolites. It is well absorbed from the upper gastrointestinal tract and it has a duration of action of four to six hours. Codeine 60 mg is equivalent to morphine 5 mg.

Dihydrocodeine (DF118)

Dihydrocodeine (DF118) is a semi-synthetic analogue of codeine with a potency value one-third greater than codeine. Dihydrocodeine 60 mg is equivalent to morphine 6–7 mg, but as with codeine, there is individual variation in the potency ratio of these drugs when compared to morphine. The usual dose of dihydrocodeine is 30–60 mg, and the clinical duration of effect is three to four hours.

A modified release preparation of dihydrocodeine tartrate is available in 60 mg, 90 mg and 120 mg tablets, with a recommended dose interval of twelve hours.

The main side effect of codeine and dihydrocodeine is constipation, but on occasion, this can be used to therapeutic advantage. Nausea and vomiting may also occur.

Dextropropoxyphene

Dextropropoxyphene is an alternative weak opioid. It is a synthetic derivative of methadone and is readily absorbed from the upper gastrointestinal tract. The usual form of administration in the United Kingdom is in combination with paracetamol (Coproxamol). Each tablet contains dextropropoxyphene 32.5 mg and paracetamol 325 mg.

The recommended dose is up to two tablets of Coproxamol four hourly. It is generally well tolerated although it may cause confusion in the elderly. Nausea, vomiting and constipation may also occur but are less troublesome than with other opioids. It is important to note that Coproxamol is a dangerous drug in overdose particularly if taken in combination with alcohol.

Strong opioids

Strong opioid analgesics form the basis of our approach to severe cancer pain. Morphine is the strong oral opioid of choice for cancer pain management. It has a half-life of two and a half hours.

Morphine – pharmacology

Morphine is a pure opioid agonist. The dose required for individual patients may vary from 20 mg per day to several hundred mg per day or more. After oral administration, morphine is well absorbed, predominantly in the duodenum and upper small bowel. There is extensive first pass metabolism. The liver is the main site of morphine metabolism and the principal metabolites found in the plasma are morphine-3-glucuronide and morphine-6-glucuronide. The conjugation of morphine with glucuronic acid shows no evidence of saturation.

The major metabolites of morphine are excreted through the kidney, and particular care must therefore be exercised in patients with impaired renal function.

Morphine-6-glucuronide (M6G) accounts for much of the analgesic activity of morphine. It is three to four times more potent than morphine when given subcutaneously. The role of morphine-3-glucuronide in analgesia is as yet unknown.

Clinical experience has consistently shown that the analgesic effect of single dose oral morphine is poor. In contrast, the regular use of oral morphine is the mainstay of our approach to cancer pain management. This difference is explained by the activity of morphine-6-glucuronide (M6G).

The analgesic activity of morphine is dependent upon activation of the opioid receptors within the central nervous system. M6G is a polar compound, which penetrates into the CNS rather slowly. The ratio of M6G to morphine in the CSF has been shown to rise tenfold when morphine is given repeatedly as compared to a single dose. M6G is a potent *mu* agonist, and is responsible for much of the analgesic effects of morphine. The increased concentration of M6G found in the CNS with continuous use of morphine is the most likely explanation for the differences observed between single dose and regular administration of morphine.[15]

Clinical use

There are four commonly used oral morphine preparations.

- Morphine hydrochloride or morphine sulphate in chloroform water. Strengths may vary from 5 mg to 200 mg per 10 ml. A four-hourly dose is required, although clinical experience suggests that it is frequently possible to omit the dose due at 1.00 or 2.00 a.m.
- Morphine Sulphate oral solution (Oramorph). This is prepared in two strengths – 2 mg per ml and 20 mg per ml. It has the advantage of offering a standardized and accurate preparation with a relatively long shelf life. In addition, it is convenient and time saving for the pharmacist. The risk of dose error, particularly when used by the elderly or visually impaired, will be significantly lessened by the introduction of single dose unit vials. The sugar content of the lower concentration (2 mg/ml) requires that extra care be taken when used by patients with diabetes mellitus.
- Morphine Tablets (Sevredol). Morphine tablets are prepared in strengths of 10 mg and 20 mg, and are useful in the management of breakthrough pain.
- Morphine Sulphate Continus (MST). This is a modified release preparation which has the advantage of a convenient twelve-hour dose interval. Tablets are available in 10 mg, 30 mg, 60 mg, 100 mg and 200 mg strengths. They have the advantage of minimizing disruption to the patient's life, thereby improving compliance. The practice of using crushed MST without loss of efficacy or change in dose interval, has been described in both children and adults.[16] However, most palliative care physicians adhere to the manufacturer's guidelines and recommend that MST continus tablets be swallowed whole. An MST continus suspension is also available, in doses of 20 mg or 30 mg per sachet. The administration interval remains 12 hours.

The choice of oral preparation must be decided for each patient, depending on individual circumstances. Explanation and reassurance regarding the treatment will help to minimize problems, and this may usefully be supplemented by providing an information leaflet.

In order to avoid unnecessary delay and embarrassment at the pharmacy, it is vital that all doctors familiarize themselves with the legal requirements relating to the medical prescription of controlled drugs. It is an offence for a doctor to issue an incomplete prescription and a pharmacist is not allowed to dispense a controlled drug unless all the information required by law is given on the prescription.

The correct dose of oral morphine is the lowest dose which achieves effective control of pain. A starting dose of 5 mg four hourly is recommended, and in elderly patients it may be necessary to start as low as 2.5 mg four hourly. The dose can then be gradually titrated against the pain response. In general, the dose can be increased by increments of 50 to 100 per cent in the lower dose ranges (less than 30 mg four hourly), and by increments of 33 per cent to 50 per cent in the higher dose ranges.

The dose of morphine is titrated to one of two clear end points:

- *Relief of pain*: Continue the morphine either as a four-hourly elixir, or if more convenient, in a twelve-hourly modified release format. Monitor and treat any side effects, and review the dose regularly.
- *Pain continues*: Unacceptable side effects. Many cancer pains are relatively or absolutely insensitive to opioids. If patients develop troublesome and persistent side effects which are not controlled by standard measures, it will be necessary to reduce the dose of that opioid or to try an alternative oral opioid. If unsuccessful, it will be necessary to explore the possibility of an alternative route of administration, e.g. spinal opioids. Consideration must also be given to the role of other approaches to pain relief, either in the form of adjuvant drugs, radiotherapy or anaesthetic techniques.

Morphine side effects

Nausea and Vomiting

Up to 30 per cent of patients will experience nausea and vomiting when the drug is first introduced. All opioids can produce nausea and vomiting by stimulation of the chemoreceptor trigger zone in the area postrema of the medulla. The prophylactic use of an antiemetic with activity at the chemoreceptor trigger zone (e.g. prochlorperazine, Haloperidol or Metoclopramide) is recommended. The role of the 5-HT$_3$ antagonists, ondansetron and granisetron in the management of opioid induced nausea and vomiting, is currently under investigation. The emetic potential of morphine is limited to about five days following dose stabilization, at which point the antiemetic can be safely withdrawn.

Constipation

All patients on regular morphine must have a laxative routinely prescribed. Constipation may present a more difficult management problem than even the control of pain. Opioids reduce gastrointestinal motility and diminish intestinal, gastric, biliary and pancreatic secretions.

Dry mouth

There is a clear association between morphine use and development of a dry mouth. This is separate to the multiplicity of other factors associated with dry mouth in cancer patients, e.g. reduced fluid intake, drugs with anticholinergic side effects, oral candida. The importance of regular mouth care and good oral hygiene cannot be over emphasized. The use of measures to promote salivary flow and artificial salivary supplements may also be indicated.

Respiratory depression

Respiratory depression is not a clinical problem in patients who are taking morphine for the relief of cancer pain. This consistent clinical observation is explained by recent animal work which has demonstrated nociceptive input to the medullary respiratory centre.[17] If pain is reduced, however, following for example a nerve block, then respiratory depression will develop unless the dose of morphine is reduced. An exaggerated fear of respiratory depression has led to a reluctance to use morphine in the control of cancer pain. This is both unnecessary and unjustified.

Drowsiness and confusion

Patients on a stable dose of morphine have normal cognitive function. A transient deterioration in mental function has been documented following an increase in dose. It is a sensible precaution to advise patients that they may feel drowsy for a few days after starting morphine or following a dose increase. They can be reassured that this will resolve after a few days.

Myoclonus

Myoclonus is a descriptive term applied to shock-like, involuntary muscular contractions, due to a variety of causes. It is a useful sign of opioid neurotoxicity and is commonly seen in the final twenty-four to forty-eight hours of life, at a time when renal function is deteriorating rapidly. Under these circumstances, there is a build up of morphine metabolites. There is scant evidence to suggest that normorphine is the metabolite primarily responsible for myoclonus.[18] When it develops, a reduction in dose is indicated and if necessary, the myoclonus can be controlled by the introduction of a benzodiazepine.

Addiction and tolerance

Addiction, an overpowering drive to take a drug for its psychological effects, does not appear to occur in patients taking opioids for cancer pain.

Tolerance, the need for a larger dose of drug to achieve the same pharmacological effect is also feared. In cancer pain, an increase in dose may well be necessary, reflecting an increase in pain consequent on continued tumour growth. This is not tolerance.

Physical dependence may develop, but if pain control improves, then it is possible to reduce the dose of morphine slowly without producing withdrawal symptoms. Indeed, if there is a dramatic reduction in pain, following a nerve block for example, then a more rapid reduction in opioid is required if respiratory depression is to be avoided.

Alternative strong opioid analgesics

Although morphine is the recommended oral opioid of choice, it will be necessary on occasion to use other strong opioids.

Diamorphine

Diamorphine (diacetylmorphine) is one of many opioid derivatives which have been synthesized from morphine. After oral administration, diamorphine is rapidly converted to 6-monoacetylmorphine and then to morphine. The principal advantage of diamorphine over morphine relates to its greater solubility. Consequently, diamorphine is the parenteral strong opioid of choice.

Some controversy exists as to the conversion ratios of oral morphine to oral diamorphine. Ratios of 1:1.5 and 1:1 are in routine clinical use. When converting from oral morphine to parenteral diamorphine, the dose of oral morphine is divided by three.

Oxycodone

Oxycodone is a synthetic derivative of morphine which may be given orally, parenterally or in suppository form. It is the strong opioid of choice for rectal use. A 60 mg suppository given eight hourly is equally potent with 30 mg of oral morphine solution given four hourly.

Dextromoramide

Dextromoramide is a strong opioid agonist with a short half life of one to two hours. It is available in 5 mg and 10 mg tablets and has a peak effect equivalent to 15 mg of morphine. Its short duration of action limits its regular use. Its main role is for breakthrough pain or as a short acting analgesic which can be taken in anticipation of some painful procedure, e.g. a dressing. It can also be given sublingually.

Phenazocine

Phenazocine is a synthetic opioid, which is five times as potent as morphine. The 5 mg tablet, which is equivalent to 25 mg of morphine, makes titration of dose somewhat difficult.

Methadone

Methadone is a synthetic opioid agonist with activity at the *mu* receptor. A single 5 mg dose of methadone is equivalent to morphine 7.5 mg. In chronic use, when the half life of methadone increases from 15 hours to two to three days, it is considerably more potent than morphine. Because of the long half life, accumulation may occur, particularly in the elderly.

Pentazocine

Pentazocine was the first mixed agonist-antagonist analgesic to be used in widespread clinical practice. It is a weak antagonist at *mu* receptors and an agonist at *kappa* and *delta* receptors. The duration of analgesia produced by pentazocine is about three hours. It has a high incidence of side effects, commonly hallucinations and euphoria. It has little role in the ongoing management of cancer pain.

Buprenorphine

Buprenorphine is a partial agonist and is 30 times as potent as morphine. Because of extensive first pass metabolism and inactivation, it is given by the sublingual route. The duration of analgesia is 6–9 hours. There appears to be a ceiling effect at about 1.2 mg per twenty-four hours. It has the potential to antagonize the actions of pure opioid agonists and therefore their concurrent use must be avoided.

Pethidine

Pethidine is a synthetic drug which is structurally unrelated to morphine. Its short duration of action (two to three hours) makes it unsuitable for use in chronic pain. One of its metabolites, norpethidine, has excitatory effects on the central nervous system resulting in tremor, agitation and convulsions. These effects are more likely to occur when there is impaired renal function.

Hydromorphone

Hydromorphone is a semi-synthetic pure opioid agonist which is used extensively in North America. The potency ratio of oral hydromorphone to morphine is approximately 7.5:1. It is more soluble than morphine which has advantages when the drug is given parenterally. It is claimed that hydromorphone causes less gastrointestinal and sedative side effects than morphine.

Alternative methods of opioid administration

As already described, the oral route is the route of choice. However, on occasion it will be necessary to use an alternative route.

Rectal administration

Morphine may be given in suppository form, However, regular four-hourly administration of suppositories is cumbersome and unacceptable to many patients. Oxycodone pectinate suppositories (30 mg), may be given eight hourly, and are a useful alternative. MST continus tablets have been used rectally on a twelve-hourly schedule. In one study of 39 patients, pain control was maintained although 11 patients required a reduction in dose due to increased drowsiness.[19]

Subcutaneous administration

The value of the subcutaneous route to deliver opioids and other drugs is well established in hospice practice. Diamorphine is the parenteral opioid of choice in the United Kingdom. It may be given intermittently by four-hourly subcutaneous injections or alternatively may be infused at a constant rate by using a syringe pump. Although continuous infusion will result in stable blood levels, this does not necessarily mean that better pain control will be achieved. The choice between four-hourly injections and a syringe pump will therefore be decided by more practical considerations, e.g. syringe pump availability, nursing time, patient/family preference.

Intravenous administration

Patient controlled analgesia, using intravenous opioids, has been shown to be a useful and effective technique in the management of post-operative pain. The role of intravenous opioids in the management of cancer pain is not so well established. Intravenous access is an obvious and important difficulty, particularly in patients who may have had a lot of chemotherapy. Administration of drugs into a central vein via a Hickman catheter will avoid the problems of gaining peripheral access. In general, the intravenous route offers no particular advantages in the ongoing management of cancer pain.

Spinal opioids

The use of spinal opioids to control post-operative, obstetrical and cancer pain has increased dramatically since spinal opioids were first administered in humans during the late 1970s. Small doses of spinal opioids can produce effective and prolonged analgesia. Ideally, spinally administered opioids would produce an optimal level of analgesia with a marked reduction in the systemic side effect profile.

As with any route of drug delivery, the dose must be individually titrated. As a starting point, the initial epidural dose is one tenth that of the previous oral dose and clinical experience suggests that it is sometimes necessary to increase this dose to one-third of the previous oral dose. Intrathecally, an initial dose of one-hundredth of the oral dose is recommended. Note however, that the size of the dose is not a useful indicator as to the clinical application of the drug.

Side effects may be mediated through central or systemic actions. Opioids administered into the epidural space may be absorbed systemically, and when injected intrathecally may spread rostrally to exert some central effects. Centrally mediated side effects of spinal opioids include pruritus, nausea and vomiting, urinary retention, sedation and late respiratory depression. It is important to note that respiratory depression is extremely rare in the setting of cancer pain management. This presumably relates to the fact that such patients will have had prior exposure to opioids, often for prolonged periods of time. Technical problems such as displacement of catheters and local sepsis are a potential difficulty. The incidence of such problems may be reduced by the use of implanted devices.

The ideal opioid for spinal administration would have a potent segmental action, without rostral spread in the CSF or beyond to the systemic circulation. In the management of cancer pain, the more lipid soluble opioids such as fentanyl and sufentanil are appropriate for continuous infusion, whereas morphine, because of its longer duration of action, is a reasonable choice for intermittent administration.

It must be acknowledged, that the specific and absolute indications for the use of spinal opioids in the management of cancer pain are as yet not defined. The role of spinal opioids will only be properly assessed by well-designed studies which evaluate the risk–benefit ratio. The palliative care physician must then evaluate the application of these new techniques to his own setting. The practical implications of administering spinal opioids in hospice units and in the community, must also be addressed.

Transdermal administration

The role of the skin as a means of delivering drugs is currently under review. Fentanyl, when absorbed transdermally, has been shown to be of benefit in the control of pain in cancer patients.[20] Fentanyl is an opioid of high potency, low molecular weight and good solubility making it ideally suited to this route of administration. Further studies are required to assess its role in the clinical setting.

Inhaled opioids

Inhaled morphine has been used in the management of post-operative pain and for the control of dyspnoea. There is however, very little data available on the absorption and pharmacokinetics of morphine when delivered by this route, and therefore its route in clinical use cannot be recommended in the management of cancer pain.

Bone pain

Bone metastases are the most common cause of pain in malignant disease. Any part of the skeleton may be involved, but the axial skeleton and the proximal limb bones are particularly susceptible to metastatic involvement. About half of all bone metastases arise from carcinoma of breast, with tumours of lung, prostate and kidney next in order of frequency.

Many bone metastases cause no pain. Sometimes, a pathological fracture may be the first manifestation of any disease. There is no good correlation between the extent of bone involvement and the severity of pain. Small localized bone metastases can give rise to excruciating pain whilst disseminated bone disease, resulting in widespread skeletal destruction, may be relatively asymptomatic.

Skeletal metastases usually result from blood borne spread. Initially, tumour emboli seed in the medullary cavity and may later extend to involve the cortex. Stimulation of osteoblastic activity, resulting in focal production of osteoid and new bone, will produce a characteristic sclerotic reaction. More commonly, stimulation of osteoclastic activity will result in bone destruction and the formation of lytic metastases. X-ray examination may show lytic or sclerotic metastases, or both.

Pain is typically localized, except where there is associated nerve involvement or damage. Pain sensitive nerve endings are located in the periosteum and joints. These can be activated by both mechanical and chemical stimuli. The relative role of mechanical pressure, caused by expanding tumour and of chemical mediators such as prostaglandins in initiating and maintaining the pain response is unknown.

Certainly, the rapid onset of pain relief which can follow radiotherapy cannot be explained by tumour shrinkage alone.

The presence of bone metastases may be suspected on the basis of a history and physical examination. The sensitivity of plain X-rays to confirm the presence of bone metastases is relatively poor,and an isotope bone scan is therefore the investigation of choice. Biopsy of a bone metastasis is generally unnecessary, but may be indicated when the primary site of tumour is unknown.

Management of bone pain

In addition to the use of standard analgesics, the following approaches may also be of benefit.

Non-steroidal anti-inflammatory drugs

Non-steroidal anti-inflammatory drugs (NSAIDs) have an important role in the management of painful bone metastases. As yet, their precise mode of action is ill-understood, but two separate mechanisms may be important, both involving inhibition of prostaglandin synthesis.

Firstly, osteoclastic activity within bone metastases is under the control of chemical mediators, including both prostaglandins and non-prostaglandin osteolysins. Secondly, although prostaglandins do not produce pain directly, they do sensitize nerve endings to substances such as bradykinin and histamine, which may result in pain transmission. It appears therefore, that NSAIDs exert their effects primarily through inhibition of prostaglandin synthesis. This is achieved by blocking the cyclo-oxygenase that catalyses the conversion of arachadonic acid to cyclic endoperoxide. This action accounts for many of the therapeutic and adverse effects of this class of drugs.

NSAIDs are classified under seven different chemical classes. There is a general consensus that the more potent the drug, the greater is its side-effect profile. It is advisable to become familiar with perhaps one or two drugs from each class (Table 3.2).

There is marked inter-individual variation in the response to all of these agents, both in terms of their therapeutic effects and their adverse effects. If symptoms are not controlled on a particular agent, there is merit in trying a drug from a different class. There is never an indication to use two NSAIDs concurrently.

The principal side effects are gastro-intestinal disturbances including ulceration and perforation; hypersensitivity reactions; blood dyscrasias, predominantly aplastic anaemia and granulocytopenia; fluid retention; cardiac failure in the elderly; acute renal failure/interstitial nephritis; hepatic dysfunction; confusion in the elderly.

If gastric toxicity is a limiting factor in the use of these drugs, then the co-administration of omeprazole or misoprostol is indicated. The H_2 receptor antagonists, cimetidine and ranitidine, have been relatively disappointing in the treatment of NSAID induced gastric ulceration.

Bisphosphonates

Bisphosphonates, stable chemical analogues of pyrophosphate, are powerful inhibitors of osteoclastic function. They are the treatment of choice in the management of humoral hypercalcaemia of malignancy. Their role in the control of bone pain associated with metastatic disease, and in reducing the incidence of fracture, is currently under review.

Steroids

Steroids are also of benefit in the management of painful bone metastases. A starting dose of Dexamethasone 8 mg is usually required, and the dose is then titrated to the lowest possible level. The side effect profile of steroids, particularly if used in relatively high doses and over prolonged periods, is such that systemic steroids cannot be recommended as a first line approach in the management of painful bone metastases.

Radiotherapy

Radiotherapy is of proven benefit in the management of bone metastases. In addition to relief of pain, radiotherapy will also help to prevent pathological fractures and will promote healing following a pathological fracture. Based on randomized prospective studies, and supported by pooled data from non-randomized studies, a mean overall response rate in excess of 80 per cent can be expected. The onset of pain relief may occur 2–3 days following treatment, and the maximum benefit is seen at 2–3 weeks.

Price et al. (1986)[21] compared a single fraction of 8 Gy with the more usual treatment of 30 Gy in ten fractions. They found no difference in the speed of onset or duration of pain relief between the two treatment regimes, and pain relief was independent of the histology of the primary tumour.[22] This is obviously of major benefit to patients, who no longer have to cope with prolonged treatment regimes, as well as having very positive implications for hard pressed radiotherapy staff and equipment.

The morbidity associated with a single fraction of radiotherapy to a long bone is virtually nil. Patients with more generalized pains associated with widespread metastases may require hemi-body irradiation. Treatment to either the upper or lower half of the body is undertaken, with a single fraction of 8 Gy.

Table 3.2   Classification of non-steroidal anti-inflammatory drugs

Group	Example
Salicylates	Aspirin
	Benorylate
Proprionic acid derivatives	Ibuprofen
	Naproxen
	Ketoprofen
Indoles	Indomethacin
Fenamic acids	Mefenamic Acid
Phenylacetates	Diclofenac
Oxicams	Piroxicam
Pyrazolones	Azapropazone

Hemi-body irradiation is associated with a higher incidence of side-effects, particularly nausea and vomiting for upper body treatment, and diarrhoea and haematological toxicity for lower body treatment. Pain relief may be expected in 80 per cent of cases, with a median time to onset of pain relief of forty-eight hours.

Surgery

Surgery is indicated in situations where there is a high risk of fracture or if a bone has already fractured. Ideally, patients considered to be at risk, should be referred for an orthopaedic opinion before such a fracture occurs.

As with any treatment, the risk/benefit ratio must be assessed, but unless a patient is in a terminal situation and clearly unfit for surgical intervention, then some form of internal fixation should be considered. Drugs are of little value in the management of the incident pain which occurs when a patient with a fracture is moved, as will be necessary in the course of basic nursing care. If surgical fixation is not appropriate, excellent analgesia will be obtained with epidural local anaesthetic agents.

Anaesthetic techniques

Depending on the sites involved, a number of anaesthetic techniques may be employed. For example, the pain of a metastasis or a pathological fracture in the neck of the femur will respond to a psoas compartment block or to epidural local anaesthetic. Rib metastases present particular problems. The lung is very sensitive to the effects of radiotherapy. Also, irradiation of the right lower rib cage may involve the liver resulting in systemic side-effects. Rowell has reported on the value of intralesional methylprednisolone as a useful alternative to radiotherapy for painful rib metastases.[23]

Liver pain

The liver is a common site for metastatic involvement by tumour. Even in the presence of diffuse hepatic involvement, patients may have no pain, and liver function tests may be normal. Liver pain is described as a dull, aching pain in the right upper quadrant, which may radiate to the right shoulder. It is typically made worse by movement, coughing or deep breathing. Episodes of more severe pain will occur if there is haemorrhage into a metastasis.

The finding of a large, irregular and sometimes tender liver extending down to the right iliac fossa, which may be associated with ascites, leaves the clinician in little doubt as to the underlying pathology. Diagnostic ultrasound remains the most useful tool for the confirmation of liver metastases. Ultrasound has the advantage of being non-invasive, and is comparatively inexpensive. CT scanning, although more accurate, is also more expensive. Liver biopsy may be required to obtain histological confirmation if this is not already available.

The liver parenchyma is notably devoid of pain sensitive nerve endings. Liver pain occurs therefore as a consequence of stretching of the liver capsule. In addition to the use of opioids, the following approaches may also be necessary.

Management of liver pain

Non-steroidal anti-inflammatory drugs

Non-steroidal anti-inflammatory drugs are the adjuvant agent of choice in the management of liver pain. The onset of action is typically within twenty-four to forty-eight hours and when successful, the response can be quite dramatic. As applies to the use of non-steroidal anti-inflammatory drugs in general, there is marked inter-individual variation in the response to different agents. It may be necessary therefore to use a system of trial and error to identify the most useful drug in any given patient.

Steroids

Dexamethasone, in a dose of 6 mg to 8 mg per day, is also of benefit. The maintenance dose should be kept as low as possible, to reduce the incidence of troublesome side effects associated with steroid use.

Coeliac plexus block

Coeliac plexus block is the most successful anaesthetic technique used in the control of cancer pain. In a retrospective analysis of 89 patients who were suffering intractable abdominal pain associated with primary and secondary tumours of liver and carcinoma of pancreas, 84 patients reported relief following a coeliac plexus block. Of these, 32 patients reported 'excellent pain relief', 39 patients reported 'good relief', and 13 patients reported 'some pain relief'.[24]

Hanna et al. recommend percutaneous coeliac plexus blockade as a useful procedure in the management of intractable upper abdominal pain secondary to malignant disease, including liver metastases.

Chemotherapy

In some chemosensitive tumours, for example carcinoma of breast, lymphoma and small cell carcinoma of bronchus, chemotherapy may be an appropriate palliative measure. Factors which will influence this decision include the general condition of the patient and their wishes, the extent of other metastatic disease, the response to previous chemotherapy regimes and the anticipated toxicity associated with the proposed regime.

Neuropathic pain

Cancer pain is mediated through a variety of different pathophysiological mechanisms. The most common form, 'nociceptive' pain, occurs by activation of physiologically normal nociceptive pathways. In general, these pains are sensitive to opioids.

In contrast, the term 'neuropathic' pain is used to describe those pains which are induced by mechanisms which cause injury or damage to the nervous system, typically by tumour compression or invasion, resulting in a functional abnormality of the nerves. Neuropathic pains are typically insensitive to opioids.

Neuropathic pains may be caused by the following mechanisms:

- Directly related to the cancer, e.g. compression or invasion by primary or secondary tumours.
- Indirectly related to the cancer, e.g. herpetic neuralgia; malignant neuropathies.
- Iatrogenic, e.g. chemotherapy induced neuropathy; radiotherapy induced neuropathy; post-surgery.

Clinically, patients will complain of an unusual but very unpleasant pain or discomfort, often in association with some of the following abnormal sensory phenomena:

- Dysaesthesia - an unpleasant abnormal sensation, whether spontaneous or evoked.
- Causalgia – a syndrome of sustained burning pain.
- Allodynia – pain due to a stimulus which does not normally provoke pain.

Simply, the description of pain in an area of abnormal sensation, 'pain in a numb area', is diagnostic of neuropathic or deafferentation pain.

Patients may also describe a shooting or stabbing component to their pain. Neurological examination may reveal motor or reflex abnormalities in addition to the sensory changes already described.

Some neuropathic pains are sympathetically maintained. This is important to recognize as these pains will respond to a sympathetic block. The benefit following such a block far outlasts the predicted duration of action of the agent used.

The main sensory disturbances associated with sympathetically maintained pain include allodynia, hyperpathia (a painful syndrome characterized by increased reaction to a stimulus) and hypoalgesia (diminished pain response to a normally painful stimulus, e.g. pinprick).

Signs of sympathetic overactivity and trophic changes may also be evident. The pain is typically described as a 'burning' pain and the affected part is usually cold to the touch. The pain does not follow a dermatomal pattern of distribution. In cancer patients, the lower limbs are involved more commonly than the upper limbs, and unusually sympathetically mediated pain may occur in the chest, head and neck.

Opioids are typically not very effective in the control of neuropathic pain. This may be explained by the theory of spinal turbulence as proposed by Sutherland.[25] In spinally mediated neuropathic pain, there is spontaneous hyperactivity of the spinal pain transmission neurones, with impulses conducted in an erratic, turbulent fashion. Opioids work in nociceptive pain, where the impulse is transmitted in a smooth laminar fashion. The origin of the impulse and the manner of its transmission, accounts for the ineffectiveness of opioids in this type of pain.

There is often a significant emotional component to a patient's distress, as they find the concept of a useless pain very difficult to understand and to accept. Any management approach must include a careful explanation to the patient regarding the nature of their pain, and realistic expectations of treatment must be agreed. Most of these patients will already have tried opioids without lasting benefit and further increases in dose will have induced an unacceptable level of side effects, without increased analgesia.

In planning treatment, consideration must be given to measures which might reduce tumour size, thereby reversing the deafferentation component. In addition, the following treatments for neuropathic pain are recommended.

Management of neuropathic pain

Antidepressants

Tricyclic antidepressants, e.g. amitriptyline, imipramine and clomipramine have a specific role in neuropathic pain which is independent of their effects on mood. They are of particular benefit for 'burning' pain. A starting dose of amitriptyline 25 mg, increasing in increments to 100 mg is usually adequate. The onset of relief may be less than one week, but Glynn recommends that any drug treatment should be given a trial of six weeks before it is considered to be a failure.[26]

Anticonvulsants

Phenytoin, carbamazepine, sodium valproate and clonazepam have all been used with success. Anticonvulsants are particularly indicated for shooting or stabbing pains. As with antidepressants, clinical experience suggests a therapeutic threshold rather than a dose-response curve.

Local anaesthetic agents

Brose and Cousins reported on the successful use of subcutaneous lignocaine in three patients with cancer related deafferentation pain which had not responded to systemic or spinal opioids.[27] Further randomized controlled studies are required to establish the precise role of this approach.

A large range of other drugs have been tried in the management of neuropathic pain. These drugs include: clonidine, dexamethasone, flecainide, mexilitine, naloxone, baclofen and l-tryptophan. Non-drug measures, e.g. trans cutaneous nerve stimulation may also be of benefit.[28] A comprehensive review of the pharmacological treatment of neuropathic pain by H.J. McQuay may be found in G. Hanks (ed.) *Cancer Surveys*, Vol. 7, London, Imperial Cancer Research Fund, 1988, pp. 141–49.

Raised intracranial pressure

Cerebral oedema is defined as an increase in brain volume due to an increase in its water content. There are several distinct types of cerebral oedema, and their patho-physiology is ill understood. Vasogenic oedema is the type of oedema that occurs in association with cerebral tumours.

CT scan will show the tumour as an area of increased density, surrounded by a low density ring of oedema. Steroids were first used in the management of cerebral oedema in 1952, and dexamethasone was first reported to be of benefit in reducing the oedema associated with cerebral tumours in 1961. Its precise mode of action is uncertain, but both an increase in regional cerebral blood flow, thereby reversing local cerebral ischaemia[29] and a reduction in regional cerebral blood volume as a consequence of vasoconstriction have both been postulated as possible mechanisms.[30]

The dose of dexamethasone varies from the conventional dose of 16 mg per day, to doses as high as 96 mg per day. The maintenance dose for each patient must be determined on an individual basis, and must be reviewed regularly. Ideally, patients will be maintained on the lowest possible dose which achieves the desired effect. As many patients with intracranial tumours will require treatment with anticonvulsants, it is important to note that anticonvulsants will reduce the effectiveness of dexamethasone and other steroids by inducing their metabolism by 6-hydroxylation.

Pain control – the role of the anaesthetist

In modern practice, anaesthetists play an increasingly important role in the management of post-operative pain, chronic benign pain, and cancer pain. There is tremendous potential for the involvement of anaesthetic expertise in palliative care units. If this symbiotic relationship is to be successful, the anaesthetist must be integrated as part of the medical team within the hospice or palliative care unit. This will involve a regular commitment from the anaesthetist to attend at the hospice and to take part in rounds and discussions on patient management. This system allows for a mutual exchange of ideas and enables each group to develop an awareness of both the potential and limitations of each other's contribution.

It is an entirely inappropriate and unfair use of anaesthetic expertise to involve the anaesthetist only in crisis management and at a point when every other approach has failed. The anaesthetist must advise on pain control in the context of a comprehensive programme of pain management and must not be viewed simply as a technician required to perform certain procedures.

The particular techniques which an anaesthetist may choose to employ will reflect his experience and training. In general, it is desirable if the procedure can be performed within the palliative care unit, in order to minimize disruption to the patient and family.

Peripheral, central and autonomic nerves can all be blocked, temporarily or permanently, depending on the choice of agent. There is now increasing interest in the use of 'drug delivery systems' and in particular, the use of spinal opioids has dramatically changed the practice of pain management in many centres.

In deciding on any management approach, there are two important steps which must be followed. The first of these is to know what can be done and the second and more difficult step is to decide what constitutes the most appropriate treatment. Henry McQuay put this most succinctly when he wrote that the single most important point is to distinguish between the phenomenon, 'it can be done' and the clinical questions, 'should it be done?' and if so, 'when and to whom?'.[31] These questions must continue to challenge palliative care physicians and nurses.

Pain control – the role of the radiotherapist

Radiotherapy has an important role to play in the palliative management of patients with advanced cancer. Ideally, the radiotherapist will work as part of the palliative care inter-disciplinary team. The radiotherapist has an important educational role and must teach others how best to use the radiotherapy services. This involves creating an awareness of the specific indications for radiotherapy in pain control, and their likely results and adverse effects. For non-radiotherapists, it is more important to know when and when not to refer than it is to understand the complexities of the various treatment regimes. This situation is best created by enabling the radiotherapist to have a regular presence on the hospice ward or palliative care unit.As applies with the anaesthetist, the radiotherapist has little to offer if involved only in crisis management.

It is an important principle of palliative radiotherapy that treatment must be undertaken without delay, and with the minimum of disruption to the patient's life. Consequently, the trend towards using lower doses of radiotherapy and in shorter fractions whenever clinically indicated, is welcomed.

Palliative radiotherapy for pain control has applications in the following settings:

- Bone metastases: Single fraction radiotherapy offers worthwhile pain relief in 80 per cent of patients with localized bone pain. More diffuse painful bone metastases may respond to hemibody radiotherapy.
- Pelvic pain due to rectal or cervical carcinoma: In patients who have not already received an optimal level of irradiation, radiotherapy can offer useful palliation of symptoms. In assessing the potential benefits of treatment however, it is important to consider the possibility of fistula formation.
- Fungating tumours: Fungating tumours can be very painful and distressing. In the case of fungating breast disease, useful palliation of symptoms can be achieved, even when the tumour is quite large.
- Skin metastases: Skin metastases, sited at or near a pressure point, are ideally suited for radiotherapy, as the lesion is so clearly accessible.
- Brain metastases: Whole brain irradiation may be appropriate in patients who are experiencing pain or other symptoms of raised intracranial pressure. Patients will require dexamethasone for the duration of their treatment and the problem of hair loss will need to be discussed and addressed prior to treatment.
- Bronchogenic carcinoma: The local pain of a primary tumour of bronchus will respond to palliative radiotherapy. In addition, the joint pain associated with hypertrophic pulmonary osteoarthropathy will be relieved by radiotherapy to the primary tumour.

Cancer pain – a team approach

It will be evident that no one individual can possess the range of skills necessary to provide a comprehensive programme of pain management. We rely therefore, on the timely and appropriate intervention of a whole group of individuals, drawn from a spectrum of medical and non-medical disciplines. The importance of developing and maintaining a coordinated and constructive approach amongst such a team cannot be over emphasized.

'We must hang together, or we will surely hang separately.'
Benjamin Franklin.

Notes and References

1. CONOLLY, M.E. 'Recent advances in the control of pain.' In: Bates, T.D. (ed.), *Clinical Oncology – Contemporary Palliation of Difficult Symptoms*, London, Ballière Tindall, 1987.
2. Cancer Pain Relief and Palliative Care. Report of WHO Expert Committee. Technical Report Series, 804. World Health Organisation, Geneva, 1990, p. 11.
3. KEARNEY, M. 'Palliative care in Ireland', *Journal of the Irish College of Physicians and Surgeons*, 1991, **20**(3), 170.
4. 'Pain', *Journal of the International Association for the Study of Pain'*, Supplement 3, 1986, S 217.
5. MELZACK, R. and WALL, P. *The Challenge of Pain*, London: Pelican Books, 1988, p. 45.
6. TWYCROSS, R.G. and LACK, S.A. 'Pain – a broader concept.' In: *Symptom Control in Far Advanced Cancer: Pain Relief*, London, Pitman, 1983.
7. SAUNDERS, C.M. and BAINES, M. *Living with Dying – The Management of Terminal Disease*, Oxford, Oxford University Press, 1983, pp. 12–13.
8. KEARNEY, M. 'Imagework in a case of intractable pain', *Palliative Medicine*, 1992, **6**, 152–7.
9. BONICA, J.J. 'Organisation and function of a pain clinic.' In: Bonica, J.J. (ed.), *Advances in Neurology*, Vol. 4, New York, Raven Press, 1974, pp. 433–43.
10. WALSH, T.D. and WEST, T.S. 'Controlling symptoms in advanced cancer', *British Medical Journal, 1988,* **296**, 13 Feb., 477–81.
11. MELZACK, R. and WALL, P. *The Challenge of Pain*, p. 40.
12. TWYCROSS, R.G. and FAIRFIELD, S. 'Pain in far-advanced cancer', *Pain*, 1982, **14**, 303–310.
13. TWYCROSS, R.G. 'Cancer pain: a global perspective.' In: Twycross, R.G. (ed.), *The Edinburgh Symposium on Pain Control and Medical Education*. Royal Society of Medicine Services Limited, London, 1989, p, 6.
14. GALER, B.S. BRADLEY, S., COYLE, N. et al. 'Individual variability in the response to different opioids: report of five cases, *Pain*, 1992, **49**, 87–91.
15. HOSKINS, P.J. and HANKS, G.W. 'Morphine: pharmacokinetics and clinical practice', *British Journal of Cancer*, 1990, **62**, 705–7.
16. GOLDMAN, A. and BOWMAN, A. (1990) 'The role of oral controlled-release morphine for pain relief in children with cancer, *Palliative Medicine*, 1990, **4**, 279–85.
17. ARITA, H., KOGO, N. and ICHIKAWA, K. 'Localisations of medullary neurones with non-phasic discharges excited by stimulation of central and/or peripheral chemoreceptors and by activation of nociceptors in the cat', *Brain Research*, 1988, **442**, 1–10.
18. GLARE, P.A., WALSH, R.D. and PIPPENGER, C.E. 'Normorphine, a neurotoxic metabolite', *Lancet* , 1990, **335**, 725–6.
19. KAIKO, R.F., HEAY, N, PAV, J., THOMAS, G.B. and GOLDENHEIM, P.D. 'The comparative bioavailability of controlled release oral morphine following rectal and oral administration.' In: Twycross, R.G. (ed.), The Edinburgh Symposium on Pain Control and Medical Education. Royal Society of Medicine Services Limited, London, 1989.

20. MISER, A.W., NARANG, P.K., DOTHAGE, J.A., YOUNG, R.C., SINDELAR, W. and MISER J.S. 'Transdermal fentanyl for pain control in patients with cancer', *Pain*, 1989, **37**, 15–21.

21. PRICE, P., HOSKIN, P.J., EASTON, D., AUSTIN, D., PALMER, S.G., and YARNOLD, J.R. 'Prospective randomised trial of single and multifraction schedules in the treatment of painful bony metastases', *Radiotherapy and Oncology*, 1986, **6**, 247–55.

22. ELOMAA, I., BLOMQUIST, C., GROHN, P., PORKKA, L., KAIRENTO, A.L., SELANDER, K., LAMBERG-ALLARDT, C., and HOLMSTROM, T. 'Long-term controlled trial with diphosphonate in patients with osteolytic bone metastases', *Lancet*, 1983, Jan. 22, pp. 146–9.

23. ROWELL, N.P. 'Intralesional methylprednisolone for rib metastases: an alternative to radiotherapy?' *Palliative Medicine*, 1988, **2**, 153–5.

24. HANNA, M., PEAT, S.J., WOODHAM, M., LATHAM, J., GOULIARIS, A. and Di VADI, P. The use of coeliac plexus blockade in patients with chronic pain. *Palliative Medicine*, 1989, **4**, 11–16.

25. SUTHERLAND, S. *Nerve and Nerve Injuries*. Edinburgh, Churchill Livingstone, 1978, 399–400.

26. GLYNN, C. 'An approach to the management of the patient with deafferentation pain', *Palliative Medicine*, 1989, **1**, 13–21.

27. BROSE, W.G. and COUSINS, M.J. 'Subcutaneous lidocaine for treatment of neuropathic cancer pain', *Pain*, 1991, 145–8.

28. McQUAY, H.J. 'Pharmacological treatment of neuralgic and neuropathic pain', *Cancer Surveys*, 1988, 7(1), 141–59.

29. REULEN H.J., HADJIDIMOS, A. and SCHURMANN, K. The effect of dexamethasone on water and electrolyte content and on rCBF in perifocal brain edema in man. In: Reulen H.J. and Schurmann, K. (eds) Steroids and brain edema. Berlin: Springer-Verlag, 1972, 239–52.

30. LEENDERS, K.L., BEANEY, R.P., BROOKS, D.J., LAMMERTSMA, A.A., HEATHER, J.D. and McKENZIE, C.G. 'Dexamethasone treatment of brain tumour patients: effects on regional cerebral blood flow, blood volume, and oxygen utilisation', *Neurology,,* 1985, **35**, 1610–6.

31. McQUAY, H.J. 'The logic of alternative routes', *Journal of Pain and Symptom Management*, 1990, **5**(2), 75–7.

Gastrointestinal Symptoms————————

Mary Baines and Nigel Sykes

Intestinal obstruction

Intestinal obstruction is caused by an occlusion to the lumen or a lack of normal propulsion which prevent or delay intestinal contents from passing distally. Obstruction occurs in about 3 per cent of patients with advanced cancer receiving hospice treatment[1] but the prevalence in advanced ovarian cancer is much higher, up to 40 per cent.

Pathophysiology

Many different factors can cause malignant obstruction in patients with advanced abdominal or pelvic cancer. Primary tumours of the large bowel can occlude the lumen in a polypoid or annular fashion. Extramural compression is caused by tumour masses or malignant adhesions. Motility disorders, leading to a functional obstruction, can be due to tumour infiltration of intestinal muscle, mesentery or coeliac plexus. Frequently, these causes coexist and, in addition, the obstruction may be at several sites.

Assessment

A careful history and physical examination will usually point to the diagnosis and the patient's general condition should also be assessed.

The pattern and severity of the obstructive symptoms of colic, vomiting, distension and bowel dysfunction must be noted. They will depend on the level and completeness of the obstruction, bearing in mind that early obstructive symptoms may be intermittent.

Abdominal X-rays are only used if the patient is being considered for surgery. They are not necessary if purely symptomatic treatment is appropriate.

Management

There are now a number of treatment options available for the patient with advanced cancer who develops intestinal obstruction. In the sections which follow the indications and results of surgery will be examined, the role of intubation evaluated and the use of drugs for symptom control described.

Surgery

Every cancer patient who develops intestinal obstruction must be considered for surgery. This includes those referred for terminal care since, even if the obstruction is due to recurrent cancer, there are individuals who will enjoy a worthwhile symptom-free period following palliative surgery. The decision to operate is not easy and the following factors should be considered:

- Age and general medical condition.
- Abdominal masses, ascites, previous radiotherapy to abdomen or pelvis, or combination chemotherapy make successful surgery less likely.
- The degree of abdominal distension is a guide to the feasibility of palliative surgery. There will be minimal distension if the small bowel is extensively infiltrated and fixed by tumour, making surgical palliation impossible.
- The patient's wishes. Treatment options should be carefully discussed and no patient referred for surgery simply to avoid a distressing death from obstruction; the correct use of drugs will prevent this.

Not surprisingly, the results of palliative surgery in the patient with advanced cancer are poor. Operative mortality in reported series is between 12 and 33 per cent. Major complications are frequent with a considerable proportion of patients remaining obstructed or reobstructing later and between 7 and 18 per cent develop enterocutaneous fistulae. Median survival is measured in months.

Gastrointestinal intubation

Nasogastric suction and intravenous fluids are used to decompress the bowel and correct fluid or electrolyte imbalance. This is of value while investigations are proceeding and a decision made about palliative surgery. A review of surgical literature shows that only between 0 and 14 per cent show a sustained response and most surgeons now recommend early surgery following adequate rehydration.

The place of prolonged conservative treatment is controversial and it should probably be reserved for the small numbers, principally with high obstruction, who fail to respond to pharmacological treatment.

Venting gastrostomy

This is a method of relieving nausea and vomiting in patients with inoperable obstruction. It is often more effective and acceptable than nasogastric drainage. As with intubation, it should be reserved for those with refractory symptoms.

Symptomatic treatment

Over the last few years it has been realized that the majority of patients with inoperable malignant obstruction can be managed well with pharmacological means. The preferred route for drug administration is by continuous subcutaneous infusion using a portable syringe driver or similar pump. Other routes are less effective or are poorly tolerated. The three major symptoms of intestinal colic, continuous abdominal pain, and vomiting, require separate assessment and appropriate medication.

Intestinal colic
- Stop stimulant laxatives, e.g. senna.
- Stop gastrokinetic antiemetics, e.g. metoclopramide. These may increase peristalsis in the small bowel.
- Diamorphine or morphine subcutaneously, with titration of dose, may be adequate without antispasmodics.
- Usually an antispasmodic is required. Hyoscine butylbromide is preferred, using from 60–200 mg/day.

Continuous abdominal pain
- Diamorphine or morphine subcutaneously, titrating the dose against response.

Nausea and vomiting
- Haloperidol 5–15 mg/day. Parkinsonian side effects may occur with higher doses.
- Cyclizine 100–150 mg/day can be used alone or added to haloperidol. Crystallization may occur.
- Methotrimeprazine 50–200 mg/day is of value in intractable vomiting. However, it causes sedation and local skin reactions.
- Hyoscine butylbromide 60–120 mg/day leads to a reduction in gastric secretions with fewer or smaller vomits.[2]
- Octreotide, a somatostatin analogue, 0.1 mg–0.6 mg/day has also been used to reduce gastro-intestinal secretions and vomiting.
- Patients eat and drink as they choose, the majority favouring small and mainly fluid meals. With adequate oral fluids, thirst is rarely a problem and the occasional dry mouth is treated with local measures such as crushed ice to suck.

In practice, the symptoms of obstruction usually coexist and a typical prescription would be: diamorphine 30 mg, hyoscine butylbromide 60 mg, haloperidol 5 mg (over twenty-four hours in the syringe driver). Using these methods, the majority of patients can be relieved of both colic and continuous abdominal pain. Vomiting is more difficult to control but can usually be reduced to about once a day with little associated nausea.

Corticosteroids have been used in these patients in the hope that their anti-inflammatory effects will open up the obstruction with resultant symptom relief. Dexamethasone 8 mg/day, by injection, is the usual starting dose. Individual patients seem to have benefited but no clinical trials have been conducted. With the intermittent nature of early obstructive symptoms, it is difficult to know if the improvement is due to the steroid treatment.

Nausea and vomiting

A number of studies have reported that between 40 and 60 per cent of patients with advanced cancer complain of nausea and vomiting. The control of these symptoms may prove difficult as there are often many contributing factors.

Pathophysiology

A knowledge of the emetic pathways and the common neurotransmitters involved is helpful in planning treatment as antiemetic drugs are effective at different receptor sites.[3]

The vomiting centre (VC) lies in the medulla and has both histamine and muscarinic cholinergic receptors. It can be stimulated in the following ways:

Table 3.3   Common causes of vomiting in the patient with advanced cancer

Chemical causes:
- Drugs, especially opioids
- Uraemia
- Hypercalcaemia
- Infection

Gastric causes:
- Gastritis or ulceration
- External pressure causing 'squashed stomach
-   syndrome'
- Carcinoma of stomach
- Gastric outflow obstruction

Intestinal obstruction
Constipation
Raised intracranial pressure
Vestibular disturbance
Cough-induced
Anxiety

- From the chemoreceptor trigger zone (CTZ) where dopamine receptors are concentrated.
- From vagal afferents from the gastrointestinal tract.
- From the vestibular centre. This, like the vomiting centre, contains both histamine and muscarinic cholinergic receptors.
- Directly, from raised intracranial pressure.
- From psychological causes, especially anxiety.

The principal causes of nausea and vomiting in advanced malignancy are given in Table 3.3

Assessment

The diagnosis of the cause of vomiting can usually be made from the following:

Medical history

In taking this, note should be taken of intra-abdominal, pelvic or cerebral spread of the tumour. Renal failure may be due to obstructive uropathy and certain histological types can cause hypercalcaemia. Drugs, especially opioids, may contribute to the problem.

Vomiting history

The volume, content, frequency and timing of vomits will quite often point to the diagnosis. For example, many patients say that they are 'vomiting' when food, and perhaps fluids, are brought up, undigested, soon after eating and never reach the stomach. This should be termed 'dysphagia' and treated appropriately. Large volume vomits, with food consumed some hours previously, indicates delayed gastric emptying. This may be due to outflow obstruction or to drugs which reduce gastric motility. Faeculent vomiting, with its characteristic smell, indicates intestinal obstruction. 'Coffee ground' vomits may be due to bleeding from tumour or ulcer. The association of headache with vomiting on waking suggests raised intracranial pressure, and the observant nurse will often notice that an anxious patient feels sick when the family visits.

Abdominal examination

The presence of hepatomegaly, tumour or faecal masses, ascites, gaseous distension and altered bowel sounds should be noted. A rectal examination must be performed.

Investigations

All patients with unexplained vomiting should have their serum urea, calcium and electrolytes checked. Radiology is occasionally used, either to clarify the diagnosis, e.g. constipation or obstruction, or before surgical treatment, if this is appropriate.

Antiemetic drugs

A large number of antiemetic drugs have been found useful and research is continuing, with the development of new agents. It is preferable to become familiar with a limited number of drugs, which are used regularly. Table 3.4 lists the recommended antiemetics, with their site of action, dosage and available routes.

Other antiemetics

Corticosteroids are used in two ways. They potentiate other antiemetics in the vomiting caused by chemotherapy and they may reduce peritumour oedema in some cases of obstructive vomiting.

Ondansetron blocks serotonin receptors in the gut and CTZ. It has proved extremely effective in the prevention of chemotherapy vomiting. Unfortunately, it remains very expensive and its role in palliative medicine has not yet been fully evaluated.

Table 3.4   Recommended antiemetics

Name	Main site of action	Neurotransmitter receptors	Dose 24 hours	Routes
Cyclizine	Vomiting centre	Histamine and muscarinic cholinergic	100–200 mg	0,I,SC
Domperidone	Upper gut Chemoreceptor trigger zone	Dopamine	30–180 mg	O,R
Haloperidol	Chemoreceptor trigger zone	Dopamine	1.5–15 mg	0,I,SC
Metoclopramide	Upper gut Chemoreceptor trigger zone	Dopamine	30–100 mg	0,I,SC
Methotrimeprazine	Chemoreceptor trigger zone	Dopamine	50–200 mg	0,I,SC

Oral = 0; Intramuscular = I; Subcutaneous infusion = SC; Rectal = R

Management

Specific treatments for some of the causes of vomiting listed in Table 3.1 are covered elsewhere in the text. Other causes are treated as follows:

- *Opioid induced vomiting.* About 30 per cent of patients starting morphine feel nauseated during the first week of treatment. Either metoclopramide or haloperidol should be given prophylactically.
- *Uraemia.* Haloperidol is usually effective, methotrimeprazine is sometimes required.
- *Squashed stomach syndrome.* Metoclopramide is used, sometimes a defoaming agent such as dimethicone is added.
- *Gastric outflow obstruction.* Treatment is started with metoclopramide. If this is ineffective it is worth trying corticosteroids using dexamethasone 8 mg daily by injection. Nasogastric suction is occasionally required.
- *Raised intracranial pressure.* Dexamethasone is the treatment of choice; if contraindicated, cyclizine is usually effective.
- *Vestibular disturbance.* Both hyoscine and cyclizine are effective.

Dysphagia

Dysphagia, difficulty in swallowing, occurs in about 12 per cent of cancer patients on admission to St Christopher's Hospice. Although 80 per cent of those with head and neck cancer have dysphagia, the relative cancer incidence in Britain means that most cases of malignant dysphagia result from oesophageal or gastric tumours.

Pathophysiology

Failure to swallow adequately not only endangers nutrition and hydration but also increases the risk of pneumonia due to aspiration. Oral tumours tend to cause dysphagia by restricting the movement of the tongue and hence the formation and initial transfer of a food bolus. Pharyngeal cancers cause obstruction but may also produce neuro-muscular incoordination by perineural spread along one or more cranial nerves and splinting of the pharynx by local presence of tumour and fibrosis. Tumours of the oesophagus or the gastric cardia narrow the oesophageal lumen and disrupt peristalsis. Oesophageal obstruction also arises from external compression caused by mediastinal lymphadenopathy.

If attempts at swallowing cause pain, dysphagia will result. Pain may arise from any of the tumours mentioned and from oropharyngeal or oesophageal infections, most of them with *Candida* or Herpes simplex.

About 30 per cent of patients who report dysphagia on hospice admission do not show evidence of swallowing difficulty on objective assessment. These patients are more likely to have a functional cause, due to anxiety or poor appetite, and respond to symptomatic treatment and a supportive environment.[4]

Assessment

The most important assessment is probably the consistency of food the patient finds it easiest to swallow. This is not necessarily the runniest available – patients with impaired peristalsis may indeed find liquids easiest to manage, but if the swallowing reflex is impaired, soft foods rather than fluids are less likely to cause aspiration. Such information is obtained by history and, if necessary, observation of test swallows. For a patient with oropharyngeal cancer, assessment by a speech therapist may provide helpful techniques to improve swallowing. The mouth should be examined carefully for infection or the presence of aphthous ulceration.

Management of malignant dysphagia

- Ensure good general pain and symptom control.
- Maintain oral hygiene.
- Provide food the patient likes, of the right consistency and attractively served.
- Steroids (Dexamethasone 4–8 mg o.d.) improve appetite and may improve dysphagia due to oropharyngeal tumour or mediastinal metastases.
- Consider insertion of an oesophageal tube, especially if prognosis is limited or if external compression is present.
- Laser treatment or radiotherapy may help dysphagia from oesophageal tumours. Intracavitary radiotherapy may offer quicker relief with less morbidity than external treatment.

In a few patients with oropharyngeal cancer it is appropriate to maintain nutrition by means of a fine bore nasogastric tube or, more discreetly, a percutaneous endoscopically placed gastrostomy. These are patients in whom the tumour is very slow-growing or who may be cured of their disease but are dysphagic as a result of their head and neck surgery. But good nutrition does not prevent aspiration, and may simply lengthen a process of increasing respiratory debility. For most patients with progressive cancers causing complete dysphagia the appropriate treatment is the control of symptoms with appropriate use of drugs as described in other sections of this book.

Constipation

Constipation is the infrequent, difficult passage of small, hard faeces. Bowel habit varies widely between normal individuals and so what is considered to be constipation by a patient will depend on their previous experience. As over 99 per cent of British people defaecate at least three times per week, a frequency of less than this is often taken as an objective indication of constipation.

About 50 per cent of cancer patients presenting to a hospice complain of constipation, but this underestimates the problem as some will already be receiving effective laxative therapy.

Pathophysiology

The principal causes of constipation in patients with terminal malignancy are listed in Table 3.5

Drugs, in particular morphine, are often blamed for constipation in cancer patients and with reason, for although there is a high underlying level of constipation among hospice cancer patients, chiefly as a result of poor food intake and impaired mobility, the proportion requiring laxatives rises from about 65 to nearly 90 per cent when strong opioid analgesia is being used. Morphine, which reduces gut peristalsis, is probably the most important single causative factor in constipation in this patient group that can be isolated.

Assessment

The history must clarify what is happening in terms of stool frequency, difficulty of defaecation and a comparison with the patient's previous experience. Stool characteristics (loose or formed, or hard pellets) indicate whether transit time is prolonged or not and are related to difficulty in expulsion.

Abdominal examination and, unless there has been a recent satisfactory evacuation, rectal examination, are important to avoid missing the diagnosis of constipation or confusing constipation with malignant obstruction.

Table 3.5   Principal causes of constipation in advanced cancer

Secondary effects of disease
  Inadequate food intake
  Inactivity
  Low fibre diet
  Weakness
  Dehydration
Direct effects of tumour
  Narrowing of gut lumen
  Spinal cord or pelvic plexus damage
  Hypercalcaemia
Drugs
  Opioids
  Drugs with anticholinergic effects, e.g. hyoscine, phenothiazines, tricyclic antidepressants
  Diuretics
  Anticonvulsants
  Iron
  Vincristine

Faecal masses felt in the abdomen are generally distinguishable from tumour masses because of indentation and crepitus felt on palpation and also because they move with time. Occasionally an abdominal radiograph is needed in order to make the distinction.

Management of constipation

- Maintain good general symptom control, enabling the patient to be mobile and to eat as well as possible.
- High fibre foods will not treat severe constipation and are unpalatable to ill patients.
- Ensure privacy for defaecation and avoid using bedpans.
- Foresee the need for laxatives and use them appropriately.

Laxatives

Laxatives are often classified according to whether their principal action is to soften the stool or to stimulate peristalsis. The laxatives most commonly used in palliative care are shown in Table 3.6, and the following is one approach to laxative therapy.

- *If intestinal obstruction is a possibility* – use only laxatives with a predominantly softening action, e.g. lactulose, sodium docusate, in order not to cause colic.
- *If there is rectal impaction with hard faeces* – soften the faecal mass using glycerine suppositories, or an oil enema retained overnight. If spontaneous evacuation remains impossible, a manual evacuation will be necessary for which sufficient sedation and additional analgesia should be provided.
- *If there is rectal loading with soft faeces* – a peristaltic stimulant, e.g. senna, may be effective alone but a stimulant/softener combination will probably be needed later and may as well be used from the outset. If there is rectal discomfort, a mini-enema may assist the initial defaecation.
- *If there is little or no stool in the rectum* – use a stimulant/softener combination and titrate the dose according to the response or the advent of adverse effects (usually colic).

Diarrhoea

Diarrhoea is the passage of frequent loose stools, but the term may be used to refer to the passage of a single loose stool, frequent stools of normal consistency or faecal incontinence. Diarrhoea is present in 7–10 per cent of hospice cancer admissions and so is a considerably smaller problem in this patient group than constipation.

Table 3.6 Commonly used laxatives

Predominantly softening

Mode of action	Examples	Usual dose range	Comments
Osmotic agents: retain water in gut lumen	Lactulose	15–40 mls bd-tds	Active principally in the small bowel. Latency of action 1–2 days.
	Magnesium hydroxide Magnesium sulphate	2–4 mg daily	Act throughout the bowel and may have pronounced purgative effect, possibly partly as a result of direct peristaltic stimulation. Latency of action 1–6 hr (dose dependent)
Surfactant agents: – increase water penetration of the stool	Docusate sodium Poloxamer (only available in combination with danthron)	Docusate 60–300 mg bd	Probably not very effective when used alone. Latency of action 1–3 days.
Lubricant agents	Liquid paraffin Glycerine (as suppositories) Arachis oil ⎫ as Olive oil ⎬ enemas		Paraffin is best used only in a 25% emulsion with magnesium hydroxide (Milpar)

Predominantly stimulant

Direct stimulation of myenteric nerves to induce peristalsis Reduce absorption of water from gut	Senna Danthron	7.5–30 mg bd 50–450 mg bd	Anthraquinone family. Danthron available only in combination with docusate or poloxamer – stains urine red/brown Latency of action 6–12 hr.
	Bisacodyl Sodium picosulphate	10–20 mg bd 5–20 mg bd	Polyphenolic family. Latency of action 6–12 hr.

Combination stimulant/softener preparations

Codanthramer standard	Danthron 25 mg Poloxamer 200 mg	per 5 ml	Suspension only.
Codanthramer forte	Danthron 75 mg Poloxamer 1 g	per 5 ml	Suspension only.
Codanthrusate	Danthron 50 mg Docusate 60 mg	per cap.	Capsule only.

Pathophysiology

The principal causes of diarrhoea in patients with terminal cancer are noted in Table 3.7. Most common of all is an imbalance of laxative therapy, usually when laxative doses have been increased to clear an accumulation of constipated stool. If laxatives are stopped for 24–48 hours the diarrhoea usually stops, after which the laxatives should be resumed at a lower dose to prevent the patient relapsing into constipation.

The next most common precipitants of diarrhoea are partial malignant obstruction and faecal impaction. Partial obstruction may produce either diarrhoea or alternating diarrhoea and obstruction. Faecal impaction is usually rectal and diarrhoea is the result of faecal material higher in the colon being broken down by bacterial action into semi-fluid form and seeping past the mass.

Assessment

A good history, including the frequency of defaecation, the nature of the stools and the duration of the complaint, often suggests the diagnosis. Pale, fatty, offensive stools indicate steatorrhoea due to malabsorption from pancreatic or small intestinal insufficiency, but profuse watery stools are a sign of colonic diarrhoea, often with an acute infective cause. 'Diarrhoea' occurring only once or twice per day may represent anal incontinence, whereas the acute onset of diarrhoea after a period of constipation, perhaps with little warning that defaecation is about to happen, suggests faecal impaction. An account of current and recent drugs is important.

Abdominal and rectal examinations should be performed to exclude intestinal obstruction or faecal impaction. Most infective episodes of diarrhoea resolve within the time taken to diagnose them and stool cultures are therefore not usually worthwhile.

Table 3.7   Principal causes of diarrhoea in advanced cancer

Drugs
    Laxatives
    Antibiotics
    Antacids
    NSAID (particularly mefenamic acid, indomethacin, diclofenac)
    Disaccaride-containing elixirs
Obstruction
    Tumour
    Faecal impaction
Malabsorption
    Pancreatic carcinoma
    Ileal resection
    Gastrectomy
Radiation

Management

Codeine, 10-50 mg four hourly, is the cheapest antidiarrhoeal drug but has marked systemic effects. The drug of choice is loperamide, which as well as having an antidiarrhoeal potency some fifty-fold greater than that of codeine is minimally absorbed and so lacks systemic opioid effects. There is wide latitude in the upper dose in adults with persistent diarrhoea. Diphenoxylate is intermediate in potency and systemic effects, but may give adverse effects due to the atropine with which it is combined to limit its abuse potential. Specific therapies include pancreatic supplements in diarrhoea due to fat malabsorption, and aspirin orally or prednisolone enemas in radiation-induced diarrhoea.

Notes and References

1. BAINES, M.J., OLIVER, D.J. and CARTER, R.L. 'Medical management of intestinal obstruction in patients wth advanced malignant disease: a clinical and pathological study', *Lancet*, 1985, **ii**, 990–3.
2. De CONNO, E., CARACENI, A., ZECCA, E., SPOLDI, E. and VENTAFRIDDA, V. 'The continuous subcutaneous infusion of hyoscine butylbromide reduces secretions in patients with gastrointestinal obstruction', *Journal of Pain and Symptom Management*, 1991, **6**, 484–6.
3. PEROUTKA, S.J., and SNYDER, S.H. 'Antiemetics: neurotransmitter receptor binding predicts therapeutic actions', *Lancet* , 1982, **i**, 658–9.
4. SYKES, N.P., BAINES, M.J. and CARTER, R.L. 'Clinical and pathological study of dysphagia conservatively managed in patients with advanced malignant disease', *Lancet*, 1988, **2**, 726–8.

Further reading

Chapters on anorexia, dysphagia, nausea and vomiting, intestinal obstruction and constipation, in:

DOYLE, D.O., HANKS, G. and MacDONALD, N. (eds). *Oxford Textbook of Palliative Medicine*, Oxford University Press, 1993.

TWYCROSS, R.G. and LACK, S.A. *Control of Alimentary Symptoms in Far Advanced Cancer*, Edinburgh, Churchill Livingstone, 1986.

Respiratory symptoms————————————————

Louis Heyse-Moore

Dyspnoea

Definitions

Dyspnoea is taken here to mean difficult distressing breathing. This definition is important because we are more concerned with relieving the distress of symptoms than of trying vainly to restore an irreversibly damaged physiology. It implies that the severity of a patient's dyspnoea is precisely what he or she says it is. It also implies that although severity of dyspnoea is usually proportional to changes in respiratory indices such as respiratory frequency or hypercapnoea, it is not always so. Thus patients dyspnoeic from the hyperventilation syndrome (HVS) may have normal lungs, while others with acidotic hyperventilation do not complain of dyspnoea.

There are then two components to dyspnoea – the first the increased effort needed to breathe, and the second the subjective distress associated.

There are a number of other respiratory patterns to be distinguished from dyspnoea. These are:

- Tachypnoea – raised respiratory frequency.
- Hyperpnoea – increased respiratory excursion.
- Hyperventilation – increased ventilation.
- Periodic breathing – waxing and waning of respiratory excursion or frequency.
- Cheyne-Stokes breathing – a form of periodic breathing where there are alternating periods of hyperpnoea and apnoea each lasting 15–20 seconds. In this case only the amplitude of respiration alters, not the frequency.
- Kussmaul respiration –hyperventilation due to metabolic acidosis.

Epidemiology

About 55 per cent of patients are dyspnoeic on admission to a terminal care unit.[1] Of patients surviving less than a day after admission, about 79 per cent were recorded as dyspnoeic in one study.[1] Thus dyspnoea becomes increasingly common nearer to death.[1,2] Further, studies will tend to underestimate incidence as iller patients more likely to be dyspnoeic may not be able to indicate their respiratory distress. Dyspnoea is severe (i.e. 3 on a scale of 0–3) in about 11 per cent of admissions.[1] There is an inverse relationship between survival and severity of dyspnoea.[1] Thus the patients' fear of dying from breathing problems may have a foundation in fact.

Men are more likely to be dyspnoeic than women (61 as against 50 per cent).[1] Age has not been found to affect dyspnoea status.

Mechanisms

Various theories have been advanced as to how dyspnoea is generated. These will be discussed only insofar as they throw light on how dyspnoea may be treated.

Length-tension inappropriateness

Campbell and Howell[3] noted that when breathing is hindered, an increased muscle effort is needed to maintain the same level of ventilation. They proposed that the imbalance developing between the demand for, and the effort of, breathing causes a misalignment between extrafusal respiratory muscle fibres and their muscle spindles. This mismatch relays via sensory nerves to the respiratory centre and is then projected to the cortex where the two signals are compared and as they do not match, perceived as dyspnoea.

J-receptor stimulation

Paintal[4] has demonstrated the existence in cats of Type J (juxta-alveolar) sensory lung receptors, sensitive to rises in pressure or volume. He postulates that it is these receptors that send a 'dyspnogenic' signal to the brain via the vagus nerve.

Diaphragmatic fatigue

Roussos and Macklem[5] demonstrated that when a subject breathing against resistance generates a trans-diaphragmatic pressure of more than about 40 per cent of maximum, the diaphragm becomes fatigued. They suggest this may play a part in the sensation of dyspnoea, since, below 40 per cent, respiration can be maintained indefinitely. Further, hypoxia shortened the time to respiratory fatigue. Hence measures to reduce airways resistance and relieve hypoxia could reduce dyspnoea. These include physiotherapy to improve efficiency of breathing, oxygen, and reducing a raised metabolic rate with antipyretics for pyrexia, tranquillizers for anxiety or transfusions for anaemia.

Hyperventilation syndrome (HVS)

HVS is common and under-recognized in advanced cancer.[6]
  Excessive ventilation leads to alkalosis and hypocapnia which causes:

- Increased neuromuscular excitability and hence tingling or muscle tremors.
- Cerebrovascular constriction and hence faintness or dizziness.

- Coronary artery vasoconstriction and hence angina or dysrrhythmias.
- The Bohr effect (a shift to the left of the oxygen dissociation curve) with reduced availability of oxygen to the tissues and thus faintness or angina.
- Catecholamine output and hence, for example, sweating and palpitations.

Dyspnoea in HVS is probably mediated through varying length-tension mismatch of respiratory muscles.[7] A vicious circle ensues with anxiety from symptoms of HVS causing increased ventilation and so increased hypocapnia and worsening symptoms.

HVS may be suspected when there are insufficient clinical findings to account for the degree of dyspnoea; a grossly irregular respiratory pattern is also suggestive.

Causes

These are legion. No detailed study of frequency of causes in advanced cancer appears to have been carried out and in many cases dyspnoea is likely to be multifactorial. Further, coincidence of pathology such as lung cancer with dyspnoea does not prove causation.

The commonest primary source for lung metastases is carcinoma of the breast.[1] Dyspnoea in one study appeared to be less common than expected in patients with colorectal carcinomas.[2]

In Table 3.8 major causes of dyspnoea in advanced cancer are listed.

Clinical features

Since dyspnoea is a symptom, only the patient can say whether he or she feels short of breath.[8] Clinical observation of, say, a raised respiratory frequency may *suggest* dyspnoea but is not diagnostic.

Patients often find difficulty in describing their dyspnoea – for example: 'I can't get enough air,' or 'My chest feels tight'. It is therefore less easy than with pain to find diagnostic pointers. However Table 3.9 lists some aspects of descriptions of dyspnoea that help.[9]

Physical signs associated with dyspnoea will be those of the underlying pathology, and often gross due to the advanced nature of the patient's illness – for example, marked stridor from tracheal compression by mediastinal lymphadenopathy.

Investigations, as always in palliative medicine, should be restricted to where they may alter management.

Table 3.10 lists some relevant tests.

The Hyperventilation Provocation Test (HVPT) consists in asking the patient to hyperventilate to see if this reproduces the symptoms of which they complain (see above). Twenty deep breaths is usually enough to reproduce symptoms.[7] Relief of dyspnoea by rebreathing carbon dioxide with a paper bag is both diagnostic and therapeutic.

Measurement

Because dyspnoea is subjective, measurement depends on the patient's own assessment rather than objective tests such as spirometry. Methods used include visual analogue scales,[10] numeric and verbal scales[6,11] and activity ratings.[12]

Treatment

Although many therapies for dyspnoea will be the same as in general medicine, some require special consideration. Palliative and symptomatic drug measures and procedures will be discussed. 'Palliative treatment' implies correcting the cause of the dyspnoea at least in part. 'Symptomatic treatment' implies reducing awareness of dyspnoea with no effect on pathology.

Table 3.8   Common causes of dyspnoea in advanced cancer

Respiratory
   Primary lung cancer
   Pleural mesothelioma
   Lung and pleural metastases
   Lymphangitis carciomatosa
   Mediastinal lymphadenopathy
   Paratracheal lymphadenopathy
   Pleural effusions
   Lung collapse or consolidation
   Pneumonia
   Chronic obstructive airways disease
   Asthma
   Pulmonary fibrosis post radiotherapy
Gastrointestinal
   Ascites
Cardiovascular
   Pulmonary embolism
   Heart failure
   Anaemia
   Ischaemic heart disease
Metabolic
   Uraemia
   Exercise
Psychogenic
   Anxiety
   Depression
   Hyperventilation syndrome

Palliative drug measures

Antibiotics

Although these may relieve dyspnoea from pneumonia in advanced cancer, they are not always indicated as they may prolong a patient's dying rather than living.

Factors to consider are:

- Patients with a reduced respiratory capacity, who cannot cough effectively, who are bed-bound or who are moribund are unlikely to respond well. A patient already dyspnoeic who develops a respiratory infection which is treated by antibiotics may on recovery be left even more dyspnoeic from further lung damage.

Table 3.9   Diagnostic pointers for dyspnoea in advanced cancer

Aspects of dyspnoea	Description	Examples of possible diagnoses
Quality	Wheeze	Asthma
	Chestiness	Pneumonia
Timing	Sudden onset	Pulmonary embolus
	Onset over hours	Pneumonia
	Over days or weeks	Pleural effusion
		Lung cancer
	Intermittent	Asthma
	Episodic over minutes and hours	HVS
Time of day	Paroxysmal nocturnal dyspnoea	LVF
	Early morning	Asthma
Positional	On one side	Check valve effect by lung tumour
Respiratory cycle	Breathing in worse	HVS
	Breathing out worse	Organic lung disease
Precipitating factors	Cold air	Asthma
	Drug induced	Cytotoxics and pneumonitis
		Opioids with pulmonary oedema
Relieving factors	Trial of salbutamol	Asthma
	Relieved by sedatives or alcohol	HVS
Associated symptoms	Pleuritic chest pain	Neoplastic pleural invasion
	Pain in C8, T1, T2 distribution	Pancoast Tumour
	Faintness, dizziness, tingling	HVS

- The wishes of the patient and his or her family must be taken into account. Sometimes, for example with an impending family event such as a wedding which the patient wishes to attend, treatment with antibiotics is appropriate. Conversely, some patients do not wish to have any treatment that might prolong their life.
- Newly admitted patients with respiratory infections are often best treated with antibiotics as it takes a while to get to know them and their families and it is only then that an informed decision can be made about therapy of future chest infections.

Hence, each case must be considered individually and if antibiotics are not given, other symptomatic measures used as necessary. Choice of antibiotic is governed where feasible by sputum culture and sensitivity. Chloramphenicol 250–500 mg oral, four hourly, is a useful wide-spectrum antibiotic because bacterial resistance is uncommon. It is active against anaerobic infections such as might occur distal to a bronchus stenosed by tumour and the risk of pancytopaenia (1:30000 courses) in patients whose median life expectancy is only about two weeks is minimal. Co-amoxiclav (Amoxycillin 250 mg and clavulinic acid 125 mg tds) is also wide spectrum and active against anaerobes.

Table 3.10 Some investigations for dyspnoea in advanced cancer

Indication	Investigation
• Is there a pleural effusion large enough to tap?	Chest X-ray
• Is there lymphangitis carcinomatosa treatable by glucocorticosteroids?	Chest X-ray
• Establishing antibiotic sensitivity in pneumonia	Sputum culture and sensitivity
• Is there reversible airways obstruction?	Spirometry
• Is there an anaemia sufficient to cause dyspnoea which would be helped by transfusion?	Haemoglobin
• Is there a treatable cardiac dysrrhythmia causing cardiac decompensation and dyspnoea?	ECG
• Is dyspnoea due to HVS?	Hyperventilation Provocation Test (HVPT) Rebreathing CO_2

Glucocorticosteroids

In high doses these may help dyspnoea in the following ways:

- Relief of bronchospasm.
- Reduction of tumour oedema in lung or mediastinal neoplasms and hence relief of airways obstruction.
- Relief of lymphangitis carcinomatosa.
- Direct antitumour effect on lymphomas affecting the lungs.
- Relief of leuko-erythroblastic anaemia.
- Prevention of lung oedema from pneumonitis during radiotherapy.

Dexamethasone 8 mg/24 hours or prednisolone 60 mg/24 hours may be used, though opinions vary as to optimum dosage, which itself may vary between individual patients.

Cytotoxics and hormones

These are not often used in palliative care. Thus a study at St Christopher's Hospice showed that only 1.6 per cent of patients were receiving cytotoxics, and 6 per cent hormones.[13]

Possible indications for palliative chemotherapy include cyclophosphamide for small cell carcinoma of the lung and cytotoxic agents such as bleomycin to be instilled into the pleural cavity after drainage of a pleural effusion. Hormones, such as tamoxifen or aminoglutethimide in breast cancer may reduce the size of lung metastases and so relieve dyspnoea.

Symptomatic drug measures

Opioids

Opioids affect respiration in several ways. They reduce the sensitivity of the respiratory centre and peripheral chemoreceptors leading to a reduced rate and depth of ventilation. They decrease anxiety, stop pain associated with ventilation such as by pleurisy, improve heart failure and, as analgesics, reduce hyperventilation due to chronic pain.

They may sometimes cause bronchoconstriction by release of histamine from mast cells in the lung, but also block bronchoconstriction from vagal stimulation.

The effects of opioids on ventilation are therefore complex and sometimes paradoxical.

Opioids are widely used in palliative care for subjective relief of dyspnoea. Fears of respiratory depression causing respiratory failure or pneumonia have not been found to be valid. Thus:

- Dyspnoeic patients taking opioids do not necessarily die quickly. Rather, the respiratory cripple may improve his mobility so much that the risks of being bed-bound (pulmonary emboli, pneumonia and pressure sores) are reduced.
- Walsh[14] investigated 20 terminally ill patients taking regular high-dose morphine. Twelve had chronic obstructive airways disease (COAD) and eight carcinoma of bronchus. Only one had a raised PCO_2. Hence

respiratory failure was not demonstrated in these patients.

- Oral opioids are probably associated with lower peaks and less rapid changes in plasma levels than if given parenterally and hence would be less likely to lead to significant respiratory depression.
- Dyspnoea may cause restlessness and increased ventilatory effort, thus leading to high energy and oxygen consumption. Opioids will reduce anxiety and hence reduce oxygen needs.
- In some patients, ventilation is set too high, as with lymphangitis carcinomatosa stimulating J receptors and so increasing the drive to breathe. Opioids will simply bring ventilation back to normal.

The same principles of opioid administration as for pain control apply. There are, however, a number of special factors to consider:

- Dosage of opioids for dyspnoea is said to be lower than that needed for pain control. This, however, does not appear to have been evaluated.
- Measurement of resting respiratory frequency is a useful way of assessing the effect of the opioid given and preventing over-dosage.
- Adjuvant medication, such as glucocorticosteroids for lymphangitis, is often useful and will allow a lower dosage of opioid to be used.
- Nebulized morphine[15] may reduce dyspnoea due to lung pathology such as lymphangitis, probably as much by a local action on opioid receptors in the lung as by a systemic effect. As with oral morphine, the starting dose is 5 mg four hourly. Its bio-availability is low. This implies the possibility of less sytemic toxicity, though knowledge of this route of administration and its advantages and disadvantages is still very limited.
- Significant respiratory depression is very rarely a problem, except in the occasional case where a nerve block has markedly reduced pain and hence reduced the respiratory stimulant effect of the pain thus precipitating hypoventilation. Naloxone is an effective antidote.

Psychotropics

These may reduce dyspnoea in the following ways:

- Alleviation of anxiety.
- Muscle relaxation – Benzodiazepines potentiate GABA neural inhibition in the brain and spinal cord[16] and so reduce muscle spindle mismatch thus reducing dyspnoea.
- Relief of depression – Depression has been shown to be associated with dyspnoea as part of its somatic presentation[9]; antidepressants lead to resolution of the dyspnoea. They may also work as anxiolytics.

With regard to specific drugs, there is conflicting evidence that diazepam 5 mg tds and 10 mg nocte reduces dyspnoea, as does promethazine 25 mg tds and 50 mg nocte. The doses used, however, are high and likely to cause unacceptable drowsiness. In the author's experience, lower doses of diazepam (e.g. 2 mg tds) may sometimes help. Alcohol has also been found to relieve dyspnoea.

Nabilone is reported as useful. It works first, through a central sedative effect and, secondly, by adrenergic and anticholinergic actions on the airways. Because of significant toxicity (such as hallucinations) the dose used should be low (e.g. 200 mcg tds) which has to be specially prepared by a pharmacist as 1 mg is the lowest strength capsule commercially available.

Atropinics

Hyoscine hydrobromide has the following effects related to dyspnoea:

- Reduction of bronchial secretions.
- Sedation. However, in the elderly it may cause the anticholinergic syndrome (excitement, ataxia, hallucinations, behavioural abnormalities and drowsiness) and so should always be given with another sedative drug such as diamorphine or chlorpromazine.
- Bronchodilatation.
- Amnesia. This is useful if the terminally ill patient survives a respiratory crisis.
  The dosage is 0.4–0.8 mg IM four hourly or 0.8–2.4 mg twenty four hourly in the syringe driver. Tachyphylaxis is said to occur but has not in the author's experience been a problem.

Local anaesthetic inhalation

These may reduce dyspnoea as follows:

- Blocking lung J receptors[17] (see page 77).
- Bronchodilatation from a membrane stabilizing effect on bronchiolar smooth muscle.

Particle diameter must be small enough (less than 4 microns) to reach alveoli. Ultrasonic or jet nebulizers fulfil this criterion. Lignocaine and bupivacaine have been used; the former tastes unpleasant and so the latter is preferred. Concentrations of bupivacaine tested vary from 0.25–5 per cent, inhaling 5 ml at a time. A four hourly regime would be reasonable clinically.

The case for these drugs remains unproven because results reported are variable, sometimes relieving dyspnoea and sometimes not. Reasons for lack of success may include:

- Using nebulizers with large particle sizes.
- Initial broncoconstriction from bronchial irritation.
- Only small amounts of the solution reach the alveoli, so their concentration may be critical in determining effect.
- Bupivacaine for non-respiratory dyspnoea (e.g. anaemia) would not be expected to work.

Unwanted effects include bronchoconstriction, pharyngeal numbness, vocal paresis and abolition of the cough reflex, though this last may be circumvented by using small particles which are less likely to fall out in the large airways, possibly from a laminar flow effect. Fasting for two hours after administration has been recommended to prevent aspiration.

Oxygen and helium

Oxygen relieves dyspnoea either physiologically by improving blood Po_2 levels and so reducing respiratory work, or psychologically, it being seen as like the breath of life. It is not usually first-line treatment for the following reasons:

- Distress caused by the cylinder and mask to the patient and family.
- The possibility of reducing anoxic drive in COAD.
- Problems of maintaining domiciliary supplies.
- Cylinder dependence – the patient can go nowhere without his oxygen.
- Dry mouth – a humidifier is therefore useful.

Helium (80 per cent) – oxygen (20 per cent) mixtures are less dense than air and so reduce the work of breathing, as with dyspnoea from malignant tracheal stenosis.

Prostaglandin inhibitors

Indomethacin 50 mg reduces breathlessness in healthy volunteers after exercise.[18] Vagal non-myelinated C fibres, including J receptors, are stimulated by prostaglandins. Thus, although the mechanism is uncertain, indomethacin may work by inhibiting these receptors.

Where pyrexia, and hence a raised metabolic rate and oxygen consumption, occurs in a dyspnoeic patient, aspirin might be expected to help by an antipyretic action. This does not appear to have been evaluated.

Relief of other symptoms

As with pain, the threshold for dyspnoea may be raised by treating other symptoms, especially anxiety, depression or isolation.

Palliative procedures

Radiotherapy

Dyspnoea from primary carcinoma of bronchus may sometimes be relieved by radiotherapy. Lung metastases, however, are more likely to be radio resistant except for lymphomas, seminomas and nephroblastomas.

Laser therapy

Lasers may be used to resect obstructing bronchial or tracheal tumours, improve ventilation and so reduce dyspnoea. Photoresection using a neodymium yttrium aluminium garnet (Nd:YAG) laser is the most popular, especially for patients who have had maximum radiotherapy, and can be repeated. Antibiotics may be needed to treat infected secretions distal to the resected obstruction. If, however, cancer has also compromised the blood supply to the segment of lung distal to the obstruction, reopening the bronchus will be ineffective and simply increase the dead space.

Stents

Silicone or expandable metal stents can be used to relieve tracheobronchial obstruction and hence dyspnoea. Metal stents are much less likely to migrate and block a bronchial orifice than silicone ones. Progression of tumour beyond the end of the tube may occur.

Pleural taps

Pleural effusions are common in patients with malignant lung or pleural tumours and may (though not always) cause dyspnoea.

Indications for drainage are:

- Where the effusion is the main cause of dyspnoea.
- If a previous tap has reduced dyspnoea.
- Before pleurodesis with a sclerosing agent such as bleomycin.
- As part of further active anti-tumour therapy.

Problems include:

- Some effusions recur rapidly.
- Toxicity and high cost of sclerosing agents.
- Very ill, frail patients may find even a simple drainage distressing.
- As drainage of more than 1.5 litres at a time runs the risk of precipitating heart failure, repeated taps may be needed to drain the effusion completely.

Hence the following protocol is suggested:

- Simple drainage.
- If rapid reaccumulation, drain to dryness with a small bore catheter, followed by instillation of a sclerosing agent.
- If the sclerosing agent is not tolerated, the catheter may be left in situ and connected to a continuous drainage bag.

Other drainage procedures

- Paracentesis will relieve the pressure of ascites on the diaphragm and so reduce dyspnoea.
- Pericardial effusion and tamponade may cause dyspnoea. Drainage is more difficult and hazardous than with pleural effusion and therefore should only be carried out in units with appropriate life support facilities in patients with longer prognoses.
- Pneumothoraces are very rarely symptomatic and therefore require no further treatment.

Blood transfusions

Anaemia is common in advanced cancer. There may be several contributory causes in one patient. Only rarely is there one treatable cause such as iron deficiency. Transfusion may sometimes help dyspnoea due to anaemia but not always. Circulatory overload is a risk in very frail patients and so packed red cells should be used. When deciding whether to transfuse, it is better to go by the symptoms rather than the haemoglobin level.

Physiotherapy

- *Clearing bronchial secretions which narrow the airways and increase the work of breathing.* Coughing exercises, postural drainage, humidified air, percussion, vibration and forced expiration may all be employed, but many of the patients are so weak that the most they can manage is gentle postural drainage and humidified air to reduce mucus viscosity.
- *Breathing exercises.* HVS and the attendant dyspnoea is helped by breathing retraining, teaching the patient to change from fast thoracic to slow diaphragmatic breathing. This helps because the ventilation–perfusion ratio is much lower at the bases of the lungs and so uptake of oxygen and excretion of carbon dioxide is relatively less than at the apices.
- *Insight therapy.* Howell[7] recommends a behavioural approach to HVS by explaining to patients the mechanisms of their dyspnoea and making them hyperventilate to reproduce their symptoms; this insight allows patients to gain control over their breathing.
- *Rebreathing carbon dioxide.* Acute attacks of HVS may be abolished using a rebreathing bag or breathing a 5 per cent CO_2 mixture.

Psychological therapies

Dyspnoea and psychological distress, such as anxiety or depression, may be closely related especially if there is a fear of choking to death. Muscle relaxation exercises and guided imagery may be useful and are simple to teach. Supportive counselling[19] is important.

Supportive procedures

Bedside fans

Cold air directed to the face, nasal mucosa or pharynx has been shown to relieve dyspnoea, probably through stimulation of the vagus nerve. Cold solutions applied to the face have a similar effect.

Overall evaluation of treatment

One study[1] found that only 36 per cent of a group of 289 home care patients obtained good relief from dyspnoea. Another found no improvement over time in dyspnoea scores in a series of 18 patients with terminal cancer.[1]

Thus although individual therapies have a higher success rate, overall control of dyspnoea lags behind that of pain.

Cough

Incidence

Cough is common in advanced cancer. In a series of admissions to St

Christopher's Hospice, cough occurred in 41.4 per cent of all admissions, 57.9 per cent of males and 27.4 per cent of females.[13] This sex discrepancy may be related to the higher rates of lung cancer in men. A lower incidence has been recorded for home care patients, (26 per cent of 334) at St Joseph's Hospice in 1980.

Pathophysiology[20]

Two types of stimuli lead to coughing:

- Mechanical irritation of receptors in the larynx, posterior wall of trachea and large bronchi.
- Chemical irritation of receptors in the acini.

The afferent fibres subserving cough travel centrally via the trigeminal, glossopharyngeal, superior laryngeal and vagus nerves to the medulla where efferent activity is coordinated, and transmitted via the recurrent laryngeal and spinal nerves.

Hence, treatment of cough will either be to remove the irritant or to reduce the sensitivity of the cough reflex pathways. In general, productive cough has a defensive function and so is best not suppressed, whereas the opposite applies for dry cough.

Causes

Luminal

- Air quality – very cold, hot or dry air stimulates coughing.
- Fumes – such as cigarette smoke, dust or irritant gases.
- Aspiration – of foreign bodies, vomit, food or liquids. This will be aggravated by diseases affecting coordination of swallowing such as oesophageal or pharyngeal tumours or motor neurone disease. The elderly are especially prone, as the sensitivity of their cough reflex is lowered.
- Haemoptysis

Mural

- Bronchial neoplasms, primary for secondary.
- Inflammatory – this includes respiratory infections anywhere along the respiratory tract, such as bronchitis, pneumonia, bronchiectasis or lung abscesses.
- Pulmonary oedema as with left ventricular failure.
- Asthma.
- Decreased pulmonary compliance as with pulmonary fibrosis.

Extramural

These include pressure on the lungs from oesophageal or mediastinal tumours or from hilar lymphadenopathy.

Other causes

- Psychogenic cough.
- Irritation of the left recurrent laryngeal nerve by tumour.

Clinical features

The description of the cough may help diagnosis as shown in Table 3.11. Occasionally, pieces of necrotic tumour may be coughed up. Investigation should be limited to situations where they may make a difference to management. Hence, a chest X-ray and sputum culture and sensitivity are most likely to help.

Complications of chronic cough include syncope, rib fractures, pneumothoraces in emphysema, and hernias.

Treatment

Many therapies for cough will be the same as for dyspnoea and have already been discussed (see Table 3.12). For these, only points of difference will be mentioned.

Glucocorticosteroids

These may help the bronchorrhoea occasionally associated with alveolar cell carcinomas.[20] Fluid restriction and anticholinergics have also been suggested for this problem.

Table 3.11 Some diagnostic features of cough in advanced cancer

Type	Description	Examples of possible diagnoses
Sound	Bovine	Abductor cord paralysis from recurrent laryngeal nerve palsy
	Brassy	Tracheal compression by tumour
	Weak	Complete vocal cord paralysis
		Myasthenic syndrome
		Cachexia
	Suppression	Severe thoracic or upper abdominal pain
Timing	Early morning	COAD
	With change posture	Bronchiectasis
	After food	Swallowing incoordination
		Malignant tracheo-oesophageal fistula
	Dry cough for years	Psychogenic
Sputum	Yellow or green	Respiratory infection
	Pus and offensive smell	Abscess or Bronchiectasis
	Bronchorrhea (> 100 ml/day)	Bronchiectasis
		Alveolar cell carcinoma

Opioids

These are cough suppressants, acting centrally on the medulla. Codeine and pholcodine are of moderate strength, and morphine or methadone are strong. There is no logic in giving morphine for pain together with codeine for cough; morphine alone will suffice for both symptoms. Dosage is as for pain control. Methadone is better avoided because of its long half-life and hence propensity for accumulation.

Bupivacaine

Since cough is stimulated by receptors in both small and large airways, it is reasonable, as well as nebulizers mentioned under treatment of dyspnoea, also to use one with a larger particle size of say 10 microns, such as the Bird nebulizer, which will allow fall-out of bupivacaine in the main bronchi.

Interpleural infusion of bupivacaine,[21] for chest pain after pneumonectomy for carcinoma of bronchus, has also been found to control a persistent cough. A possible explanation is that there is diffusion onto the hilar remnant and hence the vagus nerve, blocking the afferent limb of the cough reflex.

Psychotropics

Any sedative will help reduce cough. Promethazine is popular in cough medicines.

Water vapour inhalation

This is probably the most effective method of liquefying tenacious sputum. It may be administered nebulized by a humidifier or as an inhalation using hot water in a Nelson's inhaler. Boiling water should never be used because of the risk of scalding. Volatile oils such as menthol or benzoin may be added, are soothing and may increase sputum production.

Mucolytics

Bromhexine 8 mg tds and carbocisteine 500–750 mg tds help liquefy viscid bronchial secretions. Gastrointestinal irritation may occur.

Table 3.12   Treatment of cough in advanced cancer

Therapy	Palliative	Symptomatic
Drugs	Antibiotics Glucocorticosteroids	Opioids Bupivacaine Hyoscine Psychotropics Mucolytics Expectorants Water vapour
Procedures	Radiotherapy	Physiotherapy

Expectorants

These are claimed to increase the volume of bronchial mucus and so assist expectoration, though whether this is so is uncertain. Ipecacuanha, ammonium chloride and squill are examples and are often combined with other drugs as cough mixtures, sometimes illogically as with expectorant and cough suppressant combinations. Patients may find them helpful despite the pharmacological inconsistencies.

The movement of particles up the bronchial tree through mucociliary action has been shown to be increased by guaiphenesin and also inhaled beta-adrenergic agonists.[20]

Radiotherapy

Palliative radiotherapy can partly or completely relieve cough from an advanced primary bronchial carcinoma, though not from lung metastases unless they are highly radiosensitive.[13]

Physiotherapy

Although coughing exercises with vibration and percussion helps to clear sputum, they are beyond the capacity of many patients with advanced cancer, especially as there may be temporary bronchoconstriction after the procedure. Postural drainage with humidified air may help.

Evaluation

Investigation of the success of therapy for cough does not seem to have been carried out apart from one study on home care patients[22] where 57 per cent of 294 patients with cough enjoyed good relief of this symptom.

Haemoptysis

Causes

- Bronchial carcinoma.
- Infections – acute bronchitis, pneumonia (especially klebsiella), lung abscess or tuberculosis.
- Cardiovascular – left ventricular failure, mitral stenosis or pulmonary embolism.
- Haemorrhagic – bleeding diathesis or anticoagulant therapy.
- Epistaxis and mixing of nasal blood with sputum.

Clinical features

With haemoptyses, rusty sputum suggests pneumococcal pneumonia, sudden haemorrhage pulmonary embolus, pink frothy sputum LVF and blood mixed with purulent sputum bronchiectasis or tumour stenosing a main bronchus with infection distally.

Patients may be alarmed at seeing blood in their sputum, fearing either an imminent fatal haemorrhage, or, in those who do not know their diagnosis, that it implies life-threatening illness.

Some patients find it difficult to differentiate between retching or vomiting, and cough. A useful pointer is that any blood in vomit will be altered and dark because of stomach acid whereas in sputum it tends to be fresh.

Treatment of haemoptysis

- Radiotherapy is very effective if the patient is well enough and has not already had the maximum dose.
- Antibiotics for haemoptyses due to respiratory infections.
- Treatment of left ventricular failure with diuretics and digoxin.
- If a patient is on anticoagulants, review of their control.
- Haemostatic drugs – tranexamic acid 500 mg qds impairs fibrin dissolution by inhibiting plasminogen activation. Ethamsylate 500 mg qds reduces capillary bleeding by correcting abnormal platelet adhesion. Both of these drugs are used, though their value is unproven.
- Major life-threatening lung haemorrhages are uncommon but do occur. Cough, dyspnoea, fear and shock with a cold sweat and pallor are the main symptoms and can be relieved by an immediate injection of diamorphine 5 mg (or more if the patient is already on a higher dosage) with hyoscine 0.4–0.6 mg and chlorpromazine 12.5–25 mg. Hypotension induced by these drugs may help stop the bleeding. If the patient survives the crisis, hyoscine causes amnesia for the event.

Other respiratory symptoms

Wheeze of itself is not necessarily distressing. It is the attendant dyspnoea which requires treatment. In asthma, nebulized salbutamol, sodium cromoglycate, aminophylline and glucocorticosteroids may all be useful; the last-named can be given in high dose if necessary as long-term side effects of steroids do not apply in the terminally ill. Fixed wheeze and dyspnoea due for example to lymphangitis has already been discussed.

Stridor causes anxiety as well as dyspnoea because of the fear of choking. It is due to bronchial or tracheal compression by tumours and may be relieved by dexamethasone 8–16 mg per day followed by radiotherapy. The steroid not only reduces tumour oedema but also prevents the temporary worsening of symptoms from an initial inflammatory response to radiotherapy. Helium and oxygen mixtures may lessen the work of breathing. For the moribund patient, symptomatic relief, as described for patients with major haemorrhages, is indicated. It is important to talk through the patient's fears of asphyxiation and to reassure them that effective treatment is available. Though stenosis of the respiratory tract is common, compete occlusion is very rare.

Chest pain and hiccup are considered elsewhere. Fortunately sneezing does not seem to figure as a respiratory problem.

Notes and References

1. HEYSE-MOORE, L.H., ROSS, V. and MULLEE, M. 'How much of a problem is dyspnoea in advanced cancer?' *Palliative Medicine*, 1991, **5**, 20–26.
2. REUBEN, D.B. and MOR V. 'Dyspnoea in terminally ill cancer patients,' *Chest*, 1986, **89**, 234–6.
3. CAMPBELL, E.J.M. and HOWELL, J.B.L. 'The sensation of breathlessness,' *British Medical Bulletin*, 1963, **19**, 36–40.
4. PAINTAL, F. 'Mechanism of stimulation of type J pulmonary receptors,' *Journal of Physiology*, 1969, **203**, 511–23.
5. ROUSSOS, C.S. and MACKLEM, P.T. 'Diaphragmatic fatigue in man,' *Journal of Applied Physiology: Respiratory and Environmental Exercise Physiology*, 1977, **43**, 189–97.
6. HEYSE-MOORE, L.H. On dyspnoea in advanced cancer. DM Thesis, in preparation.
7. HOWELL, J.B.L. 'Behavioural breathlessness,' *Thorax*, 1990, **45**, 287–92.
8. GUZ, A. 'Respiratory sensations in man,' *British Medical Bulletin*, 1977, **33**, 175–7.
9. BURNS, B.H. and HOWELL, J.B.L. 'Disproportionately severe breathlessness in chronic bronchitis,' *The Quarterly Journal of Medicine*, 1969, **38**, 277–94.
10. ADAMS, L., CHRONOS, N., LANE, R., and GUZ, A. The measurement of breathlessness induced in normal subjects: individual differences. *Clinical Science*, 1986, **70**, 131–40.
11. MELZACK, R. 'The McGill Pain Questionnaire: major properties and scoring methods,' *Pain*, 1975, **1**, 277–99.
12. FLETCHER, C.M. 'The clinical diagnosis of pulmonary emphysema: an experimental study,' *Proceedings of the Royal Society of Medicine*, 1952, **45**, 577.
13. SAUNDERS, C. (ed.). *The Management of Terminal Malignant Disease*, 2nd edn, London, Edward Arnold, 1984.
14. WALSH, T.D. 'Opiates and respiratory function in advanced cancer,' *Recent Results Cancer Research*, 1984, **89**, 115–17.
15. MASTERS, N.J., BENNETT, M.R.D. and WEDLEY, J.R. 'Nebulised morphine: a new delivery method for pain relief,' *Practitioner*, 1985, **229**, 649–53.
16. GILMAN, A.G., GOODMAN, L.S., RALL, T.W. and MURAD, F. (eds). *The Pharmacological Basis of Therapeutics*, 7th edn, New York, Macmillan, 1985, 344–5.
17. LUNT, M.J., TAYLOR, J. and MELDRUM, S.J. 'A system of producing particles of controlled size from a nebuliser,' *Journal of Medical Engineering and Technology*, 1981, **5**, 138–9.
18. O'NEILL, P.A., STARK, R.D. and MORTON, P.B. 'Do prostaglandins have a role in breathlessness?' *American Review of Respiratory Diseases*, 1985, **132**, 22–4.
19. MOOREY, S. and GREER, S. *Psychological Therapy for Patients with Cancer: a New Approach*, Oxford, Heinemann, 1989.
20. WEATHERALL, D.J., LEDINGHAM, J.G.G. and WARRELL, D.A. (eds). *Oxford Textbook of Medicine*, Vol. 2, Oxford, Oxford University Press, 1983, 15.39–15.41.

21. MARSH, C.R. and HARDY, P.A.J. 'Interpleural infusion with bupivacaine for intractable cough,' *Palliative Medicine*, 1991, **5**, 349–50.
22. LAMERTON, R. *Care of the Dying*, London, Pelican, 1973, 75.

Metabolic Symptoms————————————

Robert Dunlop

The paraneoplastic symptoms of cancer

Cancer often produces symptoms by causing local damage in various organs: the pain of bone destruction or liver enlargement, breathlessness from lung infiltration, and confusion from brain metastases for example. The management of these symptoms is dealt with in the other sections of this chapter.

This section will review how cancer can affect the body generally, irrespective of the site or sites at which it is growing. The 'distant' effects of cancer are often referred to as paraneoplastic effects and a variety of syndromes have been described. Anorexia and cachexia will be considered first, in keeping with the frequency of these symptoms and their emotive significance to patients and families. The review of the metabolic effects of cancer will also discuss the management of diabetes in cancer patients. Some neurological paraneoplastic syndromes will be briefly considered.

Anorexia, cachexia

Anorexia (loss of appetite) and cachexia (the wasting of physical appearance) are common symptoms of cancer. Their paraneoplastic origin is not proven but has been inferred from the way that both symptoms may appear before a cancer is detectable and then disappear when the cancer is removed. Furthermore, the severity of these symptoms is not related to the size or location of the cancer. Some cancer patients have high levels of substances such as tumour necrosis factor which can produce cachexia when given to animals without cancer. However, the exact role of these substances as a cause of cachexia in man is unclear.

There are other causes of anorexia in patients with cancer. Many patients receiving chemotherapy or radiotherapy experience some loss of appetite, which may be associated with nausea and vomiting. Some chemotherapy agents such as cisplatinum can induce profound weight loss. These symptoms may confound patients and families who interpret them as signs of deterioration. However, if the cancer responds, the symptoms will wane over several weeks. Most oncology units are aware of the need for aggressive antiemetic therapy and provide medications when the chemotherapy is given. Home care hospice staff can improve on this by encouraging patients to start antiemetics the night before and then continue them for several days after each treatment.

Another treatable cause for anorexia is infection. Occasionally, patients develop chronic infections such as pelvic abscess with rectal cancer and lung abscess with lung cancer. Fever and a purulent offensive discharge or cough usually accompanies the systemic deterioration. A broad spectrum antibiotic such as co-amoxiclav, clindamycin or chloramphenicol can produce dramatic improvement without the need to resort to intravenous therapy.

Repeated taps of pleural effusions or ascites can exacerbate weakness and cachexia. Pleurodhesis should be considered if multiple pleural taps are required. A peritoneal shunt can be very helpful for patients with ascites from a slowly progressive intra-abdominal cancer. Cancer can produce weight loss by causing mechanical obstruction of the gastrointestinal tract.

If a treatable cause is not apparent, there are several effective palliative treatments which can be offered. Before considering these, it is important to examine the psychological issues that accompany these symptoms. Eating is one of the fundamental needs of the body; to stop eating means death. Anorexia reminds the family that they will lose the patient. The acts of preparing food and feeding someone have a nurturing component and are an important element of personhood for many caregivers. An anorexic patient quickly produces a sense of helplessness in the carer. These feelings are made worse by the emaciated appearance of patients with advanced cancer which suggests that they are dying of starvation, a sign of extreme neglect. It is little wonder that anorexia and cachexia are two of the symptoms most feared by patients and their families.

Metabolic studies have shown that there are several important differences between starvation and the cachexia of cancer (Brennan, 1981). For example, starvation victims have a reduced basal metabolic rate and whole-body glucose turnover whereas cancer patients have a higher than normal basal metabolic rate and whole-body glucose turnover. These changes are not the result of cancers using so much energy that the body starves; somehow they cause the metabolic systems in the body to waste energy. There is no evidence that providing terminally ill patients with extra nutrients prolongs life. Anecdotal cases have suggested parenteral nutrition can be detrimental because cancer growth is accelerated (Rice, 1987).

There are circumstances when alternative methods of nutritional support may be warranted. Some patients become malnourished from a direct effect of cancer, for example patients with head and neck cancers who cannot swallow. These patients can benefit symptomatically from alternative means of nutritional support such as a fine-bore nasogastric feeding tube. The indications for additional nutritional support should be reviewed with the patient and family as the disease progresses.

Very often, it is the relatives who are distressed by the patient's anorexia and weight loss. Even when the patient presents the problem, it is important to make sure that he or she is not trying to respond to the demands of the relatives. When the patient is accepting of the problem, do not be too eager to reassure the relatives but use the chance to explore the feelings of loss which the carers are trying to overcome by focusing on the issue of food. Some families adjust quickly to the patient's situation when they are given an explanation of what is happening. Many families appreciate being taught other ways to nurture the patient, such as preparing small visually attractive meals or attending to mouth cares. Strategies which ameliorate their sense of helplessness are essential to hospice home care.

Many patients cannot tolerate feeling anorexic. Their anger is often linked to a desire to beat the cancer, not to give in to its inexorable effects. Sometimes, they just do not want to be stigmatized by a gaunt appearance. These patients should be offered symptomatic treatments which can make them feel and look better. A trial of an antiemetic such as haloperidol 2 mg at night may be all that is necessary; anorexia can be an expression of low grade nausea. Very often, more potent agents are required. Corticosteroids have been the mainstay, starting with a dose of prednisone 20 mg or dexamethasone 4 mg in the morning. If the response is not satisfactory to the patient, higher doses can be used; dexamethasone 16 mg or methylprednisolone 100 mg tablet in the morning. Regular injections of high dose methyl prednisolone did enjoy a vogue but the oral route is always preferable. Corticosteroids are particularly helpful if the patient also has nausea and vomiting, nerve pain, or breathlessness. However, prolonged use can produce weakness from proximal myopathy which can exacerbate the patient's concern about becoming dependent. High dose progestagens, such as megestrol acetate 160–480 mg daily or medroxyprogesterone acetate 200 mg three times daily, are very useful alternatives. Some other drugs, notably antihistamines, can stimulate appetite but drowsiness is a limiting side effect.

Some readers will be concerned that the use of appetite stimulants will give patients a false hope and thereby delay or prevent acceptance of dying. If this philosophy is pressed onto these patients, they will often become angry and want to discontinue contact. If their choice is supported, a better rapport will be established, enabling contact to be maintained for the time when the patient does decide to let go and to help prepare the family for the 'sudden' change which occurs when patients on high-dose steroids or progestagens deteriorate. These medications lift patients off the normal downward slope of cancer and maintain them on a plateau until nearer the time of death.

Taste disturbances

Cancer patients frequently complain of altered taste sensation. Some people find that foods become tasteless and bland. More commonly, certain foods become unpalatable because their normal taste becomes heightened and unpleasant. Foods containing sugar may taste too sweet; meats may stimulate the bitter taste. Sometimes, patients complain that foods produce a metallic or other similarly unpleasant abnormal taste.

When someone complains of altered taste, the mouth should be examined to exclude correctable local problems, such as thrush or bacterial infections associated with head and neck tumours. Appropriate antifungal or antibiotic medications, with attention to good mouth hygiene, should be considered for these situations.

Usually, a local cause is not apparent, and a trial of an antiemetic or an appetite stimulant is often worthwhile. Caregivers may find that experimentation with different foods can restore the patient's enjoyment of eating. Some caregivers seem to derive pleasure from the challenge but many find it very difficult, practically and emotionally.

Fever

Fever and sweats can be a remote effect of cancer. They are classically associated with Hodgkins lymphoma but liver metastases are another common cause. Infection should be excluded. Symptomatic relief is possible with anti-inflammatory drugs and steroids.

The metabolic effects of cancer

It is important to be aware of the metabolic syndromes, particularly those which mimic the effects of advanced cancer. There have been many instances where patients have been referred to hospices in the belief that the patient is about to die. The recognition of a metabolic problem has prompted appropriate treatment and restored the patient to a good quality of life, sometimes for many weeks or months.

However, patients who are about to die from advanced cancer may develop metabolic problems as they are dying; actively treating these patients can be meddlesome and distressing. Doctors often feel compelled to treat metabolic abnormalities regardless of the whole patient, particularly in teaching hospitals where these syndromes attract considerable academic interest. Palliative care teams often face this problem.

It is not always possible to distinguish between a patient who is dying from cancer with an associated metabolic abnormality and a patient who has a reversible metabolic problem with an otherwise reasonable quality of life. Some patients will say when they 'have had enough'. They will not want any active treatments. Other patients will become agitated as they sense their deterioration and will want something done.

In general, cancer produces a gradual decline over several weeks. If the patient has been deteriorating slowly and goes into a coma which is associated with a metabolic abnormality, the patient's general condition is unlikely to respond to treatment for the metabolic problem. A sudden deterioration favours a treatable cause. Patients with advanced cancer who are near to death are often cachectic and very weak. If a patient becomes drowsy and confused but has relatively normal physical appearance and functional capacity, then a metabolic cause should be sought and treated. If the distinction is not clear, a therapeutic trial is often warranted. Treatment can always be withdrawn if the patient recovers and then expresses a wish not to have treatment.

Hypercalcaemia

Hypercalcaemia refers to a high level of calcium in the blood. It is commonly associated with multiple myeloma, breast cancer, and squamous cell lung cancers. The calcium is mobilized from bone by locally active substances produced by bone metastases or by factors such as ectopic parathormone and cytokines which circulate throughout the body to activate osteoclasts. In the latter case, bone metastases may not be evident.

Mild hypercalcaemia is often asymptomatic. Higher levels cause nausea, anorexia, vomiting and constipation, associated with thirst and polyuria. Dehydration can produce dramatic weight loss and patients frequently become drowsy, confused and eventually comatose.

Untreated symptomatic hypercalcaemia will cause the patient to die. When it is not appropriate to lower the calcium level, antiemetics are often required until coma supervenes. Occasionally, sedation may be needed if the patient becomes very agitated and confused.

If the hypercalcaemia is to be treated, the first step is to restore hydration. Some patients can achieve this by drinking more fluids; the subcutaneous route is a very safe and efficient alternative, particularly in the home care setting, when the patient is confused or vomiting. Normal saline can be infused through an intravenous administration set connected to a butterfly needle placed subcutaneously. A forced diuresis, when frusemide is used with higher volumes of intravenous fluids than are needed to correct dehydration, should not be used because there is little evidence of benefit and there is a high likelihood of causing further problems such as the distress of incontinence.

If the hypercalcaemia is only mild or moderate, oral phosphate tablets can be used. The side effect of diarrhoea can be balanced against the constipating effect of the calcium. In the longer term, patient compliance and diarrhoea can become problems. High dose oral steroids can be helpful if the underlying cancer is susceptible to their cytotoxic effect, for example breast cancer and haematological cancers. An intravenous bolus injection of a bisphosphanate such as pamidronate or etidronate will lower the calcium for several weeks. The dose can be repeated as required but it tends to become less effective. Oral bisphosphanates can maintain a lowered calcium level. Six-hourly calcitonin injections can produce a rapid response but they are usually unsuitable for long-term or out-patient use. Mithramycin is rarely used now, and antiprostaglandin agents are not effective despite their theoretical promise. Gallium is a promising new agent but the need for a several-day intravenous infusion will limit its potential.

Inappropriate antidiuretic hormone secretion

Antidiuretic hormone (ADH) is normally produced by the pituitary gland when the body needs to conserve water. Some cancers, most commonly small cell lung cancers, produce ADH constantly and cause inappropriate water retention. Patients become lethargic and confused, even frankly psychotic. Death usually results from coma. Blood tests will reveal a low level of sodium in the blood (hyponatraemia). Other tests are required to confirm the diagnosis. Rarely, some drugs which are commonly used in palliative care, such as morphine, haloperidol, amitriptyline, and carbamazepine, can produce a similar clinical and biochemical picture.

The best way to treat the syndrome of inappropriate ADH production (SIADH) is to treat the cancer. Most patients with small cell lung cancer who are referred to hospices will have failed or not be suitable for anti-cancer treatments. Restricting fluid intake to 1000 mls or less per day can produce symtpomatic improvement. If this is not effective, demeclocycline can block the effect of ADH. Urea is another alternative which at a dose of 30 g per day can promote water loss. Severe hyponatraemia may require hypertonic saline combined with intravenous frusemide but this is a very difficult option in the hospice in-patient and home care setting. When symptomatic treatment is not appropriate, sedation may occasionally be required. An anticonvulsant may also be necessary.

Cushings Syndrome

Lung cancers and a variety of endocrine tumours can stimulate excessive levels of corticosteroid. The early symptoms are muscle weakness when climbing stairs and getting up from a chair, and peripheral oedema. Some patients develop mental changes. Hypertension, hyperglycaemia, and hypokalaemia will be apparent if looked for. The other classical features of Cushings syndrome such as moon face, striae, and 'buffalo hump' only develop if the patient has a slowly growing cancer.

Treatment for the underlying cancer may be possible. Otherwise, the excessive corticosteroid production can be blocked by drugs such as aminoglutethamide, mitotane, and metyrapone. These drugs can have severe side effects, particularly nausea and vomiting, and their use requires specialist input. Despite these problems, patients with a longer prognosis can enjoy a better quality of life when the corticosteroid level is controlled. Rarely, it is appropriate to surgically remove the adrenal glands.

Hypoadrenalism

Hypoadrenalism results from low levels of corticosteroids and is not due to a paraneoplastic effect. However, it is worthy of brief mention because the symptoms are very debilitating but easily treated with oral steroids. The usual cause is sudden cessation of high-dose steroids causing the patient to experience weakness, lethargy, and the symptoms of postural hypotension. There are a number of situations when it is appropriate to stop steroids, for example when a patient with a brain tumour becomes comatose in the terminal phase. However, many doctors will reduce steroids because of concerns about their long-term effects, without taking into account the quality of life of the patient. Very rarely, metastases to the adrenal glands will produce hypoadrenalism.

Hyperglycaemia

While elevated blood glucose levels may rarely result from Cushings syndrome, they are usually due to diabetes which preceded the diagnosis of cancer or is exposed by steroid therapy. If the glucose level is high enough, the classic symptoms of diabetes occur: thirst and polyuria, tiredness, weight loss, blurring of vision, paraesthesiae, and the symptoms of infections such as oral thrush.

The management of diabetes must be modified when the patient is terminally ill. The prevention of long-term complications, which requires aggressive treatment and blood glucose monitoring to achieve euglycaemia, is not relevant. The aim of treatment should be symptomatic control, avoiding the distress of hypoglycaemic episodes and minimizing finger prick testing. Many patients will tolerate blood glucose levels in the range of 11–17 mmol/l. Restrictions on food types can often be relaxed, making for a better quality of life. Most patients have lower insulin requirements because of reduced food intake, exercise and weight caused by cancer; the clearance of insulin and hypoglycaemic drugs may be reduced if the cancer causes liver or renal impairment. Patients will usually need to change to shorter-acting insulins or tablets in lowering dosage. Treatment should be prescribed with meals so that the hypoglycaemic agent is automatically discontinued if the patient does not eat.

Diabetics who are taking steroids, particularly the high doses needed to control raised intracranial pressure, often have an increased requirement for insulin. Whenever possible, other strategies such as whole brain radiotherapy should be used for their steroid-sparing effects. Patient quality of life should not be compromised in an effort to reduce the steroid dose.

Hypoglycaemia

The usual cause of low blood glucose is excessive insulin levels in a diabetic patient. Insulin producing islet cell tumours are a very rare cause of hypoglycaemia, and some cancers such as mesothelioma, hepatoma and lymphoma can produce hypoglycaemia by using glucose. The symptoms of weakness, dizziness, nausea, confusion, sweating, and fits are very distressing and patients should not be left untreated in the expectation that they will die; death from hypoglycaemia is not inevitable and patients may be left with distressing neurological deficits. Oral glucose is usually effective but hospice in-patient units should carry glucagon in the event that the patient cannot swallow.

Carcinoid syndrome

Metastatic carcinoid tumours in the liver can produce unpleasant symptoms such as flushing, diarrhoea, and asthma. Symptomatic therapy can be sufficient: loperamide for diarrhoea, bronchodilators for asthma. The 5-HT antagonists such as ketanserin can be helpful. Regular injections of somatostatin are effective but expensive.

Non-metastatic neurological manifestations of cancer

Most neurological abnormalities in cancer patients are due to brain tumours or metastases but a number of paraneoplastic syndromes have also been described. This section is too short to permit more than a few cursory observations about these syndromes. Peripheral nerves are most commonly affected, resulting in weakness and sensory changes. Pain may be a significant problem and should be treated with medications for nerve pain rather than opioids. The brain can be affected in specific areas such as the cerebellum, or more generally, often in a patchy manner. Dementia can occur and is very distressing in younger patients. Involvement of the spinal cord can lead to paraplegia. Some patients develop a motor neurone disease.

Most of the paraneoplastic effects on the nervous system are irreversible, even if the cancer is amenable to treatment. The Eaton–Lambert syndrome, which produces proximal muscular weakness and a variety of other distressing symptoms, is one of the few syndromes which improves if the cause, usually small cell lung cancer, responds to anti-cancer treatment. The weakness of dermatomyositis may respond to steroids. Many of the paraneoplastic syndromes have an inflammatory or autoimmune basis, and a trial of high-dose steroids may be worthwhile.

References

BRENNAN, M.F. 'Total parenteral nutrition in the cancer patient', *New England Journal of Medicine*, 1981, **305**, 373–5.
BUNN, P.A. and RIDGWAY, E.C. 'Paraneoplastic syndromes.' In: De Vita, V.T.,

Hellman, S. and Rosenberg, S.A. (eds), *Cancer: Principles and Practice of Oncology*, 3rd edn, Philadelphia, Lippincott, 1989, pp. 1896–940.

RICE, M.I. and VAN RIJ, A.M. 'Parenteral nutrition and tumour growth in the patient with complicated abdominal cancer', *Australia and New Zealand Journal of Surgery*, 1987, **57**, 375–9.

Depression, Sadness and Anxiety————

Gail Hodgson

Introduction

At least 25 to 50 per cent of cancer patients (not all terminal) have sustained psychiatric morbidity in the form of anxiety states, depressive illnesses, sexual problems and organic brain syndromes. Much of this may be ignored, dismissed or accepted by family and professionals as 'understandable' and by implication tolerated, not treated or even considered as treatable.

But when does sadness become a depressive illness? How long should anger last? When does fear about the future become an anxiety state? How can these problems be managed and is treatment effective?

These are difficult questions to answer and good research is scant and controversial. There is increasing evidence that appropriate management of emotions and effective social support improves prognosis[1] and in some more controversial studies, may influence the incidence of cancer. However, there comes a time when we all must die and there is no doubt that a dignified death is a positive and even wonderful experience. It allows the grieving of those left behind to be less painful and difficult. Hence active assessment and management of the physical, psychological and social aspects of the dying is essential.

A model for understanding emotional responses

When a person is faced with an overwhelming threat, such as death, they can face intolerable fear. The threat is recognized in the higher brain centres, triggering the 'fight or flight' physiological response, with an outpouring of adrenalin. This results in the outward manifestation of anxiety, before there is a cognitive recognition of fear. To cope, function and survive, i.e. to turn off the 'flight or fight' response, humans have developed a range of psychological defence mechanisms and coping strategies (Table 3.13) which operate at an unconscious automatic level. Effective functioning of defence mechanisms and coping strategies distances the person from the threat. This allows the individual to gain control over their feelings and slow down the impact of the reality. As a consequence feelings and emotions can be expressed over a period of time, support elicited, the threat is thought and talked about and lived with. Gradually if premature death has to be faced, the perception of the reality changes to a more manageable problem which can be accepted with the consequent adaptation of life style and expectations. This process is shown diagrammatically in Fig. 3.3.

Defence mechanisms and coping strategies

Understanding these mechanisms and strategies is important as they explain many aspects of human behaviour. They are usually automatic and unconscious but are not mutually exclusive.

Regression

Is to become more child-like or revert to an earlier stage of development. When ill, normal tasks are given up and we allow others to care for us. This behaviour has survival value, eliciting extra care (physical and emotional) during times of stress. Used in excess, regression is maladaptive and leads to dependency and demanding, immature and self-centred behaviour which often results in obtaining less or inappropriate care.

Denial

Is to blot out or ignore certain realities. The use of this defence mechanism is important and we all use it, although often partially. It allows normal functioning despite grave difficulties. If denial is excessive, it becomes maladaptive. It can lead to non-compliance which may be life threatening or make symptom control difficult. Complete or excessive denial of the diagnosis with comments such as 'the biopsy report got mixed up with someone else's – mine is okay – the doctors made a mistake' means to that individual, that further treatment is unnecessary. This leads to loneliness, isolation and inappropriate planning. Doctors who deny their patient's mortality and their own helplessness, may plan inappropriate interventions, such as unnecessary surgery.

Table 3.13 Some defence mechanisms and coping strategies

Regression
Denial
Rationalization
Intellectualization
Projection
Displacement
Introjection
Repression
Withdrawal and Avoidance

Rationalization

This defence is commonly used and distances by providing an alternative explanation for the symptoms or feelings. For example, episodic vomiting explained by an everyday cause rather than advancing malignant disease.

Intellectualization

This defence distances by making the reality theoretical and so unreal. It protects against emotional pain and allows investigation of difficult issues which improves knowledge as well as allowing efficiency in spite of traumatic circumstances. Doctors tend to use this method of coping with numerous painful situations they deal with daily. It allows objectivity but used in excess can lead to cold distant relationships devoid of human feeling, often intimidating those around, isolating doctors, patients and carers.

Projection

This defence distances by pushing the problem on to others. For example, 'If the Government had banned smoking, I would never have got lung cancer.' It allows expression of anger which, in the psychologically healthy, becomes a more realistic anger at themselves and being cheated of life. Showing anger often facilitates the expression of sadness and loss. However, the excessive use of projection is maladaptive, alienating those whose support is needed most, allows avoidance of personal responsibility and in severe cases can lead to paranoid states.

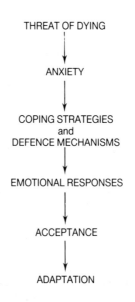

THREAT OF DYING

↓

ANXIETY

↓

COPING STRATEGIES
and
DEFENCE MECHANISMS

↓

EMOTIONAL RESPONSES

↓

ACCEPTANCE

↓

ADAPTATION

Fig. 3.3 Processes occuring when facing death.

Displacement

This defence works by displacing emotional energy away from the individual by distraction into other thoughts and activities. For example, rather than face the emotional pain of news of cancer recurrence, a mother will bury herself in a fundraising appeal for a new community centre. In excess it can lead to exhaustion, isolation and even somatization. Somatizing may occur when an individual displaces painful emotions into a bodily symptom resulting in increased or unmanageable physical symptoms, usually pain. When people who principally cope by displacement activity become medically unwell and are forced to 'stop', they may become severely depressed or anxious.

Introjection

This allows the individual to look within themselves to find solutions for their problems. This can produce change and self-help but in excess can result in self-blame, isolation and depression.

Repression

This defence is of central importance in psychoanalytic theory. However, in this context it is an unconscious suppression of painful memories. A person who has been sexually abused as a child often represses and blocks out all memory of the abuse. In later life, when faced with for example, a gynaecological cancer, a variety of abnormal behaviours may be manifest; from a detached, emotionless acceptance (complete repression) to dramatic acting out (such as repeated self-harm).

Withdrawal and avoidance

With this defence individuals withdraw from and avoid painful situations and hence have difficulties resolving problems. For example, a young man who has avoided taking responsibility for his actions, leaving jobs and relationships when they got too difficult, will have great difficulty when faced with a fast growing sarcoma which he physically cannot run away from. This situation provokes extreme anxiety and distress.

Development of defence mechanisms and coping strategies

From birth we are faced with threats to our existence. Hence, during childhood, once a child recognizes he is a separate entity (after about nine months), he becomes clinging to his mother figure, showing great distress when she is absent. At this stage the child is using the mother's security to protect him from his fears. This is known as *externalized* coping, i.e. the protector/defence is coming from a source outside the child. During subsequent years the child in a healthy family gradually learns to feel secure and to cope increasingly with independence. The child is using memories of his mother's reassurance to help him cope with his fears without her immediate presence. This is the process of *internalized* coping, i.e. the source of protection and defence against fearful threats is coming from within the child.

Conclusions

The psychologically healthy adult protects his or her psyche against overwhelming anxiety by using a variety of learnt automatic (often unconscious) defence mechanisms and internalized and externalized coping strategies, in a flexible way. The individual learns that some strategies are better used in some situations than others. The combination of defences dictates how a person copes (coping styles) and behaves. Commonly defences are not complete so fear and anxiety are part of everyday life, leading to change, ambition and so on. Mostly, effective defences distance painful realities and allow individuals to gain control over feelings of fear and come to terms with their fate. For example, the reality that any of us could die in the next few hours from an accident or cerebral haemorrhage is pushed away as a remote, unlikely possibility, using the unconscious defence mechanism of denial of death and more conscious knowledge in the form of life experience and statistical infor-mation. This allows normal functioning in the here and now, planning ahead and enjoyment of life. It also allows consideration of mortality and so it is possible to write a will or take out an insurance policy without feeling great fear.

The process of acquiring an effective range of defence mechanisms and coping strategies depends on many factors. These include:

- Personality.
- Parenting.
- Supports.
- Communication skills.
- Life experience.
- Time.

It is not difficult to predict the characteristics of copers and non-copers.

Copers

In facing premature death, those who cope with least psychiatric morbid-ity have several or all of the following:

- An intact premorbid personality.
- Maturity (not necessarily in years).
- Effective external supports (e.g. loving spouse).
- Good communication skills.
- Time.
- Good premorbid mental health.

These characteristics tend to result in a fighting spirit or appropriate denial.

Non-Copers

People who are at emotional risk and have high psychiatric morbidity often have one or more of the following:

- An immature or damaged personality.
- Poor external supports, e.g. poverty, living alone, few friends.
- Poor communication skills, e.g. deafness or learning difficulties.
- Severe or prolonged stress, e.g. chemotherapy with medical complications
- Sudden, unexpected stress, e.g. routine appendicectomy reveals widespread metastatic cancer.
- Poor premorbid mental health (or have a strong family history of psychiatric disorder)

When a person presents with these risk factors or when stress is severe, prolonged, sudden or unexpected, then even the best, most resilient effective coping strategies may be overwhelmed and more severe psychological disturbances occur. If short lived (within three months), they are known as *adjustment disorders* and most resolve spontaneously with time and support. If more persistent and pervasive then *psychiatric disorders* such as anxiety states, depressive illnesses and psychoses are likely to occur.

Individuals who use a single excessive defence, maladaptive coping strategies with stuck emotional responses, and who are unable to work through their problems, so failing to adapt to the threat of death, cause the greatest problems. They are the most difficult patients to work with and exhibit the most disturbed behaviour with or without mental illness. This particularly happens when they are unable to use that single defence, for example when complete denial is challenged by confrontation or displacement activity is no longer possible because of medical reasons (such as becoming bed-bound). The psyche becomes unprotected, the threat out of control and fear overwhelming.

Understanding these mental mechanisms allows appropriate interventions to be devised for patients, their carers and the professionals.

Assessing emotional need

It is essential that as early as possible during the course of a patient's illness, factors other than the medical pathology are addressed. These include a sympathetic but direct examination of the individual's vulnerability and assessment of their ability to cope. This requires consideration of the following:

Understanding the person in the context of their life

This means taking a psychosocial history (often 10–20 minutes well spent) which highlights their background, beliefs, understanding of the world, life experiences, philosophy, expectations and future hopes or plans. For example, a man brought up in poverty who by determination and hard work has achieved a good material life, may fear poverty and hold financial achievement as of primary importance. He considers health secondary, so the loss of his job and health is a double blow. A man from a similarly poor background, who has not achieved material wealth but has a major role in a large extended family, may be less perturbed by the loss of his job which he sees as giving him more time to spend with his family. Knowing these simple facts allows different interventions to be made. In the first case it will be important to address financial worries rapidly. This person may require brief psychotherapy to help him make the link with the past, whilst in the latter case, financial matters are likely to be sorted out within the family which will rally around.

Information about family deaths or illnesses can be invaluable. A difficult, painful death of a loved one may prime a person to have preconceived ideas and dread that their illness will be equally awful. This needs to be addressed early as does the exploration of major unresolved grief.

These feelings and facts can be elicited by asking simple questions such as, 'Tell me about your upbringing/family'; 'What have been the best/most important/difficult times/things in your life?', 'When life has been difficult/painful what keeps you going/what do you do/how do you cope?' Ask yourself these questions and see how much they tell you about your life. 'What' and 'How' questions are more useful than 'Why'. Direct questions need to be asked about major losses especially of those loved or hated. There is still no substitute for warm, empathic, non-judgemental communication where the process of being understood and listened to is therapeutic as well as informative, i.e. history taking can be very therapeutic.

Coping strategies and styles

Being patient centred

This means starting the relationship (doctor/patient, etc.) where the patient is, not where the professional thinks they ought to be. Initially this may mean accepting a level of dependence. It also means allowing control to remain in the patient's hands where possible. Where a situation is out of control, the professional should take control but hand it back to the patient as quickly as is safe.

A person's understanding of their illness and its meaning to them

A doctor may be quite sure what Non-Hodgkin's lymphoma is and means. The patient may have a completely different perception. Questions such as 'What do you understand is wrong with you?' or 'What does this mean to you?' are likely to elicit revealing information, either in a concrete reply such as 'It's cancer and it's going to kill me' or more philosophical answers.

Family and other carers

Assessing their needs and fears is often essential and as important as the patient's. This may be done formally or informally during the routine medical care. For example, not banning the children and wife from the clerking may offer an opportunity to explore family fears. A question such as 'How do you think your dad has been?' may allow the child to share a fear about their father's pain or weight loss. This often promotes the honest airing of the whole family's worry, as well as involving them in how the problem might be solved or alleviated. Sometimes it is necessary to see individual family members alone. I usually do this at least once. Again it gives the opportunity for a partner or teenage child to express fears without 'upsetting' others. Once expressed they often feel able to share their fears with the rest of the family so strengthening mutual support.

Children, even very young, know what is happening in a family or at least that 'something is not right'. They may misinterpret the atmosphere. One child told me that he thought that his father must have robbed a bank because he was away (in fact in hospital) and his mother cried a lot. Children need to be involved and told honestly what is happening, but encouraged to have as normal a life as possible, without undue responsibilities out of proportion to their age and maturity. Parents must try to avoid young children parenting them. Adults need to elicit most of their support from other adults but not to the exclusion of the children who also need to feel useful. Communication with children is considered further in Chapter 4.

Meeting emotional needs

It should be assumed that all patients feel isolated and must be offered time to be listened to and an opportunity to express their feelings. Not all will accept this. Some may need five or ten minutes now and again, others require more. Involvement in a group (support, self-help) or family treatments, which maximize self-determination, openness, constructive realism, support and promote effective coping strategies (if necessary teaching new ones), are often beneficial in terms of proven[2] and significant reductions in mood disturbance and pain. Vigorous treatment of any mental illness is essential.

Sadness and depression

There is no clear-cut distinction between sadness, transient depression (adjustment disorder) and depressive illness (also known as a depressive disorder). These may be considered as a spectrum extending from a familiar common human experience of sadness to clear-cut mental illness in the form of a depressive disorder.

Sadness

As the reality of death is faced, sadness is one of many emotions to be felt. The realization of being unable to see children or grandchildren grow up, of not seeing another spring and wondering how a loved one will cope, of missed opportunities and unfulfilled ambitions, causes the pain of sadness. This may manifest itself in tears, sighing, withdrawal, reflection and in bodily symptoms (abdominal, throat, chest discomfort/pain). Excessive activity with or without purpose or irritability may also occur. The feeling is infectious, becoming painful for onlookers who often find they want it to 'go away' or 'sort it out', and hence either ignore its presence (rationalizing that it is to be expected) or try to 'cheer up' the sufferer. This has the effect of implying to the sad person that feeling this way is 'not acceptable', further exacerbating their sense of loss and isolation.

Sadness is a 'normal' feeling but because it is a common experience, it does not mean it should be ignored. Its pain must be felt and the sufferer needs to know that their sadness is acknowledged and accepted and that their ability to cope with the distress is respected but that support is there if need be. A simple intervention, maybe a simple squeeze of a hand, a hug or comment such as 'You seem sad, do you want to talk?' will help. If the answer to such a question is 'no', this must be respected. It may be appropriate to follow up with 'Would you like me to sit with you or do you want to be alone?' or, alternatively, suggest a time when you would be available to talk. Sometimes it is appropriate to push a little (when a person has difficulty communicating) with comments such as 'Some people find it useful to talk about their feelings. . . you may find it helps you. . . even though it won't change what you have to face. . . but I'm sure you will feel less alone.' Using examples of other people's experience, such as 'many of my patients found that their fear and sadness seemed easier to bear when they talked about it', is a way of removing the focus from the individual and implying that they are not alone or unusual to feel this way. These interventions are rarely time consuming. Time is always limited so you need to state how long you have. A great deal can be achieved in five or ten minutes of intensive listening. If a person is about to open up and it looks as if they will need longer, acknowledge their need for more time and make another appointment when this can be dealt with. Most people accept this happily and are able to cope with painful feelings until they can be shared.

Regular support groups, providing an opportunity to share feelings, teaching relaxation, self-hypnosis and strategies to help patients and their families understand the illness, reduce pain and generally cope better, have been shown to be useful in reducing depressive symptoms,[3] improve compliance[4] and prolong survival.[5] Effective management of emotional symptoms of all stages of malignancy has a significant impact on all aspects of future health. It improves quality of life, reduces pain, protects against more severe psychological and psychiatric illness and increases the chances of a peaceful dignified death.

Those who use maladaptive coping strategies are likely to have problems with sadness. For example, excessive regression may result in the person adopting the sick role by taking to their bed, being very voluble in their distress and demanding of attention. This could be mistakenly diagnosed as a depressive illness. Equally, the stress of sadness may be sufficient to precipitate a depressive illness in such a vulnerable individual.

Depression

It can be difficult to decide where sadness ends and depression begins. However, it is crucial to detect pathological levels of depression.[6] What is too often assumed is that depression in the terminally ill is to be expected or is untreatable. Increasing research indicates that this is not the case and that depressive illness, even in the very terminal stages of malignancy, causes great suffering to the patient and their family and warrants very vigorous treatment. As for pain control, effective diagnosis and management of depressive illness requires training as well as serious consideration about liaison with mental health professionals, preferably a liaison psychiatry team if available.

Prevalence

Figures vary considerably between 4.5 and 58 per cent (general population prevalence is 6 per cent) depending on the patient group, severity of disability, stage of disease and diagnostic tool used.[6] Cancer sufferers appear to be no more depressed than equally physically ill people with other diseases. Hospitalized patients show greater rates, probably reflecting severe levels of medical problems or disability, with over 75 per cent meeting the criteria for depressive illness. There appears to be a continuum from no disorder to adjustment disorders with depressed or anxious mood (mild depression, 14–33 per cent), to moderate (18 per cent) and severe depression (13–24 per cent). Overall, amongst hospitalized cancer patients, with significant disability levels, over 25 per cent have a significant mood disorder.

Risk factors

Vulnerability to depression has been researched mainly in the psychiatric patient. However the following appear to be risk factors in the cancer patient:

- Past history of affective (mood) disorder or alcoholism.
- Poor pain control.
- Advanced stages of cancer, especially some tumour types, e.g. pancreatic, lung and small bowel.
- Mutilating surgery.
- Specific concurrent medical disorders, especially metabolic, nutritional, endocrine or neurological (see Table 3.14).
- Treatment with certain medications (see Table 3.14).
- Social isolation.
- Lower socio-economic status.
- Pre-morbid marital problems.
- Pre-morbid difficulty in expressing hostility (anger).

Diagnosis of depressive illness

How is depressive illness usually diagnosed? Psychiatrists look for a gradual onset of symptoms over several months or more, often following a loss (or anniversary of a loss), and seek a cluster of abnormalities in each of three modalities, psychological, somatic or biological and social behaviour.

Psychological symptoms

These include:

- Depressed mood or irritability.
- Loss of interest and enjoyment (anhedonia).
- Agitation or psychomotor retardation (mental and physical slowing).
- Cognitive change, so that the individual sees him/herself as worthless, the outside world as meaningless and the future as hopeless. This is known as the cognitive triad.

Biological symptoms

These are well known and include sleep disturbance (especially early morning wakening), diurnal mood swing (low mood in the morning), appetite disturbance, constipation and poor libido.

Changes in social behaviour

These may include decreased adaptive efficiency (indecisive), difficulties in interpersonal relationships (withdrawal, rows), increased dependence on alcohol, antisocial behaviour (especially in the young: lying, stealing, violence) and self-harming behaviours such as excessive risk taking, non-compliance and suicide attempts.

Diagnosis of depression in terminal malignancy and other life-threatening illness has a number of problems. Most research into depressive illness has taken place in psychiatric populations and often specifically excluded the medically ill. Many of the somatic symptoms of depressive illness such as anorexia, weight loss, fatigue, insomnia, constipation and pain may be due to the malignancy or its treatment. There are many organic causes of depression (see Table 3.14), which if rectified, will often lead to depressed mood improving within a couple of weeks. When an organic cause cannot be rectified or there is insufficient time, then the patient should be treated for a depressive illness.

Adjustment disorders may have all the features consistent with a depressive illness diagnosis, although the symptoms are usually milder, less pervasive and usually resolve spontaneously within three months. They are precipitated by clear events and severe stresses, such as news of recurrent malignancy. Differentiating between an adjustment disorder and a depressive illness can be difficult and may not be necessary as there is growing evidence that adjustment disorders are successfully managed in a similar way to depression.

So how is a diagnosis of depression made in a person with a terminal malignancy? Greater emphasis has to be placed on psychological and behavioural changes than on biological features, although a diurnal mood swing may be a useful indicator particularly when, despite good medical management, mood, irritability or pain are worse in the morning.

Depressive illness should be seriously considered when there are one or more of the following persistent symptoms or behaviours:

- Low mood.
- Anhedonia (loss of interest and enjoyment).
- Self-neglect.
- Self-mutiliation.
- Irritable, abusive or antisocial.
- Non-compliance.
- More impaired social and physical functioning than expected.
- Unresponsive to good pain management.
- Critical, angry or demanding.
- Agitation.
- Negative cognitions or the cognitive triad (see page 112).

If these symptoms are pre-morbidly out of character, pervasive and persist for a week or are worsening, then a depressive illness is likely.

Suicidal ideas

These occur in 10–14 per cent of newly diagnosed cancer patients and do not necessarily indicate depressive illness. They may reflect difficult social

Table 3.14   Principal organic causes of depression

Drugs
   Procarbazine HCL (30% immediate)
   L-Asparaginase (20–60% immediate, not dose related)
   Methotrexate (high IV dose) (40% on 10th–13th day)
   Vinblastine Sulphate (10–80%, dose related)
   Tamoxifen
   Antihypertensives (some)
   Digitalis
   Diuretics (some)
   L-dopa
   Cimetidine
   Metoclopramide
Cardiovascular e.g. Cerebrovascular accident, heart failure
Chronic organic brain syndromes
Brain metastases
Infections e.g. herpes zoster, hepatitis
Metabolic e.g. chronically disturbed electrolytes, calcium, glucose, uraemia
Endocrine e.g. thyroid disease
Vitamin deficiency e.g. folate, B_{12}, Thiamine
Epilepsy e.g. complex partial seizures, post ictal

---

or medical circumstances, with a fear of being a burden or of a painful death, but resolve rapidly with good medical care and effective social supports. Those who have had intense control over their lives may prefer to choose the time and place of their death rather than wait for the unknown. Given the opportunity to ventilate their feelings and regain more control over their life in other ways, suicidal intent will fade. Others face the hard reality that for them their future is bleak and intolerable. They do not have ideas of worthlessness or guilt but are experiencing great emotional pain. This group needs intensive support. Sedatives, including opiates, may be effective in relieving this grave distress. Only a small minority take their lives as a rational alternative to dying naturally, the rest are acutely distressed, depressed or isolated. Where suicidal ideas are present with a belief that death is deserved, then this is usually pathonemonic of a severe depressive illness. The cognitive triad is likely to be present. This small group present a high suicide risk and require the presence of a competent adult continuously until seen by a psychiatrist.

Risk factors for suicide include past suicide attempts, past history of an affective (mood) disorder, family history of suicide, personality disorder, recent ending (especially by death) of a close relationship, poorly controlled pain, recent knowledge of a grave prognosis, alcohol abuse and social isolation.

Asking a person about their possible suicidal ideas does not increase the likelihood of suicide. Where depressive illness is suspected, suicidal ideas should always be asked about. The subject can be broached with questions such as 'Your life is very difficult at the moment. . . have you felt that you can't go on?' This is usually enough to allow the person to start talking about their feelings, in which case details need to be sought starting with open-ended questions like 'Tell me about what you have thought' in an attempt to assess whether the person is having occasional ideas of wishing they would not wake up or has formed a suicide plan. If there is suicidal intent it is important to assess what prevents them carrying it through: 'What is keeping you going at the moment?' or 'What is stopping you harming yourself?' This can be therapeutic for the sufferer as it helps them identify their strengths and ways of helping themselves.

Closer questioning which reveals low self-esteem, ideas of worthlessness and guilt, that the past has been wasted and that the future is hopeless (even if the reality is that death is near) confirms a diagnosis of depressive illness. For example, a seventy-two year-old man with myeloma requested euthanasia. He said he had nothing left to live for with his wife dead and his children in Australia (world meaningless and the future hopeless). He was sleeping badly, waking early in pain (biological symptoms, including diurnal mood swing and medical disease), when he ruminated about what he saw as the futility of his life (worthlessness), he felt a burden to his neighbour who had to do his shopping because of his lack of interest and energy (worthlessness, anhedonia and medical illness). He functioned out of duty to make him feel less guilty. In the two years since his wife had died he had lived a quiet life alone, attending a local bowls team in the summer until pain had stopped him playing the previous summer. He was anaemic, had several blood transfusions, was seen by a hospice doctor for pain management and after four weeks on 100 mg of a tricyclic antidepressant (dothiepin) began to take an interest in the woodwork group. He took a paternal role on the ward, offering advice to younger patients (evidence of improvement of self-esteem). He no longer requested euthanasia but talked of death as 'an old friend' whom he would welcome when it came but he could now wait. He reflected that he had contemplated suicide when his back pain prevented him playing bowls. He greatly feared dependency. He became self-caring and decided to return home. With the help of the home care team, he coped alone for a further three months before accepting hospice care, where he died ten days later, still in some pain but at peace with himself. This man's story shows the importance of treating depression vigorously even in the terminal stages of disease when at some levels it appears the person has little to live for. I initially underestimated his capacity for facing his loneliness and needed the support of older and wiser colleagues who encouraged me to treat him.

Management of depressive illness

The general principles of assessment and management of emotional problems apply (see pages 109–111). Aetiological factors need to be identified as this allows a logical programme of interventions to be made. These factors can be categorized under predisposing (e.g. loss in childhood, family history of mood disorder and suicide), precipitating (e.g. recurrence of malignancy, recent loss), perpetuating (e.g. difficult unsupporting marriage, low haemoglobin, steroids) and psychodynamic (e.g. patient always been in control of household and now due to illness cannot, so the family starts to disintegrate). Management can be divided into biological, psychological and social. These will be considered in turn.

Biological

Medical state

Where possible this should be rectified and depressing medication (Table 3.14) stopped or altered.

Antidepressant drugs

Tricyclic antidepressants are still the drugs of choice in the treatment of depressive illness unless it is so severe or there is insufficient time, when electro-convulsive therapy is indicated. If there is serious cardiac disease (recent myocardial infarct or heart block) then the newer selective serotonin re-uptake inhibitors (SSRI) are useful. A tricyclic is chosen for its particular drug profile and side effects (Table 3.15). It is best to get used to using two or three drugs, one older tricyclic, one newer and one from the SSRI group.

There are some useful general principles which help in the selection, dosage and use of antidepressants. Most tricyclic drug failures are because the dose is not high enough for long enough. Most patients need at least

Table 3.15 Drug profiles

	Starting dosage mg/24hr	Therapeutic dosage* mg/24hr	Sedation	Comments
Tricyclic and related antidepressants				Reduce dose in liver and renal disease. 2–6 wk delay in therapeutic effect.
Amitriptyline	25–50 nocte	75–150 nocte	+++	O,L,IV cardiotoxic anticholinergic +++
Imipramine	10–50 nocte	75–150 nocte	+	O,L,iv
Dothiepin	25–50 nocte	75–150 nocte	++	O, useful in epilepsy, anticholinergic +
Doxepin	25–50 nocte	75–150 nocte	++	O
Lofepramine	70–140 (div)	140–210 (div)	+	O, useful in heart disease, induces liver enzymes, sweating
Trazodone	50 nocte	150–300 (nocte)	+++	O,L, useful sedative/anxiolytic in divided doses
Amoxapine	25	100–150	+++	O, some anti-psychotic effects dystonias
Selective Serotonin Reuptake Inhibitors				
Fluoxetine	20 mane	20 mane	+/–	1–3 weeks delay in therapeutic effect O, low cardiotoxicity; safe in over-dose
Fluvoxamine	50–100 nocte	100–200 (div)	+/–	transient gastro-intestinal, side effects and anxiety transient headache and restlessness
Sertraline	50 mane	50–100 mane	+/–	
Lithium Carbonate	200–400 nocte	400–1200 (div)	–	O,L, requires supervision of psychiatrist

Anxiolytics

Drug				Notes
Diazepam	6 (div)	6–60 (div)	++	O,L,IM,IV,S, long half life, prescribe 8–12 hourly
Lorazepam	1–4 (div)	1–10 (div)	+	O,IM,IV. Short half life, prescribe 6 hourly
Alprazolam	0.75–1 (div)	4–6 (div)	+	O, mild antidepressant, prescribe 8 hourly.
Midazolam		1–2 IV over 30 secs, followed 2 min later by 0.5–1. Repeat until settled, 2.5–10 usual	++	IM, IV, emergency sedation or when oral route impossible.
Buspirone	10 (div)	15–45 (div)	+/–	mild antidepressant, 2–3 week delay in onset

Neuroleptics (anti-psychotics)

Drug				Notes
Chlorpromazine (or thioridazine)	40–200 (div)	40–800 (div)	+++	lower doses anxiolytic, higher doses antipsychotic O,L,S,IM,IV photosensitivity, anticholinergic +++, dystonias +
Trifluoperazine	5–10 nocte/div	5–20	++	powerful antipsychotic, anticholinergic + dystonias ++

Notes O = oral tablet or capsule; L = liquid preparation available; IM = intramuscular; IV = intravenous; S = suppository; div divide dose.

100 mg (half in the elderly) and very little antidepressant effect is seen for two weeks, with up to six weeks being required for older tricyclics, e.g. amitriptyline. Poor compliance occurs when the two-week delay is not explained. There is also a two-week delay in the re-emergence of symptoms when the drug is stopped. Patients need encouragement to persist in taking medication. Pharmacologically dirtier drugs tend to be more potent, so it appears that amitriptyline may work when lofepramine has not, but this has to be weighed against increased side effects. The faster the increase in dose, the more severe the side effects are, but these diminish rapidly over two to three days.

Patients with prominent anxiety and agitation respond best to sedating tricyclics such as amitriptyline, dothiepin or doxepin, whilst for those with psychomotor retardation and withdrawal, imipramine or lofepramine are useful. Starting dosage depends on age and medical problems but is usually between 25 mg (older and iller) and 75 mg increasing in one to three days by 25–75 mg to a final dose of 100–150 mg (about half in the elderly or very medically frail). Rarely, doses to 300 mg may be necessary but a psychiatrist should be involved. Extreme sensitivity to side effects may require very slow increase in dosage starting, if necessary, with 10 mg of imipramine or dothiepin increasing by 10 mg per week. At this pace, high doses can be achieved; however this takes time.

Patients with serious heart disease (recent myocardial infarct or heart block) should not be started on older tricyclics but require the SSRI drugs to be tried first. They should not be deprived of an effective antidepressant treatment. If a tricyclic is chosen (e.g. lofepramine), blood pressure should be checked for diastolic rise and electrocardiogram monitored for heart block or dangerous dysrhythmias. The dose should be increased more slowly.

Side effects of most tricyclics relate to their anticholinergic effects and include dry mouth, blurred vision, constipation, difficulty in micturating, interference in sexual function (ejaculation especially), postural hypotension, sweating and increased appetite with weight gain. Less common are convulsions and paralytic illness.

Selective Serotonin Re-uptake Inhibitors (SSRI)

Drugs such as fluoxetine, fluvoxamine, sertraline and paroxetine are increasingly used by psychiatrists. They do seem to be effective in treating depressive illness. SSRI's have the great advantage of being almost free of anti-cholinergic side effects, sedation and are more rapid in the onset of action (one to two weeks). They are safer in overdose than tricyclics. The majority of patients experience transient mild symptoms of agitation and insomnia with about 10–25 per cent having gastrointestinal disturbances, a few with vomiting. These may last one to two weeks. Currently it is not possible to predict who will suffer from these side effects. They can be minimized by starting with a low, slow increase in dose taken with food. For example, starting 50 mg of fluvoxamine, increasing every two to four days by 50 mg to a total dose of 100–200 mg (latter in divided doses, 100 mg mane with breakfast and 100 mg nocte with a drink). Night sedation (e.g. zipicolone 7.5 mg to 15 mg) with daytime low dose diazepam (e.g. 2 mg tds) may be required for seven to ten days until the anti-depressant effect of the SSRI improves sleep and mood, and the side effects wear off.

Lithium

There is evidence that patients who would or do respond to ECT, also respond rapidly to augmentation of tricyclic antidepressants by lithium. Its potential toxicity (especially in the terminally ill), may preclude its use so advice must be sought from a psychiatrist before treatment.

There is some evidence that SSRIs have a similar augmenting effect when used in combination with tricyclics. However, the advice of a liaison psychiatrist should be sought prior to use.

Electro-convulsive therapy (ECT)

Such treatment is still too often considered as a last resort or not used because it is seen as barbaric. This is a great shame as in the moderately and severely depressed (especially where biological and psychotic symptoms are present) it is a safe, rapid, extremely effective therapy with fewer side effects than most antidepressants. There are no absolute contra-indicators except raised intracranial pressure, although recent myocardial infarct (MI), stroke, space occupying lesion or severe disability needs to be discussed with a senior anaesthetist and the cost benefit ratio considered. ECT should be considered as the treatment of choice where the diagnosis of moderate to severe depressive illness is clear and where the time to death is short (weeks) or where there is great distress due to depressive ruminations of worthlessness, guilt or active suicidal ideas or the person has stopped drinking (due to depression).

Treatment requires signed consent or a section of the mental health act with a second opinion (i.e. two approved psychiatrists agree on treatment) although life-saving treatment can be given under common law while the second opinion is sought. ECT is usually administered two or three times per week although this can be accelerated. The first two ECTs improve mood for two to six hours often with complete relapse in between. By the third or fourth treatment the patient's improved mood is usually sustained between treatments. Treatment continues until no further improvement is seen, usually 6–10 are required.

Psychostimulants

Massie and Holland[6] describe the use of dextroamphetamine, methyl-phenidate and pemoline as rapidly promoting a sense of well being, reducing fatigue and stimulating appetite. This may be useful where time is short. The abuse potential is limited in this patient group but the risk is of occasional increased depression, nightmares, insomnia and psychosis.

Tranquillizers

Where psychotic symptoms are present, neuroleptics are often required. Trifluoperazine is a powerful, less sedating anti-psychotic, useful where paranoid symptoms are present. 5 mg at night may be sufficient, doubling and dividing the dose if necessary (see Table 3.15). Chlorpromazine and thioridazine are also useful, being more sedating, but their anticholinergic side effects may be potentiated if used in conjunction with tricyclics. Doses of 10–25 mg four times daily are required as an anxiolytic, whilst antipsychotic doses are often higher between 50 and 200 mg qds. Dystonic reactions may occur and respond to 5 to 10 mg of procyclidine orally or intramuscularly.

Benzodiazepines

There can also be useful adjuncts when treating anxiety in depression, but are discussed in the section on anxiety (see page 123).

Table 3.16   Symptoms of anxiety

Psychic (Psychological)*
    Feelings of dread, threat and fear
    Feelings of being out of control and panic
    Irritability
    Worries over trivia
    Inner tension
    Fearful anticipation
    Repetitive obsessional thoughts

Somatic and autonomic
    Tremor**
    Palpitations**
    Difficulty breathing**
    Nausea/abdominal churning/butterflies
    Diarrhoea
    Sweating
    Frequency of micturition

General
    Poor concentration
    Initial Insomnia
    Muscle aching
    Pain
    Fatigue

Behavioural
    Hand wringing
    Angry outbursts or rows
    Restlessness
    Fear and avoidance of things and situations normally coped with (phobias)
    Clinging, repeated requests for reassurance
    Occasionally compulsive rituals such as handwashing or cleaning

*Respond to benzodiazepines
**Respond to β-blockers

Other factors

Regular nutritious food and minimizing nicotine and caffeine intake where practical reduces agitation. Good pain and other symptom control is essential. Reducing or eliminating alcohol is also useful.

Psychological

The biological treatment of moderate and severe depression is essential and central to management. However, it must not be seen in isolation. All depressed patients require psychological intervention which may range from simple support and encouragement to in-depth psychotherapy. A range of adjunct therapies, including hypnosis, meditation, self-imaging, visualization, supportive counselling, cognitive-behavioural and dynamic psychotherapy as individual or group, have been shown to be helpful in alleviating distressing emotions and depression in the psychiatric population. There is much less information regarding the terminally ill. Good studies do exist to show that a variety of group psychotherapies are effective in cancer patients but tend to be used at an earlier stage and prophylactically to prevent or ameliorate mood disorders.[3,4,5] Groups run for patients in the terminal stages can be problematical because of the deaths of group members. However, time-limited groups running eight to twelve weekly sessions are useful for the less medically ill patient and for the mild to moderately depressed. They provide support, friendship, an opportunity to talk to others who really understand without feeling a burden to close carers, engender hope and offer a forum for perceiving and tackling problems differently.

Individual psychotherapy in a range of depths and types can be useful. Where insights are required and where premorbid self-esteem is low, even a single session may enable a link or insight to be made, a fear faced or shared and extreme distress alleviated. Far more can be accomplished in a few sessions with a terminally ill patient than with a medically healthy client. When death is so close and priorities change, motivation to tackle painful issues, face truths and resolve difficulties is much greater. Where talking is difficult because of defence mechanisms, such as denial and intellectualization, or physical problems, then communication can be attempted through other media such as art or music therapy. Specialist therapists are usually required but a skilled communicator may be able to carry out therapy under the supervision of the specialist.

A cognitive behavioural psychological adjunct psychotherapy is being developed and researched in cancer patients.[7] This talking therapy helps the patient identify unhelpful thoughts (cognitions) and behaviours. This approach teaches the individual to develop a fighting spirit and alternative, more effective, coping strategies. It has been shown to be effective in alleviating cancer related anxiety and depression but is only recently being used (as yet not evaluated) in the terminally ill.[8]

Family or couple meetings can be very valuable in gathering information about pre-morbid functioning and how the family communicates (who makes the decisions, resolves arguments, etc.). Such meetings can enable communication within the family and offer a forum for information exchange and support by the professional. Conjoint or family therapy is indicated when the couple or family dynamics play a part in the aetiology (predisposing, precipitating or perpetuating factors) of the depressive illness (or other psychological disturbance). Family work can be very powerful and transform difficult situations and patients. It is considered further in Chapter 4.

Lewis[9] describes support programmes for families with a cancer sufferer, which facilitate the spouse's and children's adjustment to all the stages of the illness experience. This type of approach must become part of good, routine psychological care of those with life-threatening illness.

Social

Reynolds and Kaplan[10] showed a significant relationship between social isolation and increased mortality in cancer patients. Where social factors are important risk factors (see page 114) or in the aetiology, they should be addressed. Depressed patients isolate themselves and are lonely. Organizing regular contact at a club, day centre, hospice or support group may be sufficient. Returning to, or excessive contact with, a difficult home situation may necessitate alternatives to home or risk relapse of the depressive illness. Sometimes supporting a difficult family member may allow home stress to be reduced. For example, offering a domineering husband time to talk may take pressure off his dying wife.

Fear and anger

Beneath anger, fear is usually lurking. Both are powerful emotions causing pain and guilt. For primitive man, anger was protective, warning off an attacker and defending physical integrity. Modern man rarely has to face a hunting lion because the threat of death comes from disease from within. The threat may go consciously unrecognized, fear is suppressed together with anger, as in many cultures being angry (especially for women) or afraid (especially for men) is seen as socially unacceptable. A significant minority are unable to recognize or distinguish between these feelings. Hence it is even more bewildering, painful and frightening when emotions boil over and appear out of control. For those at the receiving end feelings can be similar. A vicious circle is easily set up with more feelings of hurt and guilt being generated. Common fears include the unknown, the manner of dying, losing control, going 'mad' or demented, being a burden and losing independence. Anger commonly occurs because patients dislike themselves for feeling afraid or vulnerable, smoking too much, not listening to health warnings, lost opportunities, insufficient religious faith or because they feel let down by God or doctors for failing to make an earlier diagnosis.

Positive management is often brief and useful in facilitating real changes to be made and relationships strengthened. Where there is anger, there is usually interest and energy. This can be turned towards fighting the disease, i.e. fighting spirit with its improved prognosis. Apathy and resignation are much more difficult to resolve. Working with an angry person may be as simple as accepting an angry outburst without complaint and without trying to justify God or doctors. This often results in a later apology with an opportunity opened by them to talk at their pace. It may be difficult to appear accepting because you also feel angry. This may be because you are picking up the patient's feelings (known as transference) or that you need to talk to someone about your feelings. Remember patients are rarely angry at you personally. If they are, it can be useful to try to resolve your differences so strengthening your relationship. If other professionals also feel angry towards a particular patient, then this is almost always a strong indicator that the patient is feeling very angry themselves or they make the professionals feel useless and helpless. Recognition of your feelings towards a patient is important clinical information. If they make you feel sad, then they are sad, if depressed then you need to consider a depressive illness (this assumes you are not depressed, sad or angry for your own reasons).

Labelling the emotion can also be useful. For example, saying 'You seem angry' may help the person to recognize that they are angry and so to talk about their feelings. Making a statement such as 'Some people I have worked with get angry when they are worrying about what the future holds or have regrets about the past' can often produce body language which will tell you if you are getting close to what is upsetting them. Knowledge of the person's background can be very useful in this respect as it is often possible to guess what is bothering him. For example, a man who had learnt to cope with an unpredictable alcoholic father by taking intense control over his adult life (running a successful business) became wheelchair bound, and made his wife's life a misery through his cynical acceptance of her care. When it was suggested to him that he had become very angry at the loss of his independence, for which he had fought so hard, he started talking about his father and his fear that he was turning out like him. Gradually, he recognized that his wife was not going to abuse him in the same way as his father had, and he accepted her help with better grace. A mobile telephone helped him maintain contact with his business. Some psychiatrists use a model for depression as anger turned inwards.

Anxiety

Some anxiety in life is acceptable as part of normal human experience. When anxiety becomes persistent and severe it becomes an illness and is classified as an anxiety state or disorder which requires treatment. Distinguishing anxiety states from depressive illness can be a problem as there is considerable overlap, although the absence of low mood and a different symptom cluster usually allow the diagnosis to be made.

Prevalence

Good data are scarce. In the general population, there is a 10 per cent life-time risk of developing an anxiety state. Clinically significant anxiety was found in 16 per cent of a general medical outpatient clinic. This figure is likely to be much higher where individuals face life threatening serious medical illness.

Risk factors

Research data are not available for the terminally ill and pre-disposing factors have to be extrapolated from the psychiatric population. These include a past history of an anxiety disorder, a positive family history, poor social supports, recent receipt of bad news, previous alcohol or benzodiazapine abuse, immature or obsessional personality, unstable environment in childhood, early experience of separation, over-protection by family or partner and experience of a distressing death of a family member or friend.

Aetiology

Anxiety occurs when defence mechanisms are incomplete or stress is overwhelming, which is often the case in terminal disease, when the threat of death is so real. Genetic factors are also important, hence the importance of family information. Psychiatrists continue to debate the usefulness of subclassifying generalized anxiety disorders (GAD) and panic disorders (PD) which includes phobias such as agoraphobia (a fear of going our or being away from home). From a clinical standpoint there is considerable overlap between subgroups and comorbidity with other disorders such as depression. Most current research neglects treatment, in particular psychological management. Furthermore, there is minimal recognition and research into the association between anxiety and medical illness. Appropriate treatments have not been formally evaluated in the medically ill. Inevitably, what is discussed below is extrapolated from diagnosis and treatment of anxiety states in the psychiatric population.

As with depressive illness, there are also organic causes of anxiety. These are not well defined in the literature but can be broadly classi-fied under headings of concurrent medical disorder (e.g. toxic such as alcohol withdrawal states, metabolic such as hypoglycaemia and hypokalaemia, endocrine such as thyroid disorders, hyperparathyroidism and hypopituitarism, neurological disease (such as stroke, brain metastases and multiple sclerosis) and secondary to some medication (such an anticholinergics and salicylates). Anxiety may be part of an acute organic brain syndrome (acute confusional state) or a chronic dementing illness (Alzheimer's), when a minor infection or constipation may exacerbate organic anxiety.

Diagnosis of anxiety state

In these disorders, excessive anxiety is the principal manifestation presenting in the psychological (psychic) and/or somatic fields (Table

3.16), often diffuse in quality in which other psychoneurotic components (such as phobic or obsessional phenomena) may be present and behaviour is altered (Table 3.16). Anxiety states may be acute or chronic. The former is usually short-lived and related to a specific situation or stress in a stable premorbid personality with no family history. Once the stress is relieved, the anxiety state remits. In the terminally ill, an acute anxiety state may start around the diagnosis and if not managed effectively will persist in even the most stable people resulting in a chronic state.

Chronic anxiety states are usually present premorbidly starting in late teens or early twenties with only 20 per cent showing improvement in three years if the disorder lasts more than six months. Social adaptation often occurs, but with each new trauma there is an acute exacerbation. These patients suffer greatly when terminally ill as the threat and stress are permanent. They require early recognition, additional appropriate support and should be reviewed frequently as they are at risk of developing a depressive illness or having a psychotic breakdown.

Somatic and general features are not useful for the diagnosis of anxiety states in the medically ill. Hence more emphasis is placed on the psychic and behavioural symptoms of anxiety (Table 3.16). Sometimes, psychic symptoms are minimal despite the presence of an anxiety state. Persistent behavioural changes such as frequent rows, demands for medical or nursing attention, non-compliance, claims that old information is unknown (poor concentration) or uncontrolled pain despite good medical management, may indicate an underlying anxiety disorder. If organic causes have been excluded, minimized and treated, then persistent and pervasive symptoms lasting a week or increasing in the absence of low mood means that an anxiety disorder should be seriously considered.

Management of anxiety states

The general principles of assessment and management of emotional problems apply (see page 109) The type and cause of the anxiety state determines its management. Individuals who have internalized coping strategies are easier and quicker to treat than those with principally externalized strategies (see page 107). This information can be obtained by eliciting how an individual coped premorbidly in a crisis or under stress. Family or close friends are often able to give this information. For example, 'She always leaned on her mum. . . went to pieces and has never been the same after she died' implies externalized coping strategies (mother), continued separation anxiety and the prediction that the person will not be easy to help.

Aetiological factors need to be identified and a logical programme of intervention made, as described for depressive illness (see page 115). Underlying medical problems need to be addressed and where possible, modified. Poorly controlled pain may transform a normally calm person into an agitated, demanding individual and good pain control is all that is required to treat the anxiety state. An elderly person, using a bottle of sherry each day, brought into hospital on becoming immobile and no longer able to buy alcohol, may become extremely agitated after twenty-four to seventy-two hours as delirium tremens starts. Detoxification is required with chlormethiazole and thiamine, if necessary augmented with chlordiazepoxide, sufficient to remove all withdrawal symptoms or provide the alcohol. Other acute confusional states (acute organic brain syndromes) need distinguishing from an acute or chronic anxiety state.

The hallmark of organic brain syndromes is the change in conscious level and disorientation. Such patients may be difficult to distinguish especially if the brain syndrome is subacute. Anxiety may be part of another psychiatric disorder such as a relapse of schizophrenia or a depressive illness. Treatment of the underlying cause alleviates the anxiety.

Biological

Good medical and pain management is essential.

Benzodiazepines

These drugs do still have a place, especially in the terminally ill with prominent psychic anxiety or where a patient has a chronic anxiety state and has been on non-escalating doses for many years. This latter group may require an increase in dose even if only temporarily. Diazepam in doses up to 40–60 mg in eight-hourly divided doses may be tolerated in those physically or psychologically addicted. Those who have not had diazepam previously should begin with 2 mg three times daily, increasing slowly. Diazepam is sedating and can be a problem in the seriously ill or elderly because it has a long half-life and accumulates rapidly. Shorter acting alprazolam is thought to be effective in treating anxiety and depression. It can be started at 0.25 mg three times daily and titrated up to 4–6 mg per day. Lorazepam is short acting, less sedating, rapidly anxiolytic (thus much more addictive) and well tolerated. It should be started as 1–4 mg divided six hourly, increased up to 10 mg in twenty-four hours if necessary. Midazolam is the drug of choice for emergency sedation or where parenteral benzodiazepine is required because the patient cannot swallow. It is non-irritant and can be used intravenously or intramuscularly (as can lorazepam). It is usually necessary to titrate the dose against relief from agitation, using slow intravenous injections of 1–2 mg over 30 seconds, followed after several minutes by 0.5–1 mg increments. 1–7 mg are required four to six hours later. Alternatively, 5–20 mg can be given intramuscularly. If the patient is able to swallow, a regular oral benzodiazepine should be started. Counselling and psychotherapy can be difficult if benzodiazepines are used in the longer term due to the amnesic effect and suppression of feelings. There is some evidence that the longer term addictive risk is lower in the terminally ill, even if used over many months. Benzodiazepines should be avoided in those with brain failure (chronic dementia).

Antidepressants

Sedating antidepressants such as trimipramine, amitriptyline, dothiepin and trazodone are increasingly used to treat anxiety states. Regretfully, the side effects are less well tolerated, especially in those with chronic anxiety. Where panic is a major part of the anxiety disorder, then imipramine is the drug of choice. Patients should start at 10 mg increasing by 10 mg per week until symptoms settle, often requiring 200–250 mg. Doses more than 150 mg should be supervised by a psychiatrist. The time scale may be impractical in the terminally ill.

Selective serotonin re-uptake inhibitors (SSRI) are being increasingly marketed for their anxiolytic effect. Whether this is treating underlying depression or is having a primary anxiolytic effect is unknown. The transient increase in agitation, insomnia and gastro-intestinal symptoms can be a problem, but where SSRIs are used in conjunction with benzodiazepines or neuroleptics for the first two weeks, are eventually well tolerated. Their true efficacy is untested.

Neuroleptics

Where there is extreme agitation with disruptive behaviour and/or an acute organic brain disorder (except alcoholic withdrawal syndrome) rapid sedation may be necessary for the safety of the patient and others. A neuroleptic is chosen for its particular drug profile and side effects (Table 3.15). 5–10 mg (occasionally increasing to 20 mg) of haloperidol can be given intramuscularly (under common law) with or without intravenous or intramuscular midazolam (augments the haloperidol and reduces the likelihood of seizures). This should be followed by vigorous investigation of an underlying cause (especially to exclude alcohol withdrawal syndrome which requires different management). Regular oral thioridazine should generally be started at a dose between 10 and 100 mg six hourly, titrating the dose to the agitation. The advice of a psychiatrist may be required. Where a patient has not responded to benzodiazepines or where there are incipient psychotic features, such as paranoid ideas or delusions, haloperidol 1.5–5 mg three or four times daily or chlorpromazine 25–100 mg (occasionally much more) four times daily or trifluoperazine 5 mg twice daily can be very effective. Where anxiety is accompanied by nausea or vomiting, these are the drugs of choice. These medications can be supplied in syrup and chlorpromazine in suppositories. If neuroleptics are required over a longer period, especially where compliance is poor or the oral route is difficult, a single intramuscular injection once every two to four weeks of depot medication should be considered. Advice from a psychiatrist should be sought.

Buspirone

This is a new treatment for anxiety and is thought to act on specific serotonin receptors. It takes two to three weeks to take effect and appears to have mild antidepressant effects. Its abuse potential is unknown although to date research indicates that there is minimal or no risk. Buspirone is started at 5 mg twice or three times daily increasing every two to three days by 5 mg to a range of 15–45 mg (30 mg in the elderly) in divided doses. Psychiatric patients normally require at least 15–20 mg for two to three weeks before its usefulness can be judged. Side effects, mainly gastro-intestinal, are usually transient and can be reduced by slowing dose increases. Care should be taken with severe liver or renal impairment and in epilepsy, where lower doses or alternatives should be considered. Because this drug is new, experience is still limited to the psychiatric population.

Beta blockers

Propanolol started 40 mg twice daily increasing to three times if necessary can be effective in controlling some of the somatic (Table 3.16) symptoms of anxiety, especially tremor, palpitations, difficulty breathing and some sweating. Psychological symptoms of worry, fear and tension are not improved. However, control of some somatic symptoms, especially when hypochondriacal fears are being triggered by physical symptoms, can be useful in convincing patients that their symptoms are due to anxiety and so prevent escalation of psychological fears. Normal precautions need to be taken when using non-cardioselective beta blockers.

Opiates

It is well known that opiates have a powerful anxiolytic effect. In some instances morphine (or an equivalent) is the most effective medication for severe anxiety states in the terminally ill. If simpler methods have not been effective, time is short and if the patient is not already on morphine for pain control, then a trial is well worthwhile. Morphine sulphate can be started in the same way as for pain control. The effects can be dramatic and it may be possible to withdraw the drug several weeks later.

Psychosocial

Use of drugs in anxiety states should never be used as a substitute for good psychological care. Acute anxiety states in a good premorbid personality often respond to simple measures such as support, an opportunity to talk about fears and ventilate feelings. This should be part of good management of all medically ill patients. Psychological management at the earlier stages of terminal illness has a considerable impact on later well being. The manner in which bad news is given has been shown to influence adjustment. This, and other communication issues are considered in Chapter 2.

Psychotherapy

This is a more intensive form of talking that assists the person to come to terms with the reasons underlying their anxiety. The cognitive behavioural approach is used most frequently, where three to four sessions with a suitably trained individual (e.g. psychologist) is usually sufficient.

Relaxation therapy

There is a large variety of techniques which help release tension. They are cheap, safe, simple to teach and are often extremely effective, giving patients an immediate tool to help themselves, regain control and self-esteem. Every ward, general practitioner's surgery and clinic should have a variety of tapes and books available for patients and their families to buy or borrow, with suitably trained individuals to advise individually or in groups. The techniques need to be practised daily and become a routine part of life. They are based on teaching individuals to control their breathing, become aware of their bodies and their thoughts, to tense successive groups of muscles then feel them relax and combine this with replacing fearful thoughts using visualization of peaceful, tranquil places. Simple ideas such as breathing in warmth and peace, then breathing out tension, pain and fear can be very effective.

Massage of part or all of the body is another method of helping an anxious person relax. It makes people aware of how tense their bodies have become. Massage, especially of the extremities (hands and feet) can be non-threatening ways of touching a frightened person, so reducing their isolation. The masseur must be suitably trained and be prepared to cope with emotional responses to their touch, such as tears or disclosure of fears regarding the future. Those who find touch threatening may allow their hair to be washed, again a non-threatening, acceptable way of offering scalp massage (effective in tension headache).

Education of patients and their relatives regarding anxiety, what helps and what hinders, is important. Involving partners, family or other carers in relaxation classes, teaching them to massage, involving them in a counselling session (not routinely), advice on available support groups and books to read can transform a helpless onlooker to an involved useful partner in care. Some therapists may record, on tape or video, their sessions with a patient who is given the tape to share with family and friends. Spouses should be encouraged to practice relaxation with the patient so emphasizing their need for care also. Teaching new strategies or maximizing old ones is also important. For example, when morbid thoughts such as 'I'm going to die in pain' are becoming intrusive, changing position or occupation can be effective and replacing the thoughts with 'I've coped with a lot of pain already, I've got through it before and I will again' (a cognitive behaviour approach). Leaving encouraging messages on small cards in strategic places such as 'Take a day at a time' can be useful. If it does nothing else, it may cause a smile.

Getting trained

All those working with dying patients would benefit greatly from undertaking workshops aimed at the psychological aspects. Even if you are not going to do intensive individual work, extra training allows greater understanding, increases confidence and ability to cope differently with the myriad of powerful emotions that face the patient, their family and other carers as well as the professional. Many of us are afraid of strong feelings. Many doctors fear or rationalize that being emotional will interfere with their objective judgement. This is one of the principal reasons for gaining more training. It allows professionals to feel and face their own emotions as well as their patients' and to survive them without burning out or losing objective judgement.

Questionnaires

There are very few which are aimed at identifying depressive illness or anxiety states in the medically ill. However, an increasingly useful and validated screening instrument for use in the terminally ill is the Hospital Anxiety and Depression Scale (HAD).[11] This is a 14-item, four-point questionnaire which is simple and quick to administer. It shows specificity and sensitivity of 75 per cent when screening for adjustment and major depressive disorders together. Questionnaires must not be used as a substitute for proper assessments and talking to patients, but they can be useful in augmenting these procedures.

Notes and References

1. SPIEGEL, D. 'Psychosocial aspects of cancer', *Current Opinion in Psychiatry*, 1991, **4**(6), 889–97.

2. SPIEGEL, D. 'Facilitating emotional coping during treatment', *Cancer*, 1990, **66**(6) Suppl., 1422–6.

3. FAWZY, F., COUSINS, N., FAWZY, N., KEMENY, M., ELASHOFF, R. and MORTON, D. 'A structured psychiatric intervention for cancer patients', *Archives of General Psychiatry*, 1990, **47**, 720–5.

4. RICHARDSON, J., SHELTON, D., KRAILO, M, and LEVIN, A. 'The effect of compliance with treatment on survival among patients with haematologic malignancies', *Journal of Clinical Oncology*, 1990, **8**, 356–64.

5. SPIEGEL, D., BLOOM, J.R., KRAEMER, H.C., GOTTHEIL, E. 'Effect of psychosocial treatment on survival of patients with metastatic breast cancer', *Lancet*, 1989, **ii**, 888–91.

6. MASSIE, M.J. and HOLLAND, J.C. 'Depression and the cancer patient', *Journal of Clinical Psychiatry*, 1990, **51**(7), Suppl 12–19.

7. MOOREY, S. and GREER, S. 'Adjuvant psychological therapy: A cognitive behavioural treatment for patients with cancer', *Behavioural Psychotherapy*, 1989, **17**(2), 177–90.

8. SANTOS, M.J.H. and GREER S. 'Adjuvant psychological therapy with a terminally ill patient: a case report', *Behavioural Psychotherapy*, 1991, **19**(3), 277–80.

9. LEWIS, F.M. 'Strengthening family supports: Cancer and the family', *Cancer*, 1990, **65**(3), Suppl., 752–9.

10. REYNOLDS, P. and KAPLAN, G. 'Social connections and risk for cancer: prospective evidence from Alameda country study', *Behavioural Medicine*, 1990, **Fall**, 101–10.

11. RAZAVI, D., DELVAUX, N., FARVACQUES, C. and ROBAYE, E. 'Screening for adjustment disorders and major depressive disorders in cancer in-patients', *British Journal of Psychiatry*, 1990, **156**, 79–83.

Confusion————————————————————

Marie Murphy

A challenge in terminal care

Confusion is a common symptom in people who are terminally ill. Dame Cicely Saunders speaks of our aim in this work as being 'To enhance the quality of living and relationships when there is only a limited time left.'[1] The period approaching a patient's death can be a time of growth and reconciliation for the patient and their family, a time for healing rifts and saying goodbye. If the dying person is confused this time may lose its meaning and become instead a time of great anguish and distress not only for the patient but also for the family and those involved in their care. Families may carry disturbing memories of their confusion with them into bereavement and this may influence their ability to cope with life and loss in the future.

Management of patients with confusion poses an enormous challenge. It raises several medical and ethical dilemmas which cause us to repeatedly question our management approach. Confusion is also 'contagious' and can lead to many problems within the team of carers. The aims and expectations of management become blurred and confusion abounds. Confused patients and their families need care in a stable environment. The caring team need a confident and united approach, otherwise patients become more muddled and the situation becomes self-perpetuating.

Definition

Confusion means different things to different people. It is useful therefore to begin by defining the term. 'Confusion is defined as a mental stage characterized by disorientation regarding time, place and person causing bewilderment, perplexity, lack of orderly thought and inability to choose or act decisively. It is usually symptomatic of an organic disorder but may accompany severe emotional stress and various psychological disorders.'[2]

Many people demonstrate bizarre behaviour or are unable to think or act decisively but it is the simultaneous presence of disorientation that confirms a confusional state.

Clinical assessment

It can be said that there are two basic confusional states. *Acute brain syndrome* or delirium is that which occurs in a previously lucid individual. It is generally reversible on treating the cause. There are many precipitating causes (Table 3.17). In delirium patients undergo a release phenomenon, i.e. they lose the control they normally exert over certain aspects of their personality. The naturally timid become terrified, the previously suspicious become paranoid. They also exhibit increased autonomic activity with restlessness, excessive sweating, a dry mouth and tachycardia. There is often an associated clouding of consciousness. It is important to identify the acute brain syndrome as the confusion may be reversible on tackling the underlying causes.

Chronic brain syndrome or dementia is a confusional state which presents with a different clinical picture. There is usually a slowly developing memory failure which the patient may initially attempt to conceal. Insomnia is often an early symptom which may lead to nocturnal restlessness and confusion as the condition advances. In contrast to delirium consciousness is usually clear, and typically these may be patients found sitting quietly in surroundings apparently unfamiliar to them with a poor short-term memory.

In practice the confusion seen in patients who are terminally ill is due to a combination of factors with some reversible features and some residual deficit in brain function.

Table 3.17　Causes of acute confusion

Organic, e.g.
Tumour, Infection, Vascular disease
Iatrogenic, e.g.
Opiates, NSAIDs, Psychotropics
Corticosteroids, H_2 Blockers, Hyoscine
Oral hypoglycaemic agents
Digoxin, Anti parkinsonian drugs
Metabolic, e.g.
$\uparrow$ urea $\uparrow$ Ca^{++} $\downarrow$ Na^+
Hepatic failure, Cardiac failure
Hypoxia
Psychological
Panic/fear, Denial of illness
General
Discomfort, e.g. pain, retention of urine
faecal impaction
Change of environment
Approaching death
Withdrawal of alcohol, benzodiazipenes, barbiturates

Analysing the cause

Why is analysing the cause important? It allows explanation to be given to the patient and their family, 'You're not mad, it's the illness that's making you like this.' It also allows a team of carers to set realistic expectations of treatment.

The history and examination are vital to the assessment of underlying causes. A patient's family may often be the ones to provide the most accurate account of the person's recent mental state and also know of any new changes in medication. Occasionally patients who have denied the presence of a terminal illness become quite paranoid as realization begins to dawn. Unable to accept that they are dying they feel that somebody is trying to kill or harm them. Questioning the family about the patient's insight and acceptance of the diagnosis should help to clarify whether emotional distress may have been a precipitating cause. Clinical examination may reveal an underlying infection, or neurological signs suggestive of intracranial disease.

Following a clinical assessment appropriate investigations can be initiated. Biochemical abnormalities are easily assessed and on occasions it may be important to carry out neuro-radiological investigations to eliminate the underlying cause.

Management

Understanding how it feels

In caring for patients who are confused it is helpful to have some insight into how it feels. A model first used in the study of schizophrenia helps to illustrate this.[3] It is proposed that our awareness is made up of stimuli from our environment, our subconscious and our bodily sensations. A filter controls entry of stimuli into our awareness and normally it is possible to determine the source of a stimulus and to choose which stimuli to attend to, e.g. focus on a flower ignoring surrounding bird song or attend to a full bladder. In confused patients it is proposed that the filter controlling input from the environment is thickened and thus they are cut off from their surroundings. In addition, confused patients have a heightened awareness of their inner world and bodily sensations. They may misinterpret events occurring around them and become frighteningly aware of their heartbeat or material from their unconscious.

A typical example of this is an elderly man who is confused and in pain from urinary retention. He may suddenly become terrified as you approach the bed. The explanation may be that he is in pain and unable to determine where the pain is coming from. He is under the misapprehension that you may be causing the pain and are now approaching to do more harm.

Confused patients are often aware of their state but unable to do anything to improve things. They feel cut off from reality and out of control. This can cause great distress which in itself can heighten their confusion.

Treating reversible causes

Once the underlying causes are established appropriate treatment can be initiated. Rehydration and bisphosphonates given intravenously can restore mental lucidity within a few days to a patient with hypercalcaemia. Withdrawal of offending medication, or the use of antibiotics for an underlying infection may also result in the restoration of mental lucidity but this can take longer to achieve. If morphine is thought to be responsible substituting an alternative opioid such as phenazocine may help. High dose steroids (Dexamethasone 16–24 mg) may improve the confusion associated with primary or secondary brain tumours but their effect is often short-lived. Other metabolic disturbances should be corrected where possible.

The aim of treatment is to reduce the distress confusion is causing to the patient and family and if possible restore the patient to mental lucidity. It may not always be in the patient's interest to actively or repeatedly treat underlying causes, and it is important to involve the entire team of carers and if possible the family and patient in the decision making.

Medication

Confused patients may cause us as carers to feel helpless, frustrated and inadequate. There is an urge to do something now to relieve the situation. The prescribing of sedative medication is usually the first action taken. This may be an appropriate measure at least initially but it is not the only answer. Medication should only be part of a broader treatment plan. Sedative medication can often make the situation worse. It enhances the confused patient's feeling of being out of control and cut off from their surroundings.

Some patients remain happily muddled with no evidence of underlying distress and do not require any sedative medication. In patients who are quietly muddled but clearly distressed a small dose of a non-sedating anxiolytic such as haloperidol may prove helpful.

Some confused patients become very agitated and hyperactive. In this situation they may prove a danger to themselves and those around them. There is an urgent need to contain the situation. Gentle coaxing and explanation may prove effective but very often the patients are 'out of reach'. They feel out of control and generally respond to a firm authoritative approach. This is an emergency situation and will require use of sedative medication to eradicate the patient's fear and agitation. It is wise to use a few drugs that you know well and titrate the dose according to the patient's response and history of previous exposure to sedation (Table 3.18). As small doses of sedative can exacerbate the feeling of loss of control in general in an emergency situation use higher rather than lower doses.

Having contained the situation one must then consider the underlying causes and decide on appropriate further management. In some situations this can mean continued administration of sedation but in smaller doses. Sadly in some instances particularly in pre-terminal confusion, the only means of containing the patient's distress may be by continuing to sedate them to a state of sleepfulness.

General measures

Confused patients misinterpret activity around them so it is important to eliminate many external stimuli. They should be cared for in quiet and well lit surroundings. Familiar faces are very reassuring, family members and as few carers as is practical should be involved in the care. Gentle re-orientation and explanation is important and may need to be done repeatedly. A daily newspaper, calendar and clock may be sufficient to re-orientate some mildly confused patients. Conversely a malfunctioning hearing aid, or loss of spectacles may be enough to cause some patients to lose their tenuous grip on reality. A change of environment, e.g. admission to hospital may be a major precipitating factor and therefore patients with mild confusion are generally best cared for within their home environment if that is possible.

In communicating with confused patients it is important to assume that they understand what you are saying. Many patients have lucid intervals or are capable of grasping some of the points covered in conversation. If a patient's thought content is very bizarre do not challenge this directly. Instead identify the mood of their conversation. An elderly confused

Table 3.18 Medication in management of confusion

Emergency treatment – parenteral route preferable	
Haloperidol 5–10 mg i.m.	
Chlorpromazine 25–100 mg i.m.	S
Methotrimeprazine 25–100 mg i.m.	E
Midazolam 2–10 mg s.c.	D
Diazepam 10 mg p.r.	A
Maintenance treatment – oral route preferable	T
Trifluoperazine 1–5 mg bd or tds	I
Haloperidol 5–10 mg nocte tds	O
Thioridazine 25–50 mg tds	N
Chlorpromazine 25–50 mg tds	
Methotrimeprazine 25–50 mg tds	
Diazepam 5–10 mg nocte	

- If phenothiazine not working add a benzodiazipene and vice versa
- Quietly muddled patient without distress requires no medication
- Mild sedation may aggravate confusion further

gentleman with brain metastases felt there was a conspiracy going on and that people were plotting to harm him, 'That sounds very frightening . . .' 'It is', 'Are you frightened?', 'I'm not frightened of death but of the dying . . . will it be very painful?' This man was comforted to hear that death would be peaceful and that we as carers would do nothing to shorten his life or prolong it unnecessarily. He continued on a mild anxiolytic and remained quietly confused until his death five days later.

It is important to give back to confused patients some sense of being in control. I recall an instance where a man with advancing carcinoma of bronchus became acutely confused. He was very agitated and attempting to harm other patients. On being approached by two familiar carers he relaxed slightly but continued to pluck imaginary items from the air and floor and was pacing about the ward. He very quickly told us that he was not going to accept any injections or other medication. We realized our powers of gentle persuasion were not working. Remembering that this patient had been a very committed union representative we suggested to him that he was now involved again in a union type negotiation. 'We're negotiating a deal here – the choices are medication by injection or tablets and you've got to decide between them, it's just like it was in the Union.' He immediately gave us his attention and appeared to recognize an area which was clearly familiar and in which he had some control. He agreed to oral medication. Haloperidol 10 mg orally was proffered – he refused it, and was reminded that he had made a deal and he had never gone back on a deal in his life. This resulted in his willingly accepting his medication and he continued to take a regular dose of haloperidol when reminded that this was the deal he had agreed to.

Using language and situations that feel familiar from the past can allow us to reach patients who are otherwise feeling lost and out of control.

Ethical dilemmas

As a group of professionals working together, managing confused patients and their families can stretch a team to its limits. In most other symptoms in palliative medicine it is possible to involve the patient in the decision making – they can make an informed decision on the best course of management with our guidance. Confusion is different. Although some confused patients clearly have insight and are in a position to be involved in treatment decisions, the majority do not. The caring team and patient's family have together to decide the best treatment options. Sometimes this decision involves sedating a patient who is already quite frail and who you know may then develop a chest infection by virtue of his sleeping and inactivity.

Confusion is a symptom and underlying it are so many factors, physical, emotional and spiritual. What will be clear from the preceding discussions is that attempts should always be made to explore these. An elderly man confused due to uraemia in association with carcinoma of prostate became increasingly agitated and paranoid. He was a practising Roman Catholic and had been visited on several occasions by the chaplain.

His family felt he wished to see the priest again. The chaplain was recalled and apparently heard the patient's confession. His agitation and paranoia immediately settled and he remained confused but peaceful until his death less than a week later. In reality, one is often left with a situation where the patient remains distressed despite the best efforts of the various disciplines involved.

Sometimes, the distress and confusion is so great that it is impossible to develop any form of spiritual or psychological link. In these instances, sedation is used to lessen the patient's distress so that more effective communication can take place. It is very gratifying when this happens but, as stated previously, it can be difficult to establish a sedating regime which allows the patient to have useful wakeful periods.

Analogies have been drawn between the use of sedatives and the use of analgesics for relief of physical pain. The dose of analgesic required is that which relieves the pain – if it renders the patient drowsy in the process this fact would not preclude its use for controlling the pain. Similarly, with sedative medication, they are used to relieve agitation and anguish and the dose required may also cause a patient to be drowsy. In this instance the symptom is the anguish and the sedative is the medication to relieve this, which may or may not result in drowsiness.

As a team caring for the patient one of the concepts that may be helpful is to assess along with the family, whether a patient's waking time is of any value to them. Are they continually distressed and muddled when awake, or are there periods of time which they still enjoy? It may in some cases, particularly in the final few days of life, become obvious that a patient is only settled when sleeping. In this instance, following discussions with team members and the family, a decision is taken to continue regular sedation so that the patient is asleep for long periods of time. This is never an easy decision and one is conscious that by remaining in a sleeping state the patient may develop a pneumonia and perhaps die sooner than might otherwise be expected. In Kennedy's guidelines on treatment of the terminally ill he states 'A doctor's obligation in treating the terminally ill is to make the patient comfortable, which includes easing his pain. If, to ease his pain, the doctor must take measures which may hasten death, this is permissible, provided the doctor's principal and primary aim is only relief of pain.'

Similarly, a dilemma arises when patients refuse medication. In an emergency situation one is legally covered to administer a sedative against a patient's wishes if they are deemed to be incapable of making an informed decision and are felt to be a danger to themselves and others.

In the continuing management of a confused patient, they may not accept medication proffered, believing in their paranoia that you are trying to harm them. In general, it is unwise to conceal the medication, e.g. in food or drink, because this may heighten the patient's mistrust if discovered. Firm coaxing by a trusted member of family or staff may suffice but if not, Kennedy in his guidelines again states that where a patient is deemed incompetent, his family can make treatment decisions on his behalf. If the decision of the family is not deemed to be in the patient's best interest, this can be overriden by the doctor involved.

While these guidelines are very helpful in theory, in practice sedating patients who are terminally ill remains a very difficult issue. The patient is the primary concern but we need also to consider the needs of their families, the other patients in the ward and staff involved in their care.

It is important that we continually question our decisions. Understanding the causes and aims of treatment is a vital part of effective care. Communication between staff involved, the patient and his family on an ongoing basis can allay much of the fear and anger that may surround the situation. Patients and families have a lot to teach us. Some situations work out as we had planned but often we are saddened at being unable to achieve what we had hoped. A retrospective look at our care of confused patients and their families may make the next confusion problem easier to manage. A rigid clinical approach does not work for patients who are confused and it is important to trust one's instincts.

Notes and References

1. SAUNDERS, C. 'Introduction.' In: Saunders, C. (ed.), *Hospice and Palliative Care – An Interdisciplinary Approach*, London, Edward Arnold, 1990.
2. Mosley's *Medical and Nursing Dictionary*, 2nd edn. St. Louis: Mosley CVs, 1986.
3. STEDEFORD, A. 'Confusion.' In: Stedeford, A. (ed.), *Facing Death – Patients, Families and Professionals*. London, Heinemann, 1988, pp. 122–6.
4. KENNEDY, I mcC. 'The law relating to the terminally ill.' In: Saunders, C. (ed.), *The Management of Terminal Malignant Disease*, 2nd edn, London, Edward Arnold, 1984, pp. 227–31.

Further reading

ADAMS, R.D. and VICTOR, M. 'Delirium and other acute confusional states.' In: Isselbacher, K.J. et al. (eds), *Harrison's Principles of Internal Medicine*, 9th edn, Japan, McGraw-Hill-Kogakusha, 1979, pp. 122–26.
STEDEFORD, A. *Facing Death – Patients, Families and Professionals*, London, Heinemann, 1988.

Mouth and skin problems———————————

Wendy Lethem

Mouth problems

Causes

Oral problems in advanced illness result from a variety of processes which may be classified broadly into three categories:

- Disease processes.
- Treatments or medications.
- Inadequate oral hygiene.

Effects of disease processes

These may be local or systemic. Malnutrition, immunosuppression, dehydration and debility all affect the mouth. Weight loss may cause ill-fitting dentures, leading to trauma, ulceration and the inability either to chew effectively or to eat comfortably. Dentures may also harbour infection. When the appetite is reduced, there is less stimulation of the salivary glands, causing reduced salivary flow and consequent reduction in moisture and natural cleansing activity, and drying is often compounded by mouth breathing. Cancer of the oral cavity itself presents local problems such as pain, ulceration, fistulae, infection and fungation.[1]

Effects of treatments or medications

Radiotherapy given locally may damage salivary glands, causing dry mouth and attendant impairment of oral functions. Taste may be altered or absent. Radiotherapy given to other parts of the body may contribute to nausea and vomiting or cause alterations in taste. Surgery or local tumour in the oral cavity may cause pain, leave ill-healed wounds or ulceration, with consequent difficulty in effective cleansing. Such wounds become foci for infection and fistulae may also develop. Chemotherapy causes damage to the epithelial cells of the oral mucosa and immunosuppression may also make the mouth particularly vulnerable to trauma and infection.[2]

Medication administered for relief of other symptoms may contribute to oral dryness: common examples are morphine, antispasmodics (e.g. hyoscine) some antiemetics (e.g. prochlorperazine and cyclizine), antihistamines (e.g. chlorpheniramine) and tricyclic antidepressants (e.g. amitriptyline). Tolerance to this side effect sometimes occurs. Antibiotics alter the balance of oral flora allowing infection by candida; corticosteroids also allow mouth infections to become established, so patients on any of these treatments should have their oral health carefully monitored.

Inadequate oral hygiene

Debilitation by illness and by the effects of treatment will not only compromise the physiological ability to counter infection but the individual's motivation and ability to counter the increased risk with stringent mouth care measures may also be minimal. At this point the patient and his carers, both family and professional, must work together to protect against oral problems.

Treatments for oral problems

The principal mouth problems encountered in terminal malignancy are listed in Table 3.19. Initial assessment of the oral cavity should take note of the conditions of tongue, teeth, palate and mucosa, the presence or absence of plaque, debris, bleeding, fistulae, ulceration, pain, infections (particularly candida), and halitosis. The fit of dentures, the amount of salivation, the individual's ability and motivation to perform their own oral care, should all be assessed. Regular oral hygiene twice a day should prevent many mouth problems but frequent and regular assessment is extremely important.

Dirty mouth/coated tongue

Unless the mouth is also ulcerated, bleeding or sore, the ideal implement for mechanically cleaning all parts of the mouth is a soft-bristled, small-headed toothbrush.[3] Tap water and toothpaste are the simplest and most refreshing agents, but a heavily coated tongue may require one of the following to help dissolve the coating:

- Sodium bicarbonate in solution. (This tastes unpleasant and should not be used with nystatin because it creates an alkaline oral environment and the potential for damage to the mucosa.)
- Vitamin C: one quarter of a 1 g effervescent tablet dissolved on the tongue four times a day.
- Hydrogen peroxide 3 per cent dilute solution (although this inhibits tissue healing).
- Sodium perborate 70 per cent (should not be swallowed and tastes unpleasant).

Table 3.19   Principal mouth problems encountered in patients with terminal malignant disease

---
Dirty mouth/coated tongue
Dryness
Infection
Pain
Halitosis
Altered taste

Until the mouth is clean, these measures should be used four or more times per day, usually after meals and at bedtime. Chemotherapy patients may require oral care every one to two hours.

Dry mouth

Thick or absent saliva is uncomfortable and makes speech and chewing difficult. Helpful measures either stimulate saliva production or replace oral moisture with substitutes:

- Stimulation of the saliva flow by sucking or chewing: ice cubes, boiled sweets, cubes of fruit, small pieces of fresh pineapple (which contains the enzyme ananase which helps break down any coating on the tongue).
- Replacement of moisture by frequent mouthwashes, preferably tap water. Avoid glycerine-containing substances as they dry the oral mucosa.
- Frequent sips of cold, clear drinks.
- Frequent use of saliva substitute aerosol spray.

Patients who are unconscious and unable to perform their own oral care must have it carried out for them regularly. The best implements for this are moistened foam sticks or gauze swabs and a gloved finger. Attendant family may be taught to do this. If a particular medication is causing dry mouth, it should be evaluated and either stopped or another which is less drying substituted.

Infected mouth

Where the person is particularly vulnerable to infection, if there are open lesions in the mouth, or where ulceration is already present, measures are needed additional to those described above, for example antiseptic mouth-washes such as povidone-iodine 1 per cent twice a day, but up to every two to four hours if necessary, or chlorhexidine gluconate 0.2 per cent solution (10 ml) twice per day. Sodium perborate and hydrogen peroxide are useful for debriding (see under 'Dirty mouth', above).

Where candida infection is present or suspected it should be treated with nystatin suspension 100 000 units/ml, 1 ml–2 ml four times daily (or four hourly) for at least one week. Alternatives are nystatin lozenges or amphotericin or miconazole gel. Very few patients can cope successfully with antifungals in lozenge form and therefore a gel or liquid form is preferable. Should these be ineffective a 7–14 day course of systemic ketoconazole 200 mg once daily usually deals with even the most resistant cases but the newer and more expensive triazole antifungals, fluconazole and itraconazole may need to be considered. Dentures harbour oral candida, so they should be removed and cleaned whenever oral hygiene measures are being carried out. They, too, should be treated with nystatin. For effective eradication of candida, dentures should be removed at night and cleaned. Non-metal dentures should be stored in disinfectant such as dilute hydrogen peroxide, while dentures containing metal should be brushed with povidone iodine and stored dry.

For herpetic ulcers on the lip use acyclovir ointment, and for ulcers inside the mouth, use acyclovir 200 mg four hourly orally for five days. Aphthous ulcers may clear more quickly when treated with tetracycline 125 mg three times a day as a mixture. The liquid should be held in the mouth for three minutes, then spat out. Infected malignant ulcers in the mouth may require systemic treatment with antibiotics.

Painful mouth

Pain may result from local trauma and/or infection or from tumour in the mouth. Mechanical cleaning may be hampered by pain. Any infection should be treated, and topical local analgesics can be used before undergoing mouthcare or eating. Useful local analgesic preparations include benzydamine hydrochloride (15 ml every one and a half to three hours) and salicylate gels.

Painful lesions may be protected by a dental barrier paste (carmellose sodium paste) after meals and at bedtime. Pain and inflammation may be reduced with the local application of the steroid triamcinolone in barrier paste base two to four times daily. (Note that steroids may be contraindicated in the presence of untreated infections.)

Halitosis

Halitosis can simply be caused by a dirty mouth, but is often due to sepsis in the respiratory or gastro-intestinal tracts, or to vomiting, especially if faeculent. Any underlying infection should be treated. Systemic metronidazole is used for anaerobic infections (e.g. 400 mg tds daily or 1 g tds rectally). It can be applied topically in the mouth if it is not tolerated systemically. A regime of careful oral cleaning, plus a refreshing mouthwash for use after vomiting, are probably the most helpful measures.

Taste alterations are dealt with on page 96.

Skin problems

The principal causes of skin problems in terminal malignancy fall into the following categories:

- Disease processes.
- Treatments or medications.
- Deficiencies in hygiene.
- Inadequate relief of pressure.

Effects of disease processes

These may be systemic or local. Generalized debility in advanced malignant disease predisposes to skin breakdown and poor wound healing.

- Nutritional status is poor, appetite is often reduced; metabolic processes are affected by tumour activity; there may be deficiencies in materials needed for wound repair, i.e. proteins, carbohydrates, some vitamins and minerals.
- Cachexia means that bony prominences exert greater pressure on vulnerable skin.
- Generalized weakness causes reduced mobility.
- Neuropathy makes patients unaware of discomfort due to pressure allowing irreversible damage to occur.
- Age reduces skin elasticity and its resistance to damage.
- Poor circulation increases risk of tissue damage and impairs healing.
- Lymphoedematous limbs are particularly vulnerable to damage, trauma, infection and poor healing.
- Incontinence (necessitates increased washing/ drying of skin), increases risk of infection if skin is broken or excoriated.
- Dehydration reduces reparability of skin and makes it more fragile.
- Diabetes damages capillaries and impairs tissue healing.
- Jaundice and malignant sweats cause itching. Scratching to relieve itch may damage skin.
- Ulceration: a tumour eroding through the epithelium forms a malignant ulcer and when infected, a fungating wound. Patients with such lesions may experience impaired self-image, embarrassment, fear and disgust.
- Fistulae may occur at the tumour site. They may discharge varying amounts of fluids such as bile, pus, serous fluid, faeces, blood, pancreatic juice, urine or a mixture of more than one of these.

Effects of treatments or medications

Some patients may experience skin reactions to chemotherapeutic agents and a few may have skin problems following radiotherapy. Alopecia may result from local radiotherapy and some chemotherapeutic agents. Steroids cause skin deterioration impairing capillary circulation and rendering it dry, friable, easily damaged and prone to infection. Some medications used in symptom control such as certain NSAIDs, e.g. fenbufen, azapropazone, and antibiotics, e.g. penicillins, cotrimoxazole, may cause rashes. Fistulae may develop after radiotherapy or surgery due to tissue damage and the poor wound healing capability of patients with malignant disease.

Effects of deficiencies in hygiene

Too much washing or use of soap can cause dry, itchy skin. Skin that is never dry and where air cannot circulate freely, as in the cleft of the buttocks or the groin, or where there is incontinence, is at risk of infection as well as being uncomfortable.

Inadequate relief of pressure

Skin already vulnerable to damage as a result of all the above is further compromised where it is subjected to sustained pressure.

Management of skin problems

Wounds, including fungating tumours and fistulae

The aims of wound care are summarized in Table 3.21 and the characteristics of the ideal would dressing in Table 3.22. Using this knowledge, a wound management regime of appropriate dressings and cleaning products can be devised according to the nature of the particular wound, and the needs of the individual patient.[4] A

Table 3.20   Principal skin problems encountered in advanced malignant disease

Wounds, including fungating tumours and fistulae
Pressure sores
Those related to skin hygiene
Lymphoedema
Rashes
Alopecia
Coincident skin disease

Table 3.21   The aims of wound care

Improve patient comfort
Prevent or reduce infection
Contain exudate or odour
Minimize or eliminate bleeding
Minimize the effect on lifestyle of either the wound itself or the dressing regime
Create a wound environment conducive to healing

Table 3.22   The ideal wound dressing

Absorbs exudate and toxins, reducing odour and/or leakage
Is impermeable to micro-organisms, so preventing secondary infection
Maintains wound surface temperature near 37°C (ideal for mitosis)
Is oxygen-permeable
Maintains moisture at wound surface
Requires minimal frequency of changing
Can be removed atraumatically, e.g. by irrigation
Inhibits bacterial growth at wound surface
May also have haemostatic properties, e.g. alginates.

large range of products is available. Local specialists such as stoma, diabetic, lymphoedema or wound-care nurses may be able to help solve particularly difficult problems.

Additional measures for specific wound management problems include:

- *Friable skin around lesion*: avoid use of adhesive tapes to secure dressings; irrigate off old dressing, hold dressing in place with bandages or tubular elastic net.
- *Excessive exudate*: negotiate acceptable regime with patient, use extra padding outside primary dressing to reduce frequency of change and prevent staining of clothes or escape of odour.
- *Infection*: anaerobic infection may be treated with systemic or topical metronidazole (400 mg orally tds or 0.8 per cent metronidazole gel topically). Antiseptic cleansing solutions help reduce numbers of pathogens from wound surface, e.g. povidone iodine 10 per cent aqueous solution. Liquid paraffin inhibits bacterial growth and may be useful in conjunction with povidone iodine on large fungating wounds and is also helpful in reducing trauma when the dressing is changed. However some of the more modern, interactive dressings, e.g. alginates, are more effective in controlling bleeding, exudate and infection. Cost may prohibit their use on very large wounds, where iodine/liquid paraffin-soaked gauze may be the most workable option.
- *Necrosis*: debriding the wound will reduce infection, exudate and odour. In patients with longer life expectancy, surgical debriding is sometimes indicated, otherwise debriding solutions or creams may be used with caution, e.g. hydrogen peroxide cream; Aserbine cream or solution, both of which contain benzoic acid, malic acid, propylene glycol and salicylic acid, the solution being more concentrated than the cream. Some hydrocolloid dressings allow desloughing of non-infected wounds and should be used in accordance with manufacturers' instructions.
- *Odour*: treat any infection and prevent leakage of exudate. Incorporate a charcoal dressing as outer element over primary dressing. An ionizer in the room may help. Stoma deodorants may be used on the outside of dressing and diversional aromas used, such as a favourite scent, air freshener or flowers. However, beware of masking wound odour with something more sickly or unpleasant, or of causing unfortunate associations between fungating wounds and previously pleasant smells.
- *Bleeding*: superficial vessels may bleed, particularly at dressing changes. Capillary bleeding usually stops within a few minutes when gauze soaked in adrenaline 1:1000 is applied. Calcium alginate dressings also reduce the likelihood of bleeding. Larger vessels which bleed may require diathermy, cryotherapy or even embolisation. Radiotherapy may be considered.
- *Pain*: NSAIDs often help relieve the pain and inflammation due to a malignant ulcer. Topical local anaesthetics may be considered. Dressing choice is important where pain is associated with dressing change.

Extra analgesia before such a painful procedure (e.g. dextromoramide 5–10 mg), may also be helpful.

- *Fistulae*: depending on the nature and quantity of effluent, the approach should aim to contain the effluent and therefore any odour, and to protect the perifistular skin from excoriation.

A wide range of stoma or fistula appliances is available, and often the best strategy for enterocutaneous fistulae is a drainable bag changed as infrequently as is feasible, while perifistular skin is protected by barrier pastes or wafers. Where a bag cannot be applied, a nurse's skills in selecting appropriate wound care products to limit leakage and odour are tested to the full to provide a comfortable and effective dressing regime.

Buccal fistulae are common in head and neck disease. Sometimes fistulae occur over areas of pressure necrosis or tumours, or at surgery sites. In such situations the use of hydrocolloid pastes or silastic foam under secondary dressings may prove the most comfortable and effective solution. Minimizing disfigurement may be an important consideration. Very small fistulae may be managed simply with external gauze pads.

Pressure sores

Prophylaxis is the key word. Patients with advanced malignant disease are at great risk of developing sores. However, should prophylaxis fail, carers should not be discouraged or feel guilty but should understand the value in terms of quality of life, of staving off pressure sore development even for a few weeks, days or months. Should sores become established, the aims of management are containment and minimizing their effect on the patient's life-style. The pain from a pressure sore may be the worst pain a patient suffers and the most difficult to control with simple analgesics. While nerve supply to the pressured skin survives, pressure relief is the most effective strategy in reducing discomfort or pain. Wound management should follow the guidelines outlined earlier.

The underlying physiological principle is that tissue damage is likely when capillary circulation is impeded by external pressure for a critical length of time. Risk assessment, initial and ongoing is important, as is observation of the skin itself, particularly the time taken for skin erythema to disappear after each turn. The patient, his family or carers and the nursing team must work together to establish an effective regime of pressure relief. A high level of dependence on nurses in achieving pressure relief may itself be one reason to admit the patient to hospital or hospice. Aids to pressure relief include variations on the following themes:

- Cushions of various kinds distribute pressure more evenly beneath the sedentary patient.
- Fleeces, natural or man made, as elbow/heel pads, on chair seats or under the patient in bed, act by reducing shearing and friction forces on the skin.
- Mattresses (inflatable or padded) act by distributing pressure more evenly over body surface.

- Pillows should be used rather than backrests to support patients in bed.
- Bed cradles keep weight of bedclothes off patients.
- Plastic drawsheets or plastic-backed incontinence sheets should be avoided wherever possible as they hold moisture in contact with the skin. However, the practicalities of caring for incontinent patients at home with limited nursing may sometimes override this consideration.
- Bed linen beneath the patient should be kept wrinkle-free.
- Avoid rubbing pressure areas; although gentle rubbing is comforting, care should be taken not to increase capillary damage/shearing by over-zealous massage. Nurses may need to advise carers about potentially harmful practices.
- Topical creams are of dubious if any value in preventing damage to the skin on pressure areas. Barrier and emollient creams help in other ways to keep skin comfortable and healthy (see below).

Skin problems related to hygiene

Dry skin is exacerbated by excessive washing or use of soap which removes from skin the natural oils which normally prevent moisture loss. Emollients may be added to bathwater, emulsifying ointment may be used instead of soap, and bathing frequency reduced. Applying emollient or other moisturizing creams of choice can help by replacing lost moisture and soothing irritation. Itching may result from dry skin or jaundice. Severe itching may respond to chlorpheniramine, 4 mg orally four to six hourly or hydroxyzine 50–100 mg six hourly. Calamine lotion is drying and should be avoided. For itching due to jaundice, cholestyramine 4 g six hourly may help but it is unpleasant to take and ineffective in total biliary obstruction. Anabolic steroids sometimes give relief.

Moisture present at the skin's surface, and/or the inadequate circulation of air, may permit fungal infections to become established, e.g. between buttocks, beneath breasts, on the perineum and in groins. In addition to careful washing, drying and regular inspection of these areas, a topical antifungal cream may be indicated, e.g. clotrimazole, miconazole or nystatin.

Sweats occur where there is malignant involvement of the liver, or due to fever caused by the cancer itself. Often worse at night, sweats may cause the patient to wake up with nightclothes and bedlinen drenched, which is disruptive to sleep and creates extra laundry for the weary carer. Apart from cooling measures such as lightweight bedlinen, the use of a fan and keeping the room well ventilated, a NSAID, e.g. naproxen 500 mg/day, or dexamethasone 2–4 mg/day, may help reduce the amount and frequency of sweating.

Incontinence, vaginal and rectal discharges necessitate meticulous washing and drying of contaminated areas. Sensitive skin may best be dried with warm air from a hairdryer if very sore. A barrier cream which contains water-repellent substances, e.g. dimethicone or other silicones, may serve to protect unbroken skin exposed to such contamination. Talc should be avoided as it tends to cake into abrasive lumps, worsening irritation or discomfort. Discharges from vagina or rectum due to local tumour may be helped by topical measures such as antiseptic douches or local corticosteroids. Tampons may help control discharge from recto-vaginal fistulae providing they are renewed regularly. In such situations local treatment, e.g. radiotherapy or laser therapy, should be considered.

Lymphoedema

The skin of swollen limbs tend to crack, become dry and permit entry of infection. Prevention of skin damage by measures which reduce swelling, such as elevating limbs, is important, while massage and compression bandaging may produce considerable reduction in size. Careful skin hygiene, avoidance of trauma and regular inspection of affected limbs for signs of damage or cellulitis are also necessary. Advice on how to avoid damaging the skin of the affected limb should include recommending the prompt treatment of cuts, abrasions or burns with a topical antiseptic, avoiding the use of razors, wearing gloves for gardening, avoiding direct heat or sunburn and avoiding wearing constrictive clothing.[5] Professionals should remember not to take blood samples from, give injections into, or take blood pressure readings on lymphoedematous limbs.

Alopecia

Usually due to chemotherapy or radiotherapy, it frequently causes self-consciousness or embarrassment. Displaying acceptance and giving encouragement to voice their feelings are perhaps the most important ways to help such patients. Concealment of the scalp using a wig, turban or hat may help. Where hair is fragile or thinned, washing should be gentle, infrequent (every four days) using a mild shampoo and brushing or combing kept to the minimum.

Coincident skin diseases

Eczma, impetigo, acne or other skin diseases may recur and require the appropriate topical treatment.

Notes and References

1. ROBERTS, H. 'Mouthcare in oral cavity cancer,' *Nursing Standard*, 1990, **4**, 26–9.
2. HOLMES, S. 'Gastrointestinal side effects.' In: *Cancer Chemotherapy*, London, Austen Cornish, 1990, pp. 178–86.
3. BENNETT, J. 'A reassessment of oral healthcare,' *Professional Nurse*, 1991, September, pp. 703–8.
4. MORRISON, M.M. 'Priorities in wound management (Parts I and II),' *Professional Nurse*, 1987, 352–5 and 402–11.
5. BADGER, C. and REGNARD, C. 'Oedema in advanced cancer: a flow diagram,' *Palliative Medicine*, 1989, **3**, 213–15.

Fractures————————————————————————————

Anthony M. Smith

In patients with advanced malignancy, fractures are not infrequent occurrences. They arise as a consequence of:

- Metastases from the original tumour.
- Other pathological causes (e.g. osteoporosis, osteomalacia, bone infection).
- Trauma (commonly, falls).

The commonest cause is metastasis. Almost any malignant tumour may metastasise to bone except the primary brain tumours. Fifty per cent of bony metastases are from breast primaries, with lung, prostate and kidney being the next commonest. Since the incidence of neoplasia is highest in the elderly, there will be a proportionately increased incidence of osteoporosis and other non-malignant pathological conditions. Falls are common in the elderly, particularly in association with the weakness and instability of advanced malignancy, and in these cases fracture does not necessarily relate to bony metastasis.

Metastases occur most commonly in the axial skeleton (skull, vertebrae, ribs, scapulae and pelvis) and proximal limb bones. However, any bone may be implicated – as, for example, a patient with a rectal carcinoma who presented with a pathological fracture in the foot!

Diagnosis of fracture

Fractures present with a history of some or all of

- Pain.
- Deformity.
- Local swelling.
- Sudden incident.
- Loss of function (e.g. paraparesis, loss of sphincter control).

The pain may have been present for a long time, slowly getting worse, with or without a recent exacerbation. It may be felt at the site of fracture or at a distance (e.g. in the hip or leg from spinal fractures, or in thigh and knee from a femoral neck fracture). Long-standing pain, worse on activity but often present at rest also, may indicate bony metastasis before fracture has occurred.

Back pain associated with sensory changes in the lower legs and weakness in one or both legs is an important presentation of spinal cord compression due to vertebral pathological fracture and requires urgent diagnosis and treatment. (See section on Emergencies in Palliative Medicine).

X-ray will confirm the diagnosis. Bone scan will identify bony metastases not yet large enough to be visualized on X-ray (and before fracture), thus identifying sites at risk, and extent of bony metastatic spread.

Prevention of fracture

Bony metastases found at bone scan, and part of a disseminated malignancy, require specific treatment if they cause pain or are at risk of fracture. The latter requires X-ray assessment to indicate the size of the lesion and the extent of associated damage to the bone cortex (thinning or partial circumference fracture) (Fig. 3.4). If there is no cortical damage, the lesion is best treated by radiotherapy for pain relief – generally by

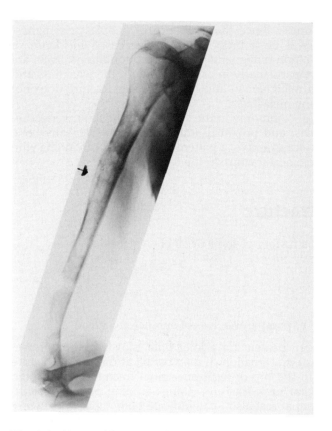

Fig. 3.4 X-ray of humerus showing multiple lytic lesions from metastastic carcinoma of breast. A partial circumferential fracture is arrowed.

a single fraction. If cortical damage is significant, however, internal fixation to support the bone (as an intramedullary nail or by plate and screw stablization) (Fig. 3.5) is wise before irradiation, which may initially cause weakening.

When a patient is known to have bony metastases, even though relatively symptom-free, there is a natural tendency to restrict activity lest fracture occur. This happens especially with metastases in the femora and in cervical vertebrae. It is important to remember the stage of the under-lying malignancy and not to prevent activities which would give the patient pleasure during his or her last weeks or months, in the hope of preventing a fracture or disability which may never occur. Thus the slow destruction of a cervical vertebra with resulting apparent instability of the cervical spine (but with fibrous or tumour tissue surrounding the spinal cord) is a very different situation from the traumatic fracture of the cervical spine in a road traffic accident where major neurological damage is an immediate result.

Immediate treatment of fracture

When a fracture occurs in a patient with advanced malignancy the urgent considerations are:

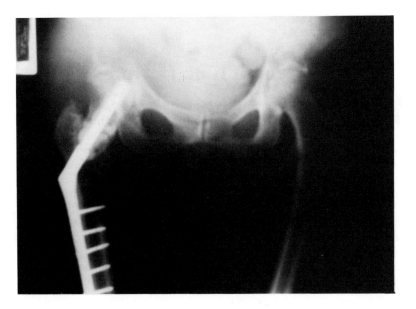

Fig. 3.5 X-ray of upper ends of femora with sliding hip screw and plate fixation of fracture of femoral neck through extensive secondary deposit from breast carcinoma. Some carcinomatous tissue has been removed and replaced with bone cement. There were extensive metastases elsewhere in the skeleton including pelvis.

- Analgesia.
- Emergency action to make comfortable.
- Confirmation of diagnosis.
- Arrangements for definitive treatment.

Appropriate analgesia will be provided by an injection of diamorphine or morphine (dose as indicated by the size and age of the patient and current opioid medication) with an antiemetic and anxiolytic (such as chlorpromazine 25 mg). Injected hyoscine at the same time has a useful amnesiant action.

If the fracture is of a limb bone, after the analgesic has had time to act, the limb may be straightened by gentle firm pulling out. It should then be immobilized with a splint or by being tied to the side of the body (for an arm) or to the other limb in the case of a leg. Even if traction is not performed, the limb should be splinted to prevent painful movement at the fracture site.

It may be useful to get a portable X-ray of a suspected long bone fracture without transfer to hospital, especially if there is doubt about the fracture or the patient is very unwell.

In most cases, however, the patient should be transferred to the local hospital for X-ray confirmation of the fracture and definitive treatment. A full note of the patient's condition and current medication should accompany the patient in a letter, along with the promise to take the patient back to a palliative care bed after treatment as soon as this is convenient for the hospital.

Definitive treatment of limb fractures

The best treatment for limb fractures is internal fixation with subsequent radiotherapy or (where internal fixation is not possible) immobilization or support for the fracture, with radiotherapy.

Appropriate analgesia will be needed. Non-steroidal anti-inflammatory drugs act at the site of pain production in the limb, but do not provide total pain relief. They are complemented by opioids, but adequate analgesia with opioids is difficult to titrate in the case of fractures because the amount needed varies rapidly with rest or movement. Hence the importance of surgical internal fixation whenever possible. We have seen such relief from pain gained by internal fixation of a fractured humerus or femur, and such recovery of hope from the simple ability to get up or move freely in bed after such a procedure, that we strongly commend surgery for long bone fractures (Fig. 3.6).

In fractures consequent on trauma, healing may be expected; unfortunately, in pathological fractures through metastases, healing does not occur spontaneously but requires, after immobilization, radiotherapy to halt bone destruction and stimulate repair processes. Radiotherapy can be given as soon as wound healing has occurred, or through plaster if the limb fracture is immobilized. A single treatment generally suffices and rarely causes systemic upset since it is given so peripherally.

Definitive treatment of limb fractures in the very ill

Where the patient is too ill to travel and to contemplate surgical or radiotherapy procedures, pain relief from the fracture may be obtained with immobilization, traction or an anaesthetic block. A portable X-ray will confirm (or refute) the diagnosis, and an orthopaedic opinion can be gained by a visit from the local specialist.

For arm and wrist fractures or lower leg fractures immobilization is achieved with plaster of Paris or lightweight casts. The limb should be well padded before application of the plaster. Lightness in weight is an advantage in the frail and elderly. Manipulation may be achieved under local anaesthetic if necessary.

For the shaft or neck of femur, plaster is unsatisfactory since the joint proximal (i.e. the hip) cannot be immobilized. For these fractures the simplest of traction systems – a straight pull over the end of the bed (see

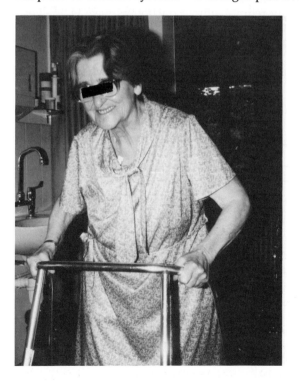

Fig. 3.6 Patient walking after internal fixation of femoral shaft fracture and radiotherapy for bone metastases.

Fig. 3.7) – will ease pain and allow better control with analgesics. Traction should not be used where it is envisaged that it will be needed for several weeks; instead, operation should be considered: time is too valuable at this stage of a patient's life to waste it on traction!

Another alternative is an anaesthetic block: an epidural or lumbar plexus block with bupivicaine can provide long-term pain relief. The block is performed with a single injection of bupivicaine 0.25 per cent with or without steroids, and the pain relief can be prolonged by inserting an indwelling catheter for regular top-ups or continual infusion from a syringe driver. Total pain relief for a femoral neck or shaft fracture can be continued for days or even weeks, at the cost of a numb leg – a price generally well accepted if explained beforehand.

Fractures of the axial skeleton

Vertebral compression fracture without long tract signs is best treated with rest and analgesia – opioids plus non-steroidal anti-inflammatory drugs – and radiotherapy. The same is true for pathological fractures of clavicle or scapula. Where there is suspicion of spinal cord compression, urgent diagnosis and treatment is essential: this is discussed in the next section.

Fractures of the pelvis may require simple traction as well as analgesia for a few days until the acute pain of the incident has subsided, and then radiotherapy. In this instance, mobilization will need to be delayed until pain is eased, and may then be started using crutches or a Zimmer frame. Sometimes a wheelchair enables the patient to begin to get around

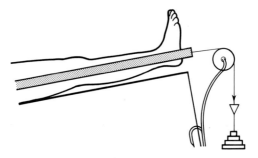

1. The leg is gently and firmly straightened and pulled.
2. Tinct. Benz. Co. is applied to the sides of the leg.
3. An extension plaster strapping is applied.
4. The leg is crepe-bandaged from ankle to top of thigh.
5. The extension cord is taken over a pulley attached to the foot of the bed.
6. Five to seven pounds weight is attached (this can be a 3 litre plastic bottle filled with water).
7. The foot of the bed is raised to provide counter-traction (as shown above).

Fig. 3.7

when the pelvis is not stable enough for weight-bearing. It is surprising how these fractures through metastases in the pelvis sometimes lead to very little pain. Where pain is a feature, however, an epidural injection of Bupivicaine and steroid provides valuable relief.

Reference

BATES, T.D., CHALMERS, J., MANNIX, K.A. and RAWLINS, M.D.,The management of bone metastases (radiotherapy, orthopaedic procedures and non-steroidal anti-inflammatory drugs), *Palliative Medicine*, 1987, 1, 117–31.

Emergencies in Palliative Medicine———

Peter Kaye

This section covers:

- superior vena cava obstruction.
- spinal cord compression.
- convulsions.
- acute haemorrhage.

Superior vena cava obstruction

Superior vena cava (SVC) obstruction is a sub-acute emergency, since it is potentially fatal but usually develops slowly. It is caused by compression (or invasion) of the SVC by tumour. The SVC is encircled by lymph nodes (anterior mediastinal and paratracheal) which drain from both sides of the thorax, and is also close to the right main bronchus. Seventy-five per cent of cases are due to a bronchogenic tumour (most commonly small cell), 15 per cent to lymphoma, 7 per cent to metastases from other cancers (breast, colon, oesophagus, testis) and 3 per cent due to benign causes (thrombosis, goitre, aortic aneurysm).

The symptoms tend to gradually worsen over a few weeks, and it is usually possible to delay radiotherapy until after a tissue diagnosis is made. Symptoms are due to venous hypertension. The SVC drains blood from the head, neck, arms and upper thorax into the right atrium. SVC compression causes tracheal oedema and dyspnoea, and also cerebral oedema with headaches (worse on bending), visual changes, dizziness, syncope or seizures. Swelling may occur of the face (especially periorbital) neck (tight collars) and hands (rings on the fingers may feel tight). Direct pressure on other structures at the thoracic inlet (trachea, recurrent laryngeal nerve) may cause stridor or hoarseness.

Signs include tachypnoea, pink eyes, periorbital oedema, non-pulsatile distension of neck veins and dilated collateral veins of the arms and upper chest. Late signs may include pleural effusions, pericardial effusions or stridor. Chest X-ray may show mediastinal widening or a right-sided hilar mass. Other investigations may be necessary if a patient presents with SVC obstruction, in order to reach a tissue diagnosis and plan treatment. Investigations may include biopsy of an enlarged supraclavicular node, sputum cytology, bronchoscopy, mediastinoscopy or even thoracotomy.

Emergency treatment is usually only needed if the patient presents late, with signs of tracheal obstruction or cerebral oedema, and involves sitting the patient upright, administering high concentration oxygen (50–60 per cent) maintaining the airway, and giving IV diuretics and high dose steroids (frusemide 80 mg and dexamethasone 20 mg) and possibly anti-convulsants. Such patients have a poor prognosis and radiotherapy may not reverse the compression at this stage. Emergency bypass surgery of the SVC may be considered.

Radiotherapy is given under cover of high dose steroids (dexamethasone 12 mg daily) to prevent initial swelling and worsening of the compression. Common regimes of treatment are 2000 cGY over five days or 3000 cGy over 10 days. Patients with Hodgkins disease might be given higher doses. Chemotherapy is as effective as radiotherapy for small cell lung cancer, lymphoma and germ cell tumours. (The right arm should be avoided for intravenous drug administration, as the blood flow is reduced.) Improvement usually begins within seventy-two hours of treatment and survival can be prolonged for several months, although the majority of patients die from progressive disease within twelve months. Symptoms of SVC obstruction often recur, when they are usually managed symptomatically as a terminal event. Dyspnoea and agitation can be controlled with a subcutaneous infusion of diamorphine and midazolam.

Failure to respond to radiotherapy suggests SVC thrombosis, which is more likely when there has been an intravenous catheter in place for drug administration. This can be diagnosed by CT scan or venogram and treatment by anti-coagulation can resolve the symptoms.

Spinal cord compression

Spinal cord compression is a medical emergency because prompt treatment within forty-eight hours can reverse neurological damage. It occurs in about 5 per cent of cancer patients, most commonly with cancers of the lung, breast and prostate (and less commonly with lymphoma, sarcoma, myeloma, and cancers of the kidney, stomach, colon or thyroid).

Cord damage usually results from direct extension of a metastasis from a vertebral body into the epidural space, but other mechanisms of cord damage include vertebral collapse, or direct spread of tumour through the intervertebral foramen (usually in lymphoma or testicular tumours) or interruption of the vascular supply.

The earliest symptom is usually thoracic back pain (95 per cent), sometimes with root irritation (causing a bilateral band of pain around the chest) worse on coughing or straining. Stiffness or weakness of the legs then occur (difficulty climbing stairs). Tingling and numbness usually start in both feet and work up the legs. Urinary symptoms (hesitancy or incontinence) and perianal numbness are late features.

On examination there is almost always localized tenderness over the thoracic spine, and there may be brisk reflexes in the legs. The plantar response may be upgoing. A clear level of sensory loss emerges later, usually somewhere between the nipples (T4) and umbilicus (T10). The sensory level is a useful clinical guide to planning radiotherapy in patients not well enough for detailed investigations. Chest X-ray may show erosion of pedicles, a collapsed vertebral body or a paraspinal mass. Other investigations (myelogram, CT scan, MRI scan) are usually only indicated if surgery is planned. Myelogram will show the entire cord and the completeness of the block. CT scan focuses on a particular level and gives good soft tissue detail, but silent lesions at multiple levels may be missed. MRI scan shows the entire cord in detail, and is the investigation of choice, but the patient must be able to lie still for thirty minutes for the procedure.

Emergency treatment can be summarized as immediate steroids and same-day radiotherapy. Dexamethasone 10 mg IV is given immediately and 16 mg daily started orally, in order to reduce spinal oedema.

Radiotherapy alone gives as good results as laminectomy plus radio-therapy and a commonly used regime is to give 3000 cGy in 10 fractions. Seventy per cent of patients who can walk at the time of diagnosis retain their ability to walk, 35 per cent of those who are paraparetic become ambulatory, but less than 5 per cent of paraplegic patients will regain the ability to walk. Unfortunately 75 per cent of patients are paralysed at presentation.

Surgical decompression is reserved for patients where the tissue diagnosis is in doubt, or if the patient's condition deteriorates during or after radiotherapy, or the tumour is radio-resistant (melanoma, renal carcinoma) or if there is spinal instability (collapse of a vertebra or extensive bone loss). The location of the compressing epidural tumour will dictate the surgical approach. Laminectomy is indicated for a posterior or postero-lateral deposit, whereas vertebral body resection and reconstruction (using methomethacrylate cement) via an anterior approach is indicated for anterior deposits. The aim of surgery is to correct any deformity by distraction of the spine, tighten lax ligaments and lessen compression. The majority of metastases occur anteriorly in the vertebral body, and the newer techniques of anterior resection followed by stabilization of the spine with Harrington distraction rods and sublaminar wiring are producing better results than posterior laminectomy. In a series of 61 patients selected for anterior resection 80 per cent achieved post-operative ambulation and 11 out of 13 paraplegic patients recovered leg functions. The presence of metal or cement does not interfere with subsequent radiotherapy.

Prognosis is better in lymphoma and myeloma. If the patient already has paraparesis, radiotherapy may still serve to rescue sphincter function (and prevent double incontinence) when treatment may still be worthwhile.

Sometimes in patients with advanced disease the most difficult decision is whether to institute emergency treatment at all, since the results of treatment are often poor and if the patient's condition is deteriorating, to embark on a course of radiotherapy may not be in their best overall interests. A discussion with the patient and relatives in order to explore their own opinions about further treatment is often the best way to decide on the correct course of management.

Compression of the spinal canal at the lumbar level causes damage to the cauda equina (because the spinal cord ends at the level of L1). The clinical picture is of flaccid weakness of the legs with sciatic pains, urinary hesitancy and perianal numbness. It can be difficult to diagnose with certainty (except at post-mortem) and myelogram can appear normal. Treatment with high dose steroids and radiotherapy is often disappointing.

Convulsions

Convulsions (fits, seizures) can occur in patients with either primary or secondary brain tumours. Convulsions due to brain tumours are not usually prolonged, and can be generalized (grand mal) or focal (Jacksonian). Emergency mangement is to lie the patient in the left lateral position to protect the airway, and to position the limbs to avoid injury. The most useful emergency medication for either grand mal or focal convulsions is a 10 mg diazepam enema given rectally. This can be repeated if necessary. The rectal route is quick and effective, and IV therapy is only necessary for the small proportion of cases where the seizure does not settle following rectal diazepam. If IV diazepam is used, it should be given as the emulsion (Diazemuls) to prevent venous irritation. Generalized myoclonic twitching can occur in the terminal phase (sometimes due to uraemia) and should be controlled, as it can be distressing to the relatives.

Oral anticonvulsants should be started to prevent the recurrence of convulsions, using phenytoin, sodium valproate or carbamazepine. Oral phenytoin, 300 mg daily, takes 4–7 days to reach therapeutic drug levels, and a slow IV infusion of phenytoin, 15 mg/kg, may be considered as a loading dose, which reaches therapeutic levels in a few hours. Measure plasma levels of drugs if convulsions are difficult to control.

A subcutaneous infusion of midazolam (Hypnovel) 15–80 mg per 24 hours can be used to control multifocal myoclonus or to prevent convulsions recurring. Midazolam is a short-acting water-soluble benzodiazepine, and it can be mixed with most of the commonly used drugs in a subcutaneous infusion, including diamorphine, cyclizine, haloperidol and methotrimeprazine.

Following a first convulsion relatives are usually frightened and need reassuring that convulsions due to brain tumours rarely affect mental function or prognosis.

Acute haemorrhage

Acute severe haemorrhage can occur in advanced malignancy due to the erosion of a major artery and may be a terminal event. Erosion of the arch of the aorta by a bronchogenic cancer can cause massive haemoptysis. Neck cancers can erode the carotid artery, and malignant nodes of the axilla or groin may erode the axillary artery or femoral artery.

With massive haemorrhage the best option is to stay with the patient, to provide companionship and a reassuring presence. This is better than rushing away to draw up drugs for injection, and leaving the patient alone. Avoid any attempts at resuscitation, which are not appropriate. The patient may die very quickly and the focus of concern then becomes the relatives and any others who may have witnessed the event (especially other patients – who can be forgotten in this situation, and who need attention and reassurance). A massive bleed is sometimes preceded by warning bleeds, and it is customary to have a red blanket (or, green surgical towels) available near such patients, which can be used to reduce the frightening visual impact of a lot of blood.

More commonly acute bleeds occur that may be quite heavy but are not immediately fatal. These can include haematemesis, rectal bleeding, vaginal bleeding or bleeding from surface malignant ulceration. Someone should stay with the patient who may be frightened. Emergency management involves controlling surface bleeding with direct pressure and controlling any distressing symptoms, especially breathlessness, with sedation. Rectal diazepam (Stesolid) 10 mg is very useful (and can be given per rectum or into a colostomy), or midazolam (Hypnovel) 5 mg can be given by intramuscular injection (into the deltoid muscle). Diamorphine will reduce dyspnoea and chlorpromazine 25–50 mg will reduce agitation. The dose of diamorphine will depend on the patient's regular dose of morphine, but if the patient is morphine-naive the initial dose will be 2.5–5 mg. Intramuscular injections may be effective, but the intravenous route may be necessary, because collapse of the peripheral circulation due to haemorrhagic shock makes intramuscular injections poorly absorbed. (Use a butterfly cannula so intravenous access can be retained in case further sedation is needed later.) The patient's pulse rate can be measured to monitor the situation, but repeated measurements of blood pressure are not indicated.

If a patient survives an episode of acute bleeding two questions may arise: how to prevent further bleeding and whether blood transfusion is indicated.

The control of bleeding is sometimes possible with radiotherapy, laser therapy, oral tranexamic acid 500 mg–1 g six hourly, or 1 per cent alum solutions for bladder washouts. It is important to note that gastro-intestinal haemorrhage in cancer patients is more commonly due to gastritis, peptic ulceration or haemorrhagic candida oesophagitis than due to malignancy.

Blood transfusion is usually only indicated if the source of the bleeding has been controlled, because otherwise transfusion simply tends to worsen the bleeding.

In conclusion, emergencies in palliative medicine are rare, but prompt recognition and correct management can greatly reduce the severity of the impact on both the patient and family. Managed badly, these emergencies can develop into a catastrophe for all concerned.

Notes and References

1. THOMAS, M.R. and ROBINSON, W.A. 'Oncological emergencies in primary care,' *Postgraduate Medicine*, 1985, **78**(4), 41–9.
2. FRANK, A.R. Spinal cord compression – an oncologic emergency, *Nebraska Medical Journal*, 1990, **75**(8), 230–5.
3. SIEGAL, T. and SIEGAL, T. 'Current considerations in the management of neoplastic spinal cord compression,' *Spine*, 1989, **14**(2), 223–8.
4. McNAMARA, P., MINTON, M. and TWYCROSS, R.G. 'Use of midazolam in palliative care,' *Palliative Medicine*, 1991, **5**, 244–9.
5. SIEGAL T. Surgical decompression of anterior and posterior malignant epidural tumours compressing the spinal cord: a prospective study. *Neurosurgery* 1985, **17**, 424–32.

Further reading

'Seminars in Oncology'. Oncological Emergencies, 1989, **16**(6), 461–594.

Other symptom challenges————

Andrew Hoy

This chapter discusses various symptoms which are frequently challenging to the clinician, but have not been considered elsewhere in this book. These symptom challenges include pruritus, sweating, weakness, haemorrhage, hiccup and the urinary symptoms of frequency and incontinence. The most fruitful approach is that of trying to define the pathophysiology before advising specific management. Only then can efficacy be maximized and toxicity minimized.

Pruritus

Causes

The neurological mechanisms underlying pruritus are similar to those for pain. Indeed pruritus is different from pain only in terms of intensity. Like pain it can be referred in a dermatomal distribution. It can also be modified by similar factors such as counter-irritation, cold, heat and vibration.

Causes may be due to local, systemic or psychogenic abnormalities. These categories are not mutually exclusive, for example hepatic disease may cause local irritation due to bile acid deposition. Thus both systemic and local measures can be helpful in management. Generally, pruritus from any cause is worse at night, with local heat and with the vasodilatatory effects of alcohol.

Local causes include dry, flaky skin which is very common in many seriously ill patients, especially if they are dehydrated; wet macerated skin that is compromised by pressure trauma and incontinence; local infection due to ulceration, scratching, scabetic infestation, poorly controlled diabetes; radiation skin reaction; intra-dermal tumour infiltration or 'en cuirasse' effect. Primary skin disorders such as eczema, psoriasis or dermatitis may be present.

Systemic causes which commonly affect terminally ill patients include renal failure; hepatic failure and cholestatic jaundice; carcinoid syndrome; thyroid disorders; iron-deficiency. Some cancers themselves are associated with pruritus, such as Hodgkin's and non-Hodgkin's lymphomas. Occasionally opioids have been the cause of centrally mediated itching. This does not happen commonly in chronic oral opioid administration.

Management

General measures include treating local infection, especially due to monilia. Dry skin can be improved by avoiding soap and long, hot baths, and applying simple emulsifying ointment or emollient creams. If the skin cannot be kept dry because of incontinence then barrier creams are helpful. If acute radiation reaction is symptomatic, then the skin should be kept completely dry, if practicable. Hydrocortisone cream (1 per cent) applied three times daily is helpful. If the skin is wet then it should be patted dry rather than rubbed, so minimizing desquamation.

Specific measures will treat correctable disease such as hyperthyroid-ism, myxoedema and iron deficiency. However, one of the most potent general causes of pruritus is cholestatic jaundice. This may well be due to inoperable obstruction of the biliary tree. In theory, if there is even minimal excretion of bile into the duodenum, then cholestyramine (Questran) given orally will prevent bile salt reabsorption via the entero-hepatic system. But this is rarely used as few patients find that they can tolerate the unpleasant taste, and the other side effects of nausea and flatulence. Pruritus associated with jaundice may respond dramatically to oral anabolic steroids in two or three days. Stanozolol 5–10 mg daily or mesterolone 25 mg tds have been used.

Pruritus associated with cancers such as lymphoma or leukaemia will respond to specific systemic anti-tumour therapy. However, when these diseases recur, it may no longer be feasible to give further systemic chemotherapy. Local, superficial radiotherapy may be helpful, particularly in the case of intradermal infiltration. A non-steroidal anti-inflammatory drug such as flurbiprofen 50 mg qds by mouth or simple aspirin is sometimes helpful for pruritus in lymphoma. Cimetidine has also been claimed to be helpful, even though the local pruritic effects are mediated by H_1 rather than H_2 receptors.

Although systemic anti-histamines are frequently promoted for pruritus, they are useful mainly when pruritus is due to allergy. There is often a cost in terms of sedation, which may be harder for an already debilitated patient to tolerate. Many preparations are available, and it is worth trying different ones to optimize treatment.[1,2]

Sweating

Causes

The temperature control mechanism is governed by the hypothalamus, with vasoconstriction and shivering as temperature raising measures, and sweating for temperature reduction. Various factors can alter the setting of thermosensitive neurones in the hypothalamus, including the presence of disseminated cancer and the secretion of tumour related humoral factors including active peptides in carcinoid syndrome. It is likely that tumour related substances also act peripherally on the sweat glands themselves.

Sweating is of significance because it may be drenching, uncomfortable and very disruptive, but it may also be a cause of fluid loss and hypovolaemia. An adult is capable of losing two litres of fluid per hour by sweating profusely. The majority of sweating is from eccrine glands under sympathetic cholinergic control. This explains why sympathetic damage results in lack of sweating of the affected distribution, and why excessive anticholinergic medication causes a dry, hot skin.

Management

The first priority is to diagnose and treat the remediable causes of sweating. If fever is present then specific infection should be identified if possible. If the cause of the fever is untreatable then it may be possible to lower it non-specifically with antipyretics and increased skin cooling by fan or damp sponging. Non-steroidal anti-inflammatory drugs (NSAID) such as naproxen 500 mg bd by mouth or simple aspirin, are effective antipyretics, but may also reduce sweating in apyrexial patients. This is almost certainly a direct hypothalamic effect.

Other more specific medication such as octreotide, initially 50 mcg bd subcutaneously, is useful in antagonising the effects of vaso-active peptides produced in carcinoid syndrome sweats. Corti-costeroids may suppress fever due to infection but they seem to be less effective than NSAIDs in suppressing the profuse sweating of apyrexial cancer patients. It is important to reduce or stop unnecessary diuretics in patients with sweating as they are at risk of symptomatic hypovolaemia and hypotension.[3]

Weakness

Causes

Weakness is the commonest of all symptoms in terminally ill patients.[4] At least 80 per cent of patients complain of it during the course of their illness. There are many causes of weakness in terminal malignant disease, and a careful assessment is necessary in order to offer appropriate treatment in the limited instances where symptomatic improvement will result.

Local or regional weakness may be due to either neuropathy, cord compression or myopathy. It may also be secondary to focal tenderness, so the presence or absence of pain is important. Peripheral nerve damage may be related to tumour, treatment, either surgery or radiotherapy, or non-metastatic carcinomatous neuropathy. A careful history must be elecited, of previous treatments, and whether there are specific features such as a myasthenic syndrome of weakness after exertion, or the rash of dermatomyositis. Proximal myopathy causing difficulty in standing up from a chair, is common after steroid administration. Spinal cord compression is nearly always associated with persistent spinal pain as well as the segmental weakness. Sensory and sphincter disturbances are often later symptoms. A prompt diagnosis is vital if there is to be a significant chance of functional improvement.

Generalized weakness may be due to medication, metabolic and electro-lyte disturbance, anaemia or tumour load. Medication induced weakness will often be associated with drowsiness. Drugs involved could be opioids, sedatives, anti-depressants or muscle relaxants, such as baclofen. Opioid weakness and lethargy usually resolve spontaneously after the first two or three days of a new dosage. However, altered renal and hepatic function may delay drug metabolism, so effectively prolonging the plasma half-life of many drugs.

Metabolic and electrolyte disturbances include hypercalcaemia, hypo-kalaemia (associated with diuretics and steroids), hyperglycaemia (steroids), hypoglycaemia (overdose of insulin due to increasing anorexia), and hyponatraemia (inappropriate anti-diuretic hormone (ADH) secre-tion). All of these disturbances can be treated and corrected, although some of them may recur. As well as the diagnosis, a decision as to the appropriateness of treatment must be made. This will usually include a knowledge of the patient's wishes and goals as well as the cost-benefit analysis of the treatment itself in terms of efficacy and toxicity.

Weakness associated with anaemia may be due to a variety of factors. Treatment induced anaemia may recover but recurrent anaemia with a leuco-erythroblastic picture is likely to be caused by widespread marrow infiltration. If the haemoglobin is less than 8 g/dl and if there are definite symptoms of anaemia palliative transfusion is worth considering.

Weakness due to 'tumour load' is multifactorial in origin and is a sign of progressive physical deterioration. It is commonly impossible to improve the symptom physically although psychological adjustment may be valuable and worthwhile.

Weakness may also be psychogenic. Depression is frequently under-diagnosed, and may mimic weakness. Anxiety and needless overactivity may cause exhaustion. Both diagnoses should be made positively and not by exclusion of other possibilities.

Management

Of the local causes of weakness, spinal cord compression is the most important to diagnose promptly.

Peripheral nerve damage may respond to local radiotherapy if the lesion is merely compressive. Similarly corticosteroids may relieve such compression also. However, established neuropathy responds much less promptly, if at all.

Drug induced weakness may be correctable with relative ease. Of the various metabolic and electrolyte disturbances, hypercalcaemia and inappropriate ADH secretion are the most treatable and are dealt with in the chapter on metabolic symptoms.

If weakness due to anaemia has responded to transfusion, then it may be worthwhile continuing to offer periodic palliation as the haemoglobin falls. However, if correction of the anaemia fails to provide improvement in weakness, then this should trigger a discussion with the patient as to the futility of further transfusion.

Depression and anxiety may respond to both psychological and pharmacological measures. Anti-depressants will take at least two weeks to produce an improvement in mood and energy. Care should be exercised when using tricyclic drugs to prescribe low doses initially if the patient is also taking opioids. Non-specific or 'tumour load' weakness may respond temporarily to dexamethasone 4 mg per day. If there is no benefit after seven days then the drug should be stopped.

Haemorrhage

Causes

Haemorrhage has either a local cause alone or occurs in association with systemic haemostatic failure.

Haemorrhage may be related to the underlying terminal illness such as local tumour necrosis, with the possibility of additional infection if there is ulceration. It may be due to the systemic effects of the disease such as thrombocytopaenia secondary to marrow replacement, haemostatic failure in liver disease or to disseminated intravascular coagulation.

Haemorrhage may also be caused by either local or systemic treatment effects. Local examples include non-steroidal anti-inflammatory drugs (NSAID) and corticosteroids causing haematemesis and hormone manipulations causing uterine bleeding. Systemic examples include depleted marrow reserve following chemotherapy, difficulty in stabilizing anticoagulant therapy in the face of metastatic liver disease or polypharmacy drug interactions.

Management

Haemorrhage may be a worrying reminder of persistent illness or rarely, if it is massive, it may be a frightening terminal event. Its management is covered in the chapter on Emergencies in Palliative Care.

Treatment for non-acute haemorrhage includes oncological, systemic and local approaches. In practice, radiotherapy is the most useful oncological treatment for tumour related haemorrhage. Palliative doses may be given to superficial tumours of the skin, breast, vulva, head and neck and lymphatic drainage areas. Bleeding from bronchial, gut and genito-urinary tumours often responds to a single fraction of radiation. Intra-cavity sources may be helpful for uterine and cervical bleeding. If previous radical radiotherapy has been given to the bleeding point, further radiotherapy is not absolutely contra-indicated, but will only be given with great caution by the radiotherapist concerned.

When radiotherapy is not possible enhanced coagulation with either systemic agents or local measures can be effective. Oral tranexamic acid 1 g tds or ethamsylate 500 mg qds can be considered. Tranexamic acid inhibits fibrinolysis, but is sometimes associated with gut toxicity. Ethamsylate increases platelet adhesion, is less toxic but also less effective. If disseminated intravascular coagulation is the cause of platelet consumption bleeding, then paradoxically, anticoagulation may need to be considered. In this case it is important to employ routine laboratory monitoring, as excessive treatment will cause unpleasant or dangerous bleeding itself.

Local measures include topical tranexamic acid and aluminium astringents. Sucralfate taken orally acts as a local astringent for bleeding points on the stomach mucosa. Bleeding from skin lesions will often respond to adrenalin (1 in 1000 solution) soaks. Similarly, visible bleeding points can be sealed by application of silver nitrate. Other tissue destructive agents such as laser, heat diathermy and cryotherapy are also useful in some circumstances.[7]

Hiccup

Causes

Hiccup is persistent spasm of the diaphragm causing discomfort and exhaustion. Hiccup is caused by irritation of any part of the complex reflex involved, which includes the vagus, phrenic and thoracic sympathetic nerves. Centrally there is no one centre coordinating hiccup, but rather an area of the brain stem including the respiratory centres, the hypothalamus and the reticular formation. Commonest causes in dying cancer patients involve gastric distension and diaphragmatic irritation. Men are affected more frequently than women.

Management

If the cause can be established, or surmised, then specific treatment can be given. Gastric distension or 'squashed stomach' may respond with a change to small frequent meals and a defoaming antiflatulent with an antacid, such as activated dimethicone and aluminium hydroxide (Asilone) qds. Metoclopramide 10 mg qds will aid gastric emptying. Another approach is to use peppermint oil as a carminative. The action is that of non-specific relaxation of intestinal smooth muscle. However, it does not have a defoaming action. As metoclopramide increases tone in the cardiac sphincter, and peppermint does the opposite it is illogical to give the two in combination. Chlorpromazine has been advocated for many years, and is effective by a central depressant effect. However, continued use causes unacceptable toxicity especially drowsiness. As a last resort, a single intra-venous injection of chlorpromazine 25 mg may be considered.

Many folk remedies for hiccup are helpful. These include swallowing granulated sugar, crushed ice or dry bread, drinking liqueur, a shock, or drinking from the wrong side of a cup. They all seem to have in common an element of pharyngeal stimulation. Twycross has suggested that this operates a pharyngeal 'gate-control' mechanism, thereby terminating the hiccup cycle.[8]

Urinary frequency and incontinence

Causes

Frequency and incontinence are closely related symptoms. Severe frequency may become incontinence, particularly at night or as the patient becomes generally weaker. Whether or not there is urinary tract tumour, infection is common in debilitated and elderly patients. There will frequently be an underlying factor which has allowed the infection to become established, such as obstruction, stasis, the presence of a catheter, or operative and parturition-related alteration of normal structure.

A vesical fistula involving the vagina or rectum will present as continual incontinence. A fistula is surprisingly easy to overlook if it is small. Infection is invariably present.

Frequency falling short of incontinence may be due to bladder irritation, in particular to detrusor instability. Agents causing detrusor hyperreflexia include infection, radiation reaction, chemotherapy such as cyclophosphamide and the presence of a catheter.

The neurological control of micturition may be disrupted by drugs such as antimuscarinics or by spinal cord compression. The neuropathic bladder is usually full, with overflow incontinence, where the sphincters cannot be relaxed and the detrusor will not contract.

Management

Infection should be treated, as it usually causes miserable symptoms but is rarely life-threatening. A suitable broad spectrum antibiotic will be needed for simple infections, but if a catheter is present and cannot be removed for a short time, then regular bladder washouts and urinary antiseptics are more appropriate. The reason is that a catheter will perpetuate infection despite antibiotics, but symptoms can be minimized with washouts.

If a fistula is present and the patient has some time to live, then urinary diversion may be considered. Conservative measures for fistulae are rarely completely effective, so a dirty, malodourous death is therefore probable without diversion.

Bladder spasm or detrusor hyperreflexia often respond to antimuscarinics, such as oxybutynin 2.5–5 mg qds or to propantheline. Toxicity is that of any atropine-like drug, and may be unacceptable. If the incontinence persists despite an indwelling catheter and the urine is 'bypassing', this usually indicates blockage or spasm, rather than a catheter which is too small. The correct management of spasm is to replace with a smaller catheter and give oxybutynin.

Catheterization is inevitable in spinal cord compression. It may be a blessing in patients with a contracted bladder due to repeated infection, surgery or radiotherapy. Many patients as they become weaker have increasing difficulty in responding promptly enough to a call to micturate. This is accentuated at night. Catheterization can sometimes be delayed by the alternative of nocturnal desmopressin intranasally 10–20 micrograms to cause nocturnal retention. Care should be exercised in the elderly patient with cardiac or renal disease.[9]

References

1. AMLOT P. Itch. (1989) In: Walsh TD (ed.) *Symptom Control*, Oxford: Blackwell Scientific Publications pp. 285–94.
2. TWYCROSS R.G. (1990) Symptom Control in Terminal Cancer. Oxford: Sobell Publications. 32.
3. AMLOT P. (1989) Fever and Sweats. In: Walsh TD (ed.) *Symptom Control*, Oxford: Blackwell Scientific Publications 195–202.
4. DUNLOP G.M. (1990) A study of the relative frequency and importance of gastrointestinal symptoms and weakness in patients with far ⁺advanced cancer: student paper. *Palliative Medicine*, **4**: 37–43.
5. GRANT R. (1989) Nonmetastatic manifestations of malignancy: neurological. *Palliative Medicine*, **3**: 181–8.
6. REGNARD C, MANNIX K. (1992) Weakness and fatigue in advanced cancer – a flow diagram. *Palliative Medicine*, **6**: 253–6.
7. REGNARD C, MAKIN W. (1992) Management of bleeding in advanced cancer – a flow diagram. *Palliative Medicine*, **6**: 74–8.
8. TWYCROSS R.G. (1992) Personal communication.
9. REGNARD C, MANNIX K. (1991) Urinary problems in advanced cancer – a flow diagram. *Palliative Medicine*, **5**: 344–8.

Physiotherapy in palliative medicine

Betty O'Gorman

The physiotherapist's role in the treatment of patients suffering from terminal malignancy is to improve, where possible, their quality of life, regardless of their prognosis, by maximizing their functional abilities and independence and to help gain relief from distressing symptoms. Many symptoms such as pain, dyspnoea, lymphoedema, general weakness and anxiety can be influenced, minimized, and at times alleviated by physiotherapy. Nevertheless, many patients labelled 'terminal' miss the opportunity to receive appropriate physiotherapy, and this may lead not only to loss of mobility but also to loss of independence and of morale.

The physiotherapist needs to work in the multidisciplinary team in order to minimize the demands and stresses that are part of this work. She has a responsibility to make an initial assessment of the patient's condition and capabilities and to pass this back to the team, as well as constantly to monitor, review and update her assessment as the patient's condition alters.

It is necessary for the physiotherapist to have an understanding of counselling techniques and a knowledge of the process of grief and loss and the patient's reactions to their disease. It is not always the ultimate grief and loss for a life that is coming to an end that has to be faced, but the ongoing losses such as the loss of the function of a limb, the loss of independent mobility, or the inability to coordinate one's body.[1]

Physical management

It is only primarily because of good medical symptom control that physiotherapy can be effectively practised in terminal care. Efficient physiotherapy will be sensitive to the patient's needs and should be able to maximize each individual's potential. A patient's goals are often simple and short term.

General principles of physiotherapy

In all treatments, the following essential guidelines should apply:

- Commence treatment as soon as posible.
- Consider the patient totally.
- Consider the safety of the patient.
- Do not make false promises.
- Be aware at all times that inappropriate, vigorous physiotherapy could cause an increase in the patient's symptoms with resulting distress.
- Be aware of the patient's own observations of his symptoms – they could indicate a change in his physical condition.
- Do not make a patient's deterioration obvious to them by their physiotherapy: do not take the patient off treatment while they are aware – scale their treatment down to their capabilities.
- Be prepared to listen to the patient.
- Consider the relatives and involve them in the patient's treatment and goals and share with them the patient's achievements.

Treatment of symptoms

Pain

Pain can be experienced by the terminally ill patient for many different reasons. As before, medication will be the major factor in the control of pain. However, physiotherapy has a substantial role to play in its control.

Some pain is the direct result of a cancerous lesion, e.g. as in bone or soft tissue, pathological fractures, traumatic fractures, neuropathic or neurogenic pain. Pain may be physical from non-malignant conditions such as osteoarthritis or rheumatoid arthritis, and indirect pain can also be experienced from joint stiffness, muscle spasm, pressure or position. As well as physical pain, there may be components of emotional, social or spiritual pain.

For all patients who are unable to move their limbs normally, regular routine exercise, both preventative and restorative, needs to be given. In order to relieve muscle spasm, maintain joint range and prevent undue pressure, regular exercise is given by the physiotherapist.

In all cases the position of the patient needs to be considered so that both local and general support is given to the body in as good a functional and anatomical position as possible. By offering good positioning and thereby aiding comfort – whether the patient be in bed, wheelchair or armchair – pain can be minimized. Pain in the chest is not necessarily relieved by physiotherapy but discomfort can often be helped by the measures given above.

The use of custom-made cushions and pillows, as well as the judicious use of slings and collars, will support limbs and the head and the neck. At times lively splints (i.e. those that allow specific movements) and orthoses are needed to support limbs. Specialized beds need to be considered in conjunction with the nursing staff.

Joint pain/nerve pain can be helped by the informed choice and use of radiant heat pads, ice, and – if metastases are not present – ultrasound.

Pain associated with bony secondaries can often be controlled at rest but may not be so on weight-bearing and attempted mobilization. The use of transcutaneous electrical nerve stimulation (TENS) can alleviate this pain and allow the patient to mobilize with carefully monitored weight bearing. TENS may be helpful for chronic pain that is neurogenic or is well localized, and sometimes relieves pruritis.

Anxiety is likely to exacerbate many symptoms, particularly pain, and the teaching of general relaxation may be helpful in alleviating this.

Dyspnoea

Dyspnoea may be present on its own or with an underlying chest infection. Dyspnoea itself is an anxiety-provoking condition. The patient will almost certainly be on the relevant drugs. The physiotherapist will assist in the positioning and general postural support of the patient, so aiding local as well as general relaxation. Breathing exercises – lateral costal and disphragmatic – will be taught in order to maximize the patient's vital capacity and to minimize the 'work' of breathing.

It is often beneficial to teach the patient formal relaxation techniques, especially shoulder girdle relaxation, on a one-to-one basis, and by using a relaxation tape the patient can practise on their own and hopefully use the tape at times of stress so that their dyspnoea will not increase. The patient's exercise tolerance needs to be monitored and influenced by encouraging them to mobilize within their capacity, to stop short if becoming breathless and regain control before proceeding, and to undertake one activity at a time, i.e. not to walk *and* talk. It is often beneficial to teach some positions of 'ease' for a dyspnoeic attack. Should the patient not be able to mobilize because of severe breathlessness, then the provision of an electric wheelchair will be of benefit.

If the patient is suffering from a chest infection, besides appropriate medication an attempt can be made to expel secretions from the lung fields. Postural drainage is inappropriate to clear secretions from the chest of a dying patient. It is usually sufficient for the patient to be treated in alternate-side lying with massage procedures of light clapping and vibration on expiration. Efficient coughing will also need to be taught. When treating the dyspnoeic patient, plenty of time needs to be allowed; the calm, unhurried approach is of great importance.

When a patient with either chest pathology and/or infections is referred for treatment, the physiotherapist needs to know whether the treatment is to be active or palliative, otherwise they may well question their own efficiency. If the physiotherapy treatment is active, the patient will be on an antibiotic and possibly also a mucolytic agent, and nebulized drugs themselves can be active or palliative. If the treatment is to be palliative there will certainly be no antibiotic and there is not the same pressure to disturb the sleeping patient. Sometimes what begins as an active treatment changes to a palliative one if the patient does not improve. Physiotherapy will continue as long as the patient is being helped. If secretions in the lung fields become a problem, causing distress and noisy respiration, then appropriate medication will be given rather than physiotherapy.

Oedema

Oedema may be postural, lymphoedematous, cardiac, renal or venous, so appropriate diagnosis is essential. Postural oedema is often found in the patient with weakened muscles or paralysed limbs. It can be influenced by the provision of an elastic support, such as shaped Tubigrip or elastic support hose. As well as elastic supports, massage will often be of benefit as well as limbs being supported and not allowed to be dependent. It is helpful to take standard measurements weekly in order to monitor the reduction in the oedema.

Lymphoedema secondary to cancer is more difficult to influence and manage. The British Lymphology Interest Group (BLIG) have stated the following minimum standards of care:

1. Skin care.
2. External support/compression in the form of hosiery.
3. Exercise programme.
4. Self-massage.

(The last of these, however, may be inappropriate in palliative care.)

Out-patients can be offered a thrice-weekly treatment of massage, multi-layered compression bandaging and exercise for a two–three week period. At times it is appropriate to admit the patient for a concentrated daily treatment programme, as above, in order to attempt to influence the oedema. Following a reduction or containment in the size of the limb, an elastic compression garment will need to be provided and worn constantly in order to contain its size. In addition, a pneumatic compression pump may be used. Advice on the care of the skin and exercise must be given. For the terminally ill patient, it may be that treatment will oscillate between bandaging and a compression garment, and at times a combination of both in order to contain, if not reduce, the swelling as the condition deteriorates.

If lymphorrhoea is a problem, it can often be alleviated by the multi-layered compression bandaging. If there is much more leakage from the skin, some form of plastic-backed padding will have to be used in order to keep the bandaging dry.

The regime of treatment is complex and the reader is referred to specialist texts[2,3,4] for details.

Musculo-skeletal

General weakness

General weakness is often caused by a combination of factors and events. The disease process itself may cause weakness because of the inability to eat properly, prolonged bed rest or immobilization, which in themselves can lead to generalized weakness. The patient may not have been encouraged by professional carers to maintain their mobility, and at times over-anxious caring families may contribute to the patient's becoming inactive and therefore weakened.

For patients who are generally weak and whose mobility and independence is threatened, a simple scheme of active leg exercises and the provision of an appropriate walking aid may be all that is required. If the patient has actually lost his mobility through weakness, then appropriate measures will be as before, but a little more time will perhaps be needed to restore the patient's independence.

It is often best to mobilize a patient as soon as possible. When quadriceps contract against gravity, standing with assistance (if necessary) will be attempted, followed by walking. When the patient is mobile, attention can be paid to any other weak areas and they can then be exercised accordingly. The use of a rollator walking frame, especially for the generally weak patient or those with pathology in the arms, thorax or upper spine, is preferable to a walking frame. This will allow the normal walking pattern to continue without the need to lift a frame.

Those patients who remain only just mobile need encouragement from a physiotherapist, sometimes a scheme of active leg exercises and possibly assessment for a walking aid. Any scheme of active exercise that the patients are asked to repeat on their own needs to be written down because of poor short-term memory and also so that the relatives may be involved.

General or local stiffness

Prolonged inactivity can lead to general stiffness, especially as patients often suffer from malignant multiple pathology. There may also be associated non-malignant multiple pathology.

Patients suffering from both general and potential local stiffness need regular exercises. Any limb that is paralysed or that the patient is unable to move unaided needs to have regular preventative exercise. Primary or secondary bone tumours may result in a pathological fracture needing operative repair, and will need appropriate exercise in order to maximize mobility and maintain independence.

Exercise is also needed for any non-malignant condition that is present, e.g. osteoarthritic joints or spine, rheumatoid arthritis, neurological conditions – multiple sclerosis or previous polio – amputations, etc.

If a patient presents with a stiff joint, then the appropriate manual therapy techniques, i.e. the 'gentler' procedures, may be used, in conjunction with the use of heat, ice, or (if there are no metastases present) ultrasound on the affected joint.

Aids to daily living (ADLs)/wheelchairs

The early provision of ADLs such as rollator walking frames, light touch switches for call systems and television, and adapted cutlery will aid the patient's independence. When walking is an exercise rather than a means of getting about, the provision of a self-propelled or electric wheelchair will offer some degree of independence.

Further reading

1. McATEER, M. 'Some aspects of grief in physiotherapy,' *Physiotherapy – Journal of the Society of Physiotherapy*, 1989, **75**(1), 55–8.
2. REGNARD, C., BADGER, C. and MORTIMER P. 'Lymphoedema – advice on treatment', Beaconsfield, Bucks, Beaconsfield Publishers.
3. GRAY, R. 'The management of limb oedema in patients with advanced cancer', *Physiotherapy – Journal of the Society of Physiotherapy*, 1987, **73**(10), 504–6.
4. BADGER, C and TWYCROSS, R. *Management of Lymphoedema – Guidelines*, Sir Michael Sobell House, Churchill Hospital, Oxford, 1988.

Psychosocial dimension of palliation

Barbara Monroe

> Cancer can affect a family in much the same way as it affects a body – causing deterioration if left untreated.
>
> Colin Murray Parkes

Dying patients are facing loss at every level; physical health, independence, career and status, normal family life, predictability and future plans, motivation and meaning. They will experience a draining diminution in their self-confidence and in their belief in their ability to control their own lives. These losses will be experienced in parallel by their families and carers. Everyone will express their grief through a powerful, unfamiliar and frightening mixture of confused emotions including shock, denial, anxiety, anger, guilt and sadness. In the face of such pressures both patient and family may retreat into a conspiracy of fear and denial with individuals holding on to agonizing burdens. Frightened people distance themselves from one another and may find themselves isolated just when they most need support and intimacy. Professionals can impose further losses on patients and families through their own poor or uncertain communication. Patients and their families have similar needs; to receive clear, factual information at a speed they find acceptable, to express and share their feelings, to explore spiritual pain – 'Why me, Why him, Why now?' They need to consider their options and to exercise choice, reasserting their own sense of dignity and self-worth by making decisions and regaining control wherever possible. The purpose of this chapter is to examine how professionals can assist patients and their families to achieve these objectives.

Why family?

A terminally ill patient is not just an individual with problems and symptoms, but a member of a family whose reactions interlock with his. It is therefore important to make the patient *within* his family the unit of care. Understanding the family can help in understanding the patient and his pain. Making the family part of the caring team offers the possibility of encouraging and using their strengths and resources rather than simply cataloguing the difficulties they face. The patient and family also belong to a community within society and this entire social network also contains resources that can be marshalled to help meet the consequences of the patient's illness and death. Finally, and most importantly, good palliative care includes the dimension of preventive health care. The way professionals help a family to manage the illness and death of one of its members can have a profound impact on both their health in bereavement and their capacity to cope with a whole variety of future crises.

What is the family?

The family is a network of attachments and belonging, a complex system that changes over time. It has a past and a future that exert pressures on the present and its exists within a social and cultural context. In palliative care the term 'family' means more than a blood relationship with the patient. It refers to those relationships that are significant for the patient and to other networks in which the patient is significant. Thus friends and neighbours may be more important than biological links and a diagnosis of terminal disease will reverberate not only amongst the biological family but also, for example, amongst the patient's work colleagues, his fellow members of the squash club and his church congregation.

What are the problems?

Over time families develop patterns of relating to one another, adopting certain fairly fixed roles and following accepted codes of behaviour in order to fulfil the tasks they face and cope with the problems that confront them. Families create a sort of balance for themselves, even if to outsiders their system appears unstable. In some families for example, it is normal to argue all the time and such regular evidence of apparent conflict does not in fact imply impending disintegration. However the crisis of terminal illness brings particular pressures to bear on the family which may threaten its balance.

The medical journey that ends with terminal care will probably have created a breakdown in communication in the patient's family. The patient and family will have seen a series of different professionals who will have told them all different things at different times. The transition to palliative care will itself have created uncertainty and ambiguity. These factors will all make communication difficult and will all add to the feelings of helplessness already engendered by the patient's physical deterioration.

Both patient and family will also be experiencing social isolation as friends and neighbours retreat, uncertain of what to say or do. Comforting routines of interaction at work and leisure will be shattered as the illness progresses. Familiar roles will have to be renegotiated and the panic of assuming new roles dealt with. A young dying mother may have the pain of relinquishing some of her parenting role to a visiting mother-in-law, who senses resentment and feels powerless to address it. In turn the patient's husband is both packing lunch boxes for the first time and considering the frightening future of life as a single parent with all its emotional and practical problems. His dying wife is worrying too, about his motivation and abilities; can she trust him with her children?

On top of all these changes everyone will be experiencing personal confusion as they face the anguish of painful and conflicting feelings: 'I'm so sad my husband is dying. I'm so angry that he's leaving me with three children and no money.' Both family and patient will want to protect themselves and one another from further hurt. It may begin to seem safer to avoid talking about difficult emotions. In addition the loyalty that most families engender can make it hard to express sadness or to plan for a future without the patient. In the face of such separating forces the task of the professional should be to keep people together wherever possible.

Professionals and families

The families that professionals in palliative care meet are anxious and confused. Family anxiety is often mirrored in the professional carers who may be frightened about how to respond to the emotional agendas between patient and family and worried that seeing them together will get out of control, make things worse or simply take too long. However what is often needed is a shift in attitude rather than an increase in resources. Professionals do not own the patient and family nor are they personally responsible for solving their problems. Empowerment, acceptance and self-awareness are important components in the appropriate set of professional attitudes. Families come in all shapes and sizes and professionals must avoid judging them against their own internal vision of what behaviour is normal and appropriate in 'the family'.

It is important for professionals in palliative care to work within a team culture. Patients and families choose who they want to talk to and from whom they find help most acceptable. It is often easier to have a difficult conversation with a family if two colleagues are present to support one another or if someone is available to talk to following such a meeting. However coordination of the professional team visiting the family is vital if they are not to be swamped and confused. Too little help reduces their options, too much help delivered by a whole range of concerned and worried professionals can leave the family exhausted and deskilled, convinced that the problems are beyond their power to resolve. The mother of a dying child spoke of the time absorbed by the visits and sometimes conflicting advice of the GP, the district nurse, the Macmillan nurse, health visitor, hospital psychologist and so on, and said despairingly, 'I need to do it *my* way.'

Professionals should set against their anxieties an appreciation of how much they can help the patient and family to achieve, even within a very limited time scale. The heightened emotion accompanying potential loss will make the family more open to interventions and to change. Most families want to say important things to one another, to be involved in patient care, to plan for the future, both short and long term; it is just that they do not know how to begin and what to say. In order to make decisions and to recognize the need and the opportunity to complete unfinished business everyone will need information about what usually happens and about what their options are. For example what services might be available to support the patient's return home or what responses to expect from a bereaved teenager. The presence of a concerned professional can help to generate safety and confidence in a situation that feels out of control. The power of one meeting in which everyone hears the same information at the same time cannot be overestimated. Most families will manage well with just a little help. Asking to meet the patient and family together models openness and the possibility of truth as something to be shared rather than to be feared. The issues are already present in the family and their capacity for action may be released by naming them. The dying mother who does not want to be a burden on her daughter but is desperate to go home, her daughter's guilt and anxieties about her own responsibilities and commitments, if shared openly, are the material from which effective compromises can be made.

Assessment

A clear assessment is vital to identify properly what the patient and the family's needs are and how best to meet them. Such an assessment will have four main perspectives; the individual, the family, their physical and their social resources.

The individual

It is necessary to discover something about the experiences and personality of the patient before his illness in order to establish how his life has changed since the illness. What was his job and its satisfactions? How does he view his family? Who is important to him within it? Who does he worry about most, and who or what is currently supporting him? What are the implications of the illness for the patient? Does it leave him with any practical or emotional unfinished business? How does he view the illness; is it, for example, a release or a punishment? How has he dealt with stress and crisis in the past? Enquiries must also be made about the patient's aims; for example, does he want to attend a daughter's wedding, seek some relief for an exhausted, caring wife, want to die at home or in a hospital or hospice?

The family

The patient must be placed within the context of his family and some attempt made to understand how it usually works, the normal patterns of support, conflict and communication.

Consideration of the following questions may assist an understanding of the impact of terminal illness on family life.

- What roles does the patient usually play in the family, both practical and emotional? Is he for example the wage-earner, the chief worrier, the peacemaker? What gaps will be left? Who in the family might move or be moved to fill them in? For example teenagers are sometimes unfairly expected to fill a dying parent's roles. Also remember that in a desire to protect the patient, the family may be prematurely removing roles from him, further depriving his life of meaning.
- How do the personal histories of other family members affect the patient? A husband who watched his father stand helplessly by as his mother died in pain will approach his own wife's death with increased anxiety.
- At what stage in their lives are family members? The husband of a dying woman may be frightened about a lonely retirement, her mother may feel guilty that her daughter is dying before her, her teenage son may be anxious that his father will try to keep him at home for company. If left unexplored such differences in life-cycle perspectives can reduce the family's ability to communicate.
- How have the family coped with previous crises? They will have developed problem solving mechanisms. They may need putting back in touch with these and reminding that they are survivors.
- What other changes are the family facing at the moment; a redundancy, a wedding or pregnancy, a rebellious teenager, a change of job or accommodation?
- What are the common family myths? All families create stories about themselves and their members that can have the force of rules restricting change and growth, 'Men in the Jones' family never cry. Martin is a difficult and uncommunicative teenager.' It is important to understand these stereotypes in order to challenge them effectively.
- What is the effect of the illness on any intimate partnership? One of the impacts of terminal illness on a couple is the loss of a future in which to put things right. Quiescent dissatisfactions or quarrels may suddenly loom large. The narrowing social circle of the patient may place enormous pressures on a relationship that relied on emotional distance and now finds itself too close for comfort. Furthermore, many partnerships derive their success from bringing together different but mutually satisfying emotional cultures. The objective, practical, but emotionally inhibited husband may have many needs successfully met by his warm, scatty outgoing

wife, whilst meeting her needs for order and security. However this happy partnership may founder in the uncharted waters of terminal illness as the dying wife wants to talk to her husband about her feelings and he resists, never having developed the skills and confidence to do so.

- Are there other vulnerable individuals within the family such as dependent elderly or disabled relatives or young children? Terminal illness may be the final burden that topples a delicately balanced system of nurture and support.
- It is not usually possible to support everyone in a family. Who is the key person who, if helped, will be able to support the others?

Physical resources

An assessment must include the family's physical resources as unmet physical needs may become their biggest concern. The family who are threatened with eviction for rent arrears because their dying father cannot work will find it difficult to concentrate on other needs. A proper financial assessment is vital. A washing machine for the exhausted carer of a patient with night sweats may be of more value than extra counselling support. It is essential to evaluate what aids to daily living are available, what housing adaptations might be required and to consider who will provide them. Sometimes the most effective work for a family may be to introduce them to other agencies and to act as their advocate. The timely provision of a day centre place, meals on wheels, domestic help, a nursery place, may avoid or delay the requirement for inpatient care.

Social resources

The family themselves must be looked at within the context of their community and social network. Further consideration of the importance of understanding the family's ethnic, cultural and religious background and their impact on the patient and his illness will be found in David Oliviere's section in Chapter 4 on the cross-cultural principles of care. Enquiries should be made about formal and informal helping systems available to the family within their community, such as schools, churches, neighbours and employers. Families often already have access to people who can help them but may need outside help to identify or mobilize this, for example the scoutmaster who has a good relationship with their child, a sympathetic teacher, the church group who can offer a rota of care, the employer who would like to offer financial assistance.

Meeting with families

The conclusion from a proper assessment may be that the patient and family have adequate coping mechanisms and are well supported within their community. They need only a regular opportunity to hear information and to ask questions together. Doing nothing may also be the right decision in less satisfactory circumstances. It is not possible to solve all the problems of the past during the period of a terminal illness. The patient or family may need their defences against a long history of relationship difficulties and emotional pain. The sensitive provision of physical care may be sufficient to maintain dignity, where an attempt to solve misunderstandings or isolation may be feared and resented. It is, however, always proper to offer the opportunity for further help, to accept its rejection quietly and to remember that people sometimes change their minds.

Patients and families also need to be heard as individuals as well as having the opportunity to talk together. Meeting family members on a one-to-one basis may well be an important prelude to work within the whole family. Individual difficulties and perspectives may need to be understood before their communication and potential resolution is sought within a wider group. For example, the elderly wife of a dying husband may need to express her fears of waking to find him dead beside her before she can listen to his urgent desire to return home from hospital. Further discussion of individual communications will be found in Chapter 2.

Helping families to communicate can achieve very rapid results. The cliché of the deathbed reconciliation is a real image. For example, exploiting the shared love of a dying parent can help to restore relationships between family members who have not spoken to one another for years and help the patient to see some meaning in his death, as well as releasing additional practical resources to cope with the illness. Late is always better than never. Children told of the terminal nature of a parent's illness only twenty-four hours before the death will be helped by having been involved, by being judged significant enough to be included in something of such importance to the family.

Preparation

Preparation and structure help professionals to feel confident when meeting with family groups. Confidence is catching. Five minutes deliberation before a meeting will be amply repaid. Consider:

- What do you know about individual objectives within the family?
- What do you want to achieve?
- What could go wrong? What would be your emergency strategy if the 'worst' did happen?
- How do the family see you? Have they met you or one of your profession before? What were their impressions? Do you need to make a clear or alternative statement of your role?
- Who should attend the meeting? Which family members should be there? Should the patient? At the start or later? Do you need a colleague? It is often helpful to work in pairs, for example a doctor and a social worker. The doctor might begin with a factual overview

of the illness and its history, the social worker then has a platform from which to explore the family's differing responses. The absence of important members needs mentioning early on to avoid their silent 'shadow' dominating proceedings.

- Who should start the session and how? Think of two or three specific phrases to get the meeting started with the right tone and direction.
- Be aware of your language, adapt your style to that of the family. Try to pick up and use any key words that you are aware of in the family. Try to avoid judgemental vocabulary. It is difficult to behave positively towards someone defined as 'hysterical', whereas 'out of control' implies some responsibility on the part of the professional to help them regain it.

Structure the session

You are in charge. You have the right to enforce your rules. Well-defined boundaries make people feel safe. Make it clear that everyone has the right to speak without interruption and to speak for themselves. You may want to suggest that people change where they are sitting in order to facilitate discussion. At home, it is appropriate to request firmly that the television be turned off 'as we are going to be talking about some important issues and I will find it easier to concentrate on what you say'. Remember that time boundaries are important. 'We've got about half an hour together today.' It may seem off-putting to let people know how long you can spend with them, but in practice it often helps them to know how much emotional string they have time to unravel. Reliability, turning up when you say you will, and undivided attention are much more significant factors in developing trust and communication than the length of time spent. Equally it implies respect and returns responsibility to the family to give them a warning about the approaching end of a meeting. 'We've got about five minutes left now – what else is there that it is important for you to say?'

The role of the professional

Families are not just a group of individuals and it is important not to conduct a series of one-to-one interviews with the professional at the centre doing all the work. The family should do most of the talking. The aim is to help them to solve their problems in a way they feel reasonably comfortable with, not to sort everything out for them. Externally imposed solutions never stick and you will not always be there. If the family find balance only with and in your presence, you have become part of the problem rather than helping them find an answer. A neutral attitude on the part of the professional is important. It is not necessary to approve of what people say or do, but they do need to know individually that the feelings behind their words or actions are understood.

The professional working with families has three main tasks; to ensure a clear and adequate flow of information, to acknowledge emotional pain and facilitate its expression and sharing, and to help people discover and act upon what is important to them. The following points describe some of the methods that may assist in achieving these tasks.

Find out how the family define the problem

Use direct, open-ended questions:

- 'What is the worst thing at the moment?' This is probably different for everyone and it will help them to begin to understand each other's perspectives.
- 'What worries you most about the illness?'
- 'What do you want most from your husband/wife?'
- 'What is helping most at present? What else would help you cope?'
- 'What else do you need to know about your illness/treatment?'
- 'Do you have questions about where things are likely to go from here?'

Adopt an open style

Family reaction will provide a guide to pace, also check on it directly: 'Does this feel comfortable? Are we going too fast?' Help the family to explain themselves to one another by asking them to clarify their stories and feelings: 'It sounds as if. . ., Are you saying. . ., Can you help me to understand that a bit better, Can you tell me a bit more about that? Let me see if I can sum up. . .' Do not worry about always finding the 'right thing' to say, it will prevent you listening accurately. Pay attention to your 'gut reaction'. If you get it wrong, say so; mistakes openly acknowledged are usually forgiven. 'I'm sorry, I obviously got that wrong, can we start again?' If you do not know what to say, say so, everyone will be struggling with uncertainty and it will help to acknowledge this. Use simple 'feeling' words, 'sad, angry, frightened', they help people to say difficult things.

Normalize, anticipate fears and problems

Try to remind the family that they have managed difficult situations in the past. 'Have you coped with that before? How? Have you felt that before – when?' Reinforce their achievements in the current crisis: 'You have helped the children enormously by involving them. I know it's been hard.' Some problems will require information on a practical level, others will be helped by the professional assuming their potential existence: 'A lot of people worry about/find that/wonder whether. . .' It's hard to say what you want to when you're visiting someone in hospital.' Recognize and permit differences in the family: 'The illness will be affecting you all differently . . . John wants to go off on his own, Peter wants you all to stay together and talk.' Also point out similarities, 'The important thing is that you all love your Mum and you want to do the best for her.' Stating the obvious aloud can be an enormous relief: 'I think what everyone in this family is worrying about is how you will manage when Mum isn't here to look after you all.' Sometimes little else is necessary from the professional. It is important when enough has been said and when to go and perhaps leave the family alone with their tears.

Encourage change

Define the problem in a positive form, then you can attempt to challenge it. 'You love your children and you want to protect them. I wonder if they perhaps sense that something serious is happening?' Help people to see things slightly differently by offering them a safer framework within which to work. 'It is always right to hope for the best, but planning for the worst creates a safety net which you can then forget about.' 'It is like taking out an insurance policy; it does not mean you want or expect to die, just that if the worst happened those you love would be looked after.' Try to offer people a dignified way of standing down, giving up a particular hope does not mean giving up all hope: 'I can see that it is important to you to look on the bright side. Is there ever a moment . . . ?'

If you want people to act differently make them practise the changes while you are present. 'He won't listen to me . . .' 'Then talk to him now.' Help families, and couples in particular, to focus and agree on concrete specific changes, preferably around what to start, rather than stop, doing. 'You find his visits very supportive – you wonder if he could manage more . . .', is more likely to be successful than 'she wonders why you can't come to see her more often'. Ensure that couples hear what one another feel and want by picking out important sentences, 'Did you hear that. . . ? He said. . .'

External advisers can help the family and patient to explore what it is reasonable to expect from one another and to negotiate changing roles. 'Your wife needs your permission to take a break.' 'He needs you as a wife and friend – you can't be if you're always exhausted by nursing.' Families will have experienced a dramatic change in what is achievable and may need help to adjust expectations, to segment problems and to focus on one or two difficulties at a time that can be tackled in a chaos that threatens to overwhelm. Successful action depends on realistic goals.

Stand back

Try to notice what is going on in the family, *how* they talk to each other as well as what is being said. Share your perceptions with the family. Do not get too obsessed with the detail of history taking. Emotional truth matters more than unravelling the minutiae of past relationships which can act as a distraction to the family. Bring unspoken feelings into play: 'You say you are alright, but you look so very tense.' Gently challenge non-involvement and try to recognize over-protection or conflict.

Anger within the family can be very threatening to professionals. It is necessary to avoid a defensive posture and to allow its expression. It often represents the energy people need to take action. It is helpful to name and recognize anger, 'Something has happened to make you very angry,' and then to remember that it usually masks more painful feelings. Naming these feelings, 'It sounds very lonely too', can provide the necessary pivot for the meeting to begin to address the sources of conflict and for family members to recognize their shared anguish. Anger is frightening for the family too. The professional may need to set limits either by using a firm, slow tone of voice, or by suggesting stopping the meeting for a period 'while we all cool down'.

Allow silence and stay with the feeling of the family without making premature attempts to make it all better. You cannot put things right and an uncomfortable silence can represent important thinking and feeling time. It can also generate the emotional depth and tension sometimes necessary to achieve change. Take risks, say the unsayable, you will not be putting ideas into people's heads and you may help them to concentrate on what can be achieved. Dare to challenge and to confront. For example, to a husband and dying wife who are bickering over a relative 'Is this really how you want things to be?' Challenging discrepancies between what people actually do and what they say they want to achieve, can help them to clarify their problems and find new ways of thinking and behaving.

Collusion represents a particular challenge. It is essential to respect and validate the reasons why family members want to protect the patient and to explore their fears. 'How has he taken bad news in the past? How do you think he will react? Most patients know most of the truth.' Find out what it is costing the relative not to tell the patient and suggest a talk with the patient to assess their view of how things are going. Then stand firm. You will not lie to the patient, nor will you force the truth upon him.

Summarize

It helps to create a sense of security if the meeting ends with a review of what has been said in terms of both feeling and content; where the meeting started and what has now been decided, what important themes have emerged. It may be valuable to rehearse how other people not present will be informed of any changes.

Case study

This case study is intended to illustrate the impact of terminal illness on the family and methods of intervention. It also demonstrates the value of the family tree. Family trees can provide:

- A clear, shorthand, easily updated recording tool.
- A visual image of gaps and losses past, present and anticipated, roles and patterns of communication.
- A safe, non-threatening and unintrusive way of gathering information about the family.
- A visual image of security; who has died, but who remains, especially for children.

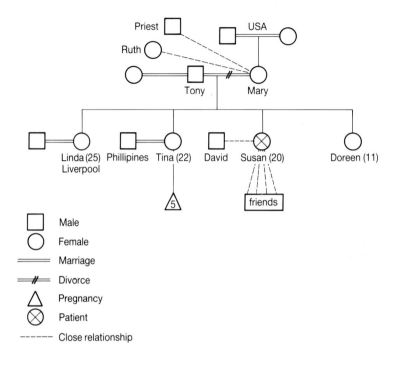

Priest
USA
Ruth
Tony   Mary

Linda (25) Phillipines Tina (22) David Susan (20)   Doreen (11)
Liverpool

5

friends

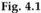 Male
Female
Marriage
Divorce
Pregnancy
Patient
Close relationship

Fig. 4.1

Introduction

Susan was a twenty year-old girl with a sarcoma of the right thigh, chest secondaries and involvement of the pericardium. She knew that she had cancer and that the disease had metastasized. She had been diagnosed two and a half years previously and had received four lots of surgery and radiotherapy following diagnosis and triple recurrence. She was referred to the hospice home care team by the treating hospital with a problem of severe, sporadic chest pain. The possibility of further chemotherapy had been raised with Susan but not fully discussed. The team secured the general practitioner's consent to their involvement.

Assessment

Individual

Susan wanted to find someone who would talk openly to her about chemotherapy and its prospects. She said that she was tired but could not give up for her mother's sake. She expressed anxiety about the whole family and great distress at the recent breakup of her relationship with her boyfriend David. Above all she felt completely helpless.

Family

Susan's parents were divorced. Her father had remarried. Two of her sisters, Tina aged twenty-two and Doreen aged eleven, were living at home with her and her mother. Tina was five months pregnant and her husband was serving abroad in the American Army. Everyone in the family was affected by Susan's illness. Tina was exhausted with trying to support her mother and concerned for her pregnancy. She worried that her sister was jealous and resentful about the prospect of impending birth as she faced her own death. Doreen felt excluded and was bored with all the attention lavished on Susan. She had received little direct information about Susan's illness. Mary's parents and Linda were said to feel frustrated at their distance and inability to help. Mary was exhausted. She was alternately sad and angry and was struggling to hold the family together. Tony, Susan's divorced father, was finding it hard to express his sadness for Susan within his new family. The family seemed unable to communicate with one another. In their efforts not to hurt one another they had stopped sharing their feelings.

Physical

A full financial assessment was made and several benefits were obtained for the family. The house was well adapted for Susan's care at home. As the illness progressed the family were offered a night nurse.

Social

Susan had had a wide circle of friends and an active social life. However the stresses and upheaval of her illness and treatment had isolated her from her friends and they had become embarrassed about the distance between them. Mary was well supported by her close friend Ruth and the whole family were visited regularly by the Roman Catholic priest.

Intervention

There were several individual meetings with family members both to allow them to express their emotional pain and to try to understand what was happening. Some people were properly seen only on an individual basis. For example, Susan's boyfriend David needed to express his guilt over what he saw as his 'desertion' of Susan and to have it set in the more normal context of a casual boy/girl relationship. Susan's father needed to grieve the loss of his first marriage and his closeness to Susan before he could accept her transition from active to palliative treatment. He had

been forcefully urging her to accept chemotherapy. Various family group-
ings were also seen together by various members of the multidisciplinary
team.

Encouraging communication and the confidence to act

On discussion Susan made it clear that she did not want further chemotherapy, but felt guilty about 'giving up' and anxiety that her mother
wanted her to live for as long as possible. She agreed to a meeting with
the social worker and her mother to check this out. Mary cried and told her
daughter that she wanted a good life for her, not endless hospitalizations.
They were sad together and then began to plan for a future which included
Susan dying at home if at all possible. Shortly after this Susan and her
mother went on a weekend trip to visit relatives. Sharing their feelings
had given them the confidence to take control and for Susan to decide
what she wanted to do with the time she had left.

Shared information

Susan's family needed preparation for her death, what to expect in
terms of symptoms, what to do when she died, when should the
funeral director be contacted, how long could they keep Susan at
home afterwards? Mary was shown how to help Susan avoid pressure
sores. Families can find confidence if they are taught the skills of caring.
Doreen and Mary were helped to talk together about Susan's illness and
her teacher was involved.

Strengths and resources

People need help to understand themselves and others, to be given
permission to do what they can and to stop worrying about what they
cannot manage. Susan's mother needed to know that it was alright to
restrict visitors when she was exhausted. Tina encouraged Susan's friends
to make a rota for visiting and a system for loaning her tapes of favourite
pop music. Susan's mother was her best nurse and needed to be told
regularly. Doreen took on the role of helping Susan with her meals. The
team helped Tina to contact the Army and request her husband's return to
the UK. This family had many strengths and a good community network
that simply needed reactivating.

Normalizing, anticipating problems and fears

Susan's mother needed permission to be at once desperately sad and angry
at the limitations Susan's illness was placing on her life. Susan needed to
talk about letting go and its appropriate place in the history of her illness.
The issue of Tina's pregnancy was openly discussed with her and Susan,
and Susan was able to express her delight in it. Tina later found comfort
in helping the nurse to wash Susan's body and to lay it out after death in

the bridesmaid's dress Susan had worn to Tina's wedding. This had been Susan's request to Tina.

Adopting an open style

After a few weeks of good symptom control Susan began to experience ever more frequent episodes of severe central chest pain that were very difficult to control. She was chesty, bedbound and oedematous. Professional teams can demonstrate wholeness for the family by the way they work together and share responsibility. The home care consultant joined a nurse and the GP in a meeting with Susan and the whole family to answer questions about her intractable pain and the various courses of action available. There was an open discussion about whether or not she should be admitted to the hospice, whether she could stay at home, what she wanted, what her mother could manage. The team's joint presence in the home seemed to generate a feeling of confidence in an otherwise chaotic and difficult situation. Susan's pain remained difficult to control but she died peacefully at home, where she wanted to be, with her family around her four weeks after the onset of her acute cardiac pain.

The team

Coordination of the professional team was vital if Susan and her family were not to feel swamped and muddled. It was important to work with the family's existing support systems in complementary, not parallel, activity and to be aware of the risk of professionalizing the family out of control. This problem needed active management and was not always easy.

Sexuality

The area of sexuality often represents a particularly difficult topic for professionals to approach. Embarrassment, fears of intrusion and uncertainty over language can all mean that this area of palliative care remains unaddressed. However intimacy, the ability to communicate and receive love, of which sexual intercourse itself is only one part, is a vital human need. Palliative care declares a commitment to quality of life for patients and their families and this must include a willingness to help them with their sexual needs. This involves remembering that the physical environment in which care is provided can itself deny intimacy, for example privacy, the opportunity to have a hair-do, to be helped with make-up, the reassurance of touch and a cuddle. Concerns about body image need addressing, 'Before the cancer I felt young and sensual. Now I'm a fat, bald, one breasted old woman', as do more direct pleas. Consider for example the woman with cancer of the cervix who sadly declares, 'My husband just doesn't seem to love me any more.'

Professionals need to be able to encourage patients and their partners to discuss issues of sexuality, to respond to their cues and to continue the conversation with a reasonable degree of comfort. To do so they will need to feel at ease with their own sexuality. The guidelines for such conversations are exactly the same as for other family encounters. Professionals already possess the necessary skills, what they need is the confidence to shed their inhibitions. More than anything else couples need to know that it is acceptable to talk about the problems and it is often easier to do so with a sympathetic outsider.

Graded, open questions help: 'How has your illness changed your work/home/life as a couple/ability to get close to one another physically?' It also helps to normalize problems: 'People often have questions they would like to ask about the sexual side of life.' Most people are tired and sexually unaroused after surgery and chemotherapy or radiotherapy. Many people find it hard to kiss and cuddle in the artificial environment of a hospital. Some will be helped by suggestions of alternative ways of getting close, such as massage. Fears should be anticipated and myths explored. 'Is cancer contagious?' 'Sex might cause pain or damage.' 'Can I accept her changed body?' Many anxieties about what a partner thinks of an altered body image are exaggerated and are certainly worsened by the avoidance of professional carers. A couple may be helped by expressing their mutual fear and revulsion for a colostomy in front of one another, whether it will smell or burst and what to do if it does. Above all, wherever possible, information about the potential physical and emotional consequences of surgery or treatment should be given in advance. Cancer changes the way people feel about themselves and each other. The losses it imposes can be alleviated by confronting them. Most people respond with gratitude to a straightforward and sympathetic approach. A sense of humour will usually assist with any difficult moments and is often greeted with relief by patients and their partners.

Children facing bereavement

The care offered to the family by professionals is incomplete without consideration of the needs of children facing bereavement. Terminal illness causes enormous changes within the family and children quickly sense that something very serious is happening. However many adults, parents and professionals alike, in their desire to protect children actually succeed in isolating them, excluding them from the family concerns and leaving them alone with their fantasies. Children cannot ultimately be protected from the truth. They will be sad. If they are involved in the impending death, the adults around them can offer them support in their sadness. Ideally children will receive preparation before the death: an opportunity to ask questions, to receive reassurance and to express feelings.

Children facing bereavement have similar needs and emotions to adults, but may express them differently. For example, the quiet child who becomes aggressive at school, the child who refuses to go to school or wets the bed, are all expressing grief through their behaviour rather than in the words with which adults are more familiar. Children can sometimes upset adults by seeming casual or callous, like the little boy who greeted his brother's death with the announcement, 'I always wanted my own bedroom anyway'. Such behaviour does not mean that they are not also very sad.

Work with parents

It is vital that professionals treat parents as colleagues. They are not helped by staff who take over from them. They know their own children best and the aim must be to help them to help their children. Children need the understanding of their families who will be around long after the professionals have disappeared. It is often necessary to work with parents on their own before children's needs can be addressed. A couple who cannot openly acknowledge impending death between themselves are not well placed to help their children.

Parents also need encouragement to widen their child's support network by involving other adults close to them, rather than feeling they have to do everything themselves. Teachers, clergy, youth club leaders, a close relative, may all help to offer the child another listening ear. Schools have a special part to play in helping children as they often represent a kind of second family and a haven of routine and safety away from the confusing emotions of a grieving family. Parents may welcome the help of professionals in contacting teachers and discussing children's needs. Teachers too, will appreciate discussion of a situation which may be unfamiliar to them.

It is impossible not to communicate

Many parents have good reasons for their reluctance to share information about illness and death with their children. They are anxious about what their children understand about death and about what words to use. They worry that saying the wrong thing will make an already difficult situation worse. They themselves will be grieving and will worry about their ability to maintain control. Children also want to protect their parents. They may try to obey an unspoken rule of 'not talking about it' by pretending that nothing is happening. External helpers need to reassure parents that they understand and share their concerns for their children. However they must also gently remind parents that there is not a choice about whether or not to tell children. Children are aware of changes in routine, they will read the emotions around them, respond to body language and overhear conversations. What is at issue is whether they will receive consistent and regularly updated information from their parents whom they trust, or misleading and sometimes contradictory snippets of information from a variety of sources.

Professionals need to acknowledge with parents that it is not easy to talk to children when what you say is going to hurt them: 'This is probably the

most difficult thing you are ever going to have to do.' Parents may appre- .
ciate advice about explanations of death and vocabulary appropriate to
their child's age and about the kind of reactions they may anticipate. They
may want lists of appropriate books to read with their children[1] or leaflets
on childhood grief[2] to read for themselves in order to gain some intellectual mastery over an emotionally unfamiliar subject. For many parents
this will be sufficient and they will want to speak to their children alone.
Others will welcome sharing the task with a professional. The suggestion
that parents and their children meet with a doctor, nurse or social worker
to answer questions about the illness may be reassuring. Parents want to
do what is best for their children and they learn fast. Being part of just one
direct conversation between a child and a professional can help to give
them the confidence to continue for themselves. Wherever possible the
suggestion should be made that children be included in important family
meetings. Teenagers may appreciate the chance for a separate meeting
with the nurse or doctor when a parent is dying. Staff should always make
a particular effort to introduce themselves to children and to offer routine
and simple explanations about equipment such as syringe drivers.

The environment

Institutions can assist parents by creating an environment that positively
welcomes the presence of children, perhaps a designated area with small
chairs and a toy box. Videos and tapes will amuse older children and toy
medical kits, puppets and telephones can help younger children to act
out their concerns and to ask questions. Children will respond positively
to being shown where they display their pictures and cards by the bed.
Some children find conversation difficult and will respond to suggestions
that they bring their homework in or tell the patient about their feelings in
a letter.

Children's understanding of death

It is important to know something about the development of the concept of
death in children in order to communicate with them at an appropriate and
therefore effective level. Theorists generally suggest that children under
the age of five see death as absence, often temporary or reversible, with
five to nine year-olds seeing death as violent and permanent, and nine
to eleven year-olds beginning to develop a full death concept with
elements of inevitability and universality.[3] However, research by Richard
Lansdown,[4] a psychologist at Great Ormond Street Hospital, indicates that
many much younger children understand more about death than adults
are prepared to accept. Of course, this is not a comfortable idea. It places
less responsibility on adults to believe that young children are incapable
of understanding death.

When seven year-old Martin's father was admitted to a hospice with a
terminal brain tumour, his mother told medical staff that he did not know

what was actually wrong with his father, just that he was ill. She agreed that Martin could ask the doctor any questions about his father's illness. He did: 'Can you stop the bad thing in Daddy's brain? Will it grow inside the rest of his body? Can Daddy come home?' If Martin had not received simple and honest answers to his questions he would have made up his own.

Children's needs

Information

Information needs to proceed at the child's pace and should be clear, simple, truthful and repeated. The child will need to know what has happened and why, and what will happen next. It is helpful to link explanations to things children have noticed already. 'What have you noticed that's different about Mummy?' 'She sleeps a lot and her hair has fallen out.' This allows the opportunity to validate the child's experiences, to assess his level of understanding and to correct any misapprehensions. It is important to answer the question that is actually being asked. 'What happens to you when you are dead?' may be a request for information about coffins and funerals, rather than a question about the existence, or not, of heaven. Some explanations of death are confusing. 'Daddy has gone to sleep' can lead to the response 'I shall stay awake all night.' The team need to be aware of the family's own belief system and not offer explanations that conflict with it. Information should be simple and factual. 'When someone dies their body stops working.' Ideally children should be given information gradually. 'Daddy is very ill. Daddy is so ill the doctors aren't sure they can make him better. Daddy is so ill that he is going to die.' It may be useful to make a 'scrapbook'[5] for children to complete with their parents' help as a less threatening way of beginning difficult conversations. 'Draw a picture of Mummy. Which bit of her is ill? Who is helping to look after her?'

Reassurance

Children facing the death of a parent need reassurance about their own continuing care. They will have all sorts of practical anxieties. 'Who will take me to school? Will I still be able to go to football practice on Fridays?' It can be an enormous relief to them and their parents when these painful issues are openly addressed. Bereaved children need to know what will not change in their world, as well as what will. Children also need explicit reassurance about the fact that cancer is not contagious, that neither they nor other relatives are likely to become ill and die. Children need to know that their own behaviour or thoughts could not have caused the death. Young children in particular sometimes believe that they can make things happen by thinking about them and saying them out loud, 'I hate you and I wish you were dead.'

Children learn to mourn and to grieve healthily by observing others.

They are often uncertain about what is allowed and need to see others crying, especially their parents. They may also need reassurance about the behaviour of adults around them: 'I'm sorry I was cross, I'm not angry with you. I'm just terribly sad because Granny has died.'

Professionals can help parents by reminding them of their children's needs for extra security and routine. A teenage girl ran away from home after her father's death because her mother stopped telling her off when she got in late at night. The girl felt that no one cared about her now her father was dead. Her mother had been trying to be gentle with her.

Expression of feelings

Children's grief is neither expressed nor answered simply through words. Parents may need help to anticipate, understand and accept their children's altered and often difficult behaviour especially when they themselves are grieving. Poor concentration and low tolerance of frustration are normal. For example, without help, a man whose wife has died may interpret his children's unruly and erratic behaviour as evidence of his own failure as a parent rather than an expression of their grief. Parents need telling not to be too hard on themselves. Children need a clear acknowledgement of their loss. They need a chance to say goodbye, like the little girl who came to visit her dying father and left her toy rabbit with him 'to look after him'. Encouraging children to express their feelings is not the same as telling them how to feel. 'Be brave now and don't upset your mother', denies a child's right to grieve.

Parents are often anxious about funerals and whether or not their children should attend. Professionals can help them give their children information in advance about what to expect so that the child and family can decide together what they feel comfortable with. Funerals allow children to recognize that a change has taken place and to see that other people loved the dead person and are sad just as they are. 'The funeral is when everyone who cared about Mummy will get together to say goodbye. Mummy's body will be put in a special box called a coffin.' It will usually help to suggest that a friend or relative be particularly responsible for the child at a funeral where the death very closely involves the parent. If children do not attend the funeral, they should be told as soon as possible afterwards what happened and offered a later visit to the church, crematorium or grave.

All children will be helped by having a memento of the person who has died. It could be a watch, a photograph, some tools, a piece of jewellery or a book. It will provide reassurance that life does go on and a tangible reminder of the existence of the dead person and their importance. Practical involvement in patient care such as watering the flowers or assisting with drinks will also help children's positive memories after the death.

Professional pain

Working with children facing loss involves professionals in considerable pain. Part of the anguish results from the knowledge that the situation cannot be 'made better'. Professionals need to share their feelings of helplessness with their colleagues and to remind themselves, as well as the parents they meet, that children have an amazing capacity to deal with the truth. Offered it with love they can survive and respond to the challenges of bereavement.

Grief and the family

Before death

Bereavement begins before the death of the patient and much can be achieved by providing help in advance. Professionals should try to assist families to create good enough memories for the future. Family members need incorporating into the caring team to whatever extent they feel comfortable. It is easy for them to feel excluded by others' professional skills and they may like to participate in practical nursing tasks such as washing the patient or moistening lips and so on. It is important to discuss with each individual whether or not they wish to be present at the time of death and to give them information about what to expect and what to do, so that their fears do not predetermine their decision. For example, how will symptoms be controlled and what will happen immediately after death. An explanation of the shift from oral to parenteral medication and why the pattern of breathing is changing will help to alleviate anxieties. All information should be offered in advance and repeatedly. Families under stress may worry about the possibility that injections or a failure to eat or drink are contributing to the patient's deterioration. Explanations are necessary if these are not to become troublesome stumbling blocks in bereavement.

Everyone needs a chance to say goodbye. If professionals maintain a sense of dignity and identity for the patient even when he is unconscious, relatives will feel encouraged to say what they need to. Suggestions about the value of holding hands, stroking the hair and a reminder that although the patient is unable to show any response he may well be able to hear, are all helpful.

However much it is anticipated, death is always a profound emotional and sometimes physical shock for relatives. Privacy is important. The time of death represents an opportunity for the family to unite in grieving and receiving comfort and staff need to be careful not to intrude. Ritual may later help both to comfort and to contain shock and panic; prayer, a cup of tea, assistance with important telephone calls.

After death the body should be treated with care, and respect paid to practices required by religion and culture. Family members should be offered the opportunity to assist with washing and dressing the body if they wish to do so. It is important to remember the part that this death will play in the grieving of other patients and their families. They need to be told promptly and sensitively that the death has occurred.

Grief

Grief is the personal experience that follows a loss. It is a normal human journey, not an illness, but it lasts much longer and is much more painful than most people expect. Mourning is a process unique to the individual experiencing it. It has no set pattern but does contain a recognizable and to some extent predictable series of feelings, behaviours and physical sensations.

Consider for example this list written by a man three weeks after the death of his wife from motor neurone disease.

1. The strange feeling of waiting for something to happen.
2. The feeling that my wife is around somewhere which is immediately replaced with the painful reality that she is dead.
3. Lack of initiative to do anything constructive. I feel I should but I lack the physical or mental impetus.
4. Deep fear that I might not see her ever again.
5. Sorrow about all the things I didn't say to her.
6. My eating and sleeping habits have become abnormal.
7. I find it difficult to talk to my friends and family because they don't seem to understand.

The following is an excerpt from a letter written to a bereavement counsellor by a widow with a young son, a year after the death of her husband.

> I ache for him. I miss him so badly the pain of it is quite unbearable sometimes. I pine for the life we had before he died; I pine for what could have been. I feel so totally alone; no direction, no future, just an empty void of weeks and weekends, filled with nothingness, endlessly spread before me. I feel anger and resentment. These people safe in their lives, telling me 'you'll get over it, it's nearly a year now'. I don't want this life that my husband's death has brought me.

William Worden's[6] tasks of mourning provide a helpful framework for understanding the process of mourning. He speaks of four tasks: to accept the reality of loss, to experience the pain of grief, to adjust to an environment in which the deceased is missing and finally to reinvest emotional energy. However it is important to remember that grief is not linear and that people do not move consecutively from one discrete stage to another. It really is a matter of 'two steps forward and one back'. The way to begin to understand someone's grief is to know something about their personality, their relationship with the deceased, their previous losses and response to them, their social and cultural supports. The interplay between society and the mourner can help grieving or make it harder, for example the common notion in Western societies that men do not cry.

Grief is something that people 'do', not just something that happens to them. It involves pain and effort because the reality that has come to be taken for granted, and the sense of meaning and identity it conveys, are totally disrupted and new relationships and meanings have to be found. Avoiding grief carries a price in terms of withdrawal from relationships, physical symptoms and compulsive behaviours. It is therefore essential that palliative care professionals offer at least some kind of emotional first aid to help families and individuals begin the process of mourning.

Brief interventions

A great deal can be achieved in a brief one-off meeting shortly after the death. This may take the form of a family returning to the ward the day after the death of their relative to meet a nurse who cared for him, or it may be a somewhat later visit to the home by a district or Macmillan nurse or a family doctor. Such a visit represents a difficult task for both the professional and the bereaved. As Colin Murray Parkes observes: 'Pain is inevitable in such a case and cannot be avoided. It stems from the awareness of both parties that neither can give the other what he wants. The helper cannot bring back the person who is dead and the bereaved person cannot gratify the helper by seeming helped.'[7] However the bereaved do need to be heard and understood. The visit marks an important change of focus from the patient to the family, an acknowledgement of their pain and sorrow and a recognition of their right to be cared for.

Such a visit has several objectives: to encourage and answer questions about the illness and death, to help grief, to assess risk and refer on where appropriate and to permit goodbyes for both family and staff. A clear structure will help the professional to avoid the danger of this becoming a purely social visit. A deliberate slowing of the pace of speech and good eye contact will help to cut through embarrassment and uncertainty.

Letting go of the past

Encourage questions about the illness and death and go over the facts clearly. People cannot let go of something they have not understood. 'Would an earlier admission have helped? What was the effect of the last injection? Why did the doctor talk about carcinomatosis, I thought he had cancer of the stomach?'

Accepting the reality of death

Where appropriate ask about the funeral and comment on photographs. Use the past tense and try to say the word 'dead'. Hearing and saying this is one of the first and most painful hurdles for the bereaved. Handing over the patient's property also helps to reinforce reality, however uncomfortable it may feel for the professional. Similarly, families should be given the opportunity to read the death certificate for themselves.

It helps to mention any opportunity to view the body early in the meeting so that the family do not have the anxiety of wondering if they have to request this. Ask them if they have seen someone who is dead before and offer a description of the body and the room containing it. They will need to know that the body will be cold, whether it will be in a bed or a coffin, whether it will be directly visible when the door is opened or whether there is an ante room. Individuals differ about whether or not they wish to view the body and everyone in the family should be encouraged to make an individual choice, with a staff member offering to accompany those wishing to view. Verbal goodbyes or an embrace can be stimulated by the professional gently touching the body and suggesting, 'Perhaps there are things you would like to say? Would you like me to leave you alone for a while? It's hard to say goodbye, to leave him here . . .'

Receiving information

Relatives need clear and practical advice about such matters as how and where to register the death, how to arrange the funeral and what to do with pension books. They may welcome an opportunity to voice anxieties, 'I think he wanted to be cremated, but I'm not sure I can go ahead with that.' People under stress forget easily and information should be written down, most helpfully in the form of a standard leaflet. The same is true for the telephone number of a local bereavement service which might well be included in a simple leaflet explaining some of the unfamiliar emotions and sensations of grief.

Beginning the remembering

It often helps the bereaved if a professional shares a personal memory of the dead person and expresses their own sadness. Grieving is about remembering and it may feel safer to begin the process if someone else indicates its appropriateness.

Recognizing grief

Family members may need to share some of their immediate experiences encouraged by remarks like: 'How are you yourself?' 'It's hard to imagine he's really dead.' They will need some preparation for the otherwise bewildering emotions of bereavement. For example, they will want to know that 'if only's' are inevitable and to be reassured that hearing the dead person's voice does not mean they are going mad. Families must be encouraged to give one another permission to grieve in their own way and their own time. 'You may find that some of you will cry and for some of you tears won't come immediately, this will not mean that one of you cares and one of you doesn't.'

Unacknowledged differences in grieving can be a source of family tension.

Feeling that they did what they could

It is important that the professional recognizes the family's role in patient care, leaving them with a validation of their achievements. 'It was wonderful that you managed to look after him at home for so long.'

Acknowledging past losses

Professionals can let the family know briefly and simply that they recognize past losses and their reawakened power to hurt. Few others may think to mention this. 'I can imagine this is reminding you of your Dad.' Members of the family who are not present at the meeting should also be remembered. For example, if children are not present, their need to grieve should be discussed.

Achieving an ending

Endings are important for families and professionals. The family are losing not only the patient but often regular contact with professionals to whom they may have become very close. Listening patiently and seriously to family expressions of gratitude helps them to re-establish a separate identity and sense of integrity. It is essential to be clear about whether it really is goodbye. Ambiguous messages that imply that future contact will be welcomed, yet leave the family vulnerable to resentment if it takes place, will create dependency and leave individuals diminished. Tell people what your relationship with them has meant and then make a clear and considered statement:

- 'You can come back to me at any time.'
- 'I would like to see you again on.'
- 'If things get difficult do think about contacting your GP or a local bereavement service.'

Do not make promises that cannot be kept.

Assessing for risk in bereavement

Most people will successfully accomplish the tasks of grief with the help of their family, friends and local community. Grief should not be viewed as an illness requiring professional intervention. Indeed, over-enthusiastic contacts by professionals can actually stifle support that exists within the family's own network. However, many professionals will want some system of attempting to identify those who will be particularly vulnerable in bereavement. The following list indicates circumstances that may complicate grief. In any assessment it is important to distinguish between facts and opinions.

The death itself

- Was it expected, did the family feel prepared?
- Were the family present?
- Did they perceive the death as peaceful?

After the death

Facts

- Are there children or dependent family members – meaning the person has little time to grieve?
- Have there been other recent deaths in the family?
- Have there been other major losses in the last year, e.g. house move, redundancy?
- Are there major financial problems?
- Is the bereaved person seriously ill, particularly with cancer or heart disease?
- Is the bereaved person taking tranquillizers, antidepressants, more alcohol than usual?
- Is the bereaved person requesting help? If so, respond.

Opinions

- Is the bereaved person particularly sensitive to separation, particularly angry or guilty?
- Does the bereaved person have a psychiatric history?
- Is the bereaved person considered to be a suicide risk, past or present?
- Does the bereaved person find their family unhelpful?
- Was the care of the patient very stressful?
- Was the bereaved person especially distressed at the patient's change of body image or personality?

(Note that the uncertainty and delay of a referral to the Coroner usually suggests the benefit of follow up.)

Following such an assessment the professional needs to balance any risk factors with a perception of the strengths and resources available to members of the family. What was encouraging about the way they handled the illness and death? Have they coped adequately with previous crises? Who is special to them in the community? Are they expressing emotion appropriately? The palliative care professional should then place the whole assessment within the contexts of time and culture and pay close attention to their own 'hunch' about the individual's capacity to cope.

Many reactions that are to be expected in the period immediately following a death will cause greater concern if they persist a year or so later, although it is very difficult to place rigid time scales on what is appropriate. Examples would be; an inability to change the room of the dead person, radical changes in life style, imitating the dead person or experiencing similar physical symptoms to them, persistent guilt, low self esteem or euphoria, not believing the death.[8] The continuation of such reactions would suggest the need for professional help in bereavement.

Bereavement services

It is important for palliative care professionals to be realistic about their own capacity to provide bereavement care. Such services, whether provided by the professionals themselves or by trained and supervised volunteers are costly and time consuming. It may be more effective to concentrate on good preparatory work before the death in the form of information and emotional support for the family and then to focus on making good collaborative links with pre-existing local bereavement services. Bereavement leaflets, anniversary cards and memorial services are other simple and effective forms of help for the family. There is also evidence that one-off bereavement evenings at the institution for several families together are much welcomed. Staffed by professionals, often at about three months after the death, such meetings offer families another opportunity to say goodbye and the chance to see that others are finding the experience of grief as powerful and painful as themselves.

When does grief end?

There is an important sense in which individuals remain permanently vulnerable to their losses, but the following list will provide some clues about grief resolution:

- Can the bereaved accept that the person has died?
- Can he remember the whole person, their irritating features as well as those much loved?
- Can he talk about the dead person without becoming overwhelmed?
- Is there evidence that the bereaved person is reasserting himself, practically and emotionally?
- Is the bereaved person reintegrating with family and community, building a new personal and social life and looking to the future?
- Is he sleeping, eating and attending to physical and mental health and appearance?
- Ask the bereaved person how he feels – he usually knows.
- Consider how you feel when you leave him, his feelings will be infectious, are you more worried or more optimistic?
- Remember that it will not be 'better', bereavement is not like a dose of 'flu.

The cost to the professional carer

Working with those experiencing loss is painful. Professionals coming close to the anguish of others find it difficult to maintain their own sense of balance. Their natural reaction will be to try to reduce pain for others. However as professionals they know that they cannot take the pain away and that the successful conclusion of their work is a dead patient whose family and friends have begun to grieve and to recognize and experience the inevitable suffering their loss will cause them. Too much care, too much nurturing and enfolding, can be intrusive and prevent patients and families from asserting themselves and discovering the growth that may come from exploring their own dejection and despair. The tension between the personal emotional reaction to protect and the professional response makes very special demands on staff. Only people committed to caring will survive in palliative medicine, on the other hand their professional expertise will require that they do not over-engage in their patients' emotional problems. Thus the organizational requirement to support staff with the emotional content of their work is very important. Professional carers also have an individual responsibility to pay attention to the task of looking after themselves. These issues will be explored more fully in Chapter 7.

Notes and References

1. For example: *Someone Special has Died*. London: St Christopher's Hospice, 1989, COULDRICK, A. *When your Mum or Dad has Cancer*. Oxford: Sobell Publications, 1991, *Your Parent has Died*. London: St Christopher's Hospice, 1991.
2. For example: COULDRICK, A. *Grief and Bereavement: Understanding Children*. Oxford: Sobell Publications, 1988.
3. KANE, B. 'Children's concepts of death', *Journal of Genetic Psychology*, 1979, **134**, pp. 141–53.
4. LANSDOWN, R. 'The development of the concept of death in childhood', *Bereavement Care*, 1985, **4**(2), pp. 15–17.
5. For example: 'My Book about. . .' London: St Christopher's Hospice, 1989.'
6. WORDEN. J.W. *Grief Counselling and Grief Therapy*, 2nd ed, London, Routledge, 1991.
7. PARKES, C.M. *Bereavement: Studies of Grief in Adult Life*, 2nd ed, Harmondsworth, Penguin, 1986.
8. LAZARE, A. *Outpatient Psychiatry: Diagnosis and Treatment*. Baltimore: Williams and Wilkins, 1979.

Further reading

GROLLMAN, E. *Talking about death*, 3rd ed. Boston: Beacon Press, 1990.
HILDEBRAND, J. 'Working with a bereaved family', *Palliative Medicine*, 1989, **3**, 105–11.
JEWETT, C. *Helping Children Cope with Separation and Loss*. London: Batsford, 1984.
KIRSCHLING, J.M. (ed.) *Family-based Palliative Care*, Howarth Press, New York, 1990.
PINCUS, L. *Death and the Family*, London, Faber, 1976.
SMITH, NICK 'The impact of terminal illness of the family', *Palliative Medicine*, 1990, **4**(2), 127–5.

Cross-cultural principles of care———————

David Oliviere

The 'art and science' of palliative care lies in considering every aspect of people's lives which may be important in providing 'total care'. An integral part of this consideration is the person's culture. Each patient or family displays a different set of mores, patterns of relationship and verbal and non-verbal reactions to situations. These responses are partly defined by cultural patterns learnt from babyhood and evolved by exposure to other cultural influences.

'No one can ever be categorized solely in terms of their cultural and religious background, but there has been a heightened interest in how these factors may, sensitively understood, much enhance the quality of care'.[1]

Culture

Inherited values, ways of behaving, beliefs, styles of living, tastes and rituals all make up culture and are shaped by it. According to Helman:[2]

> Culture is a set of guidelines (both explicit and implicit) which individuals inherit as members of a particular society, and which tells them how to view the world, how to experience it *emotionally*, and how to *behave* in it in relation to other people, to supernatural forces of gods, and to the natural environment. It also provides them with a way of transmitting these guidelines to the next genera-tion – by the use of symbols, language, art and ritual. To some extent, culture can be seen as an inherited 'lens', through which individuals perceive and understand the world that they inhabit, and learn how to live within it.

Culture can be experienced as a basic set of rules – some very explicit; others quite subtle – about different aspects of living and, of course, dying. Some of these 'rules' are rejected, reinforced or amalgamated with other sets of rules during one's lifetime.

Many Western societies are now 'multi-cultural' and 'multi-faith'. Religion and culture are often inextricably linked and give 'meaning' to body and mind. Their understanding in making the person what they are is imperative. Even though many people from ethnic minority groups do not practise specific religious rituals or engage in active worship, their traditions and culture are shaped by a Christian, Hindu, Jewish, Muslim or other religious background. For some patients and relatives, the approach of death initiates new and richer meaning in their religious rituals and traditions. For others, these will be less meaning-ful. (See Fig. 4.2.)

Recent National Health Service guidelines encourage the introduction of local standards of care to ensure respect for the religious and cultural beliefs of each patient.[3]

Respect for the person whatever their complex make-up has always been important in palliative care. In order to understand the patient and their family as well as their wishes, we must understand their culture as well as ours.

Basic to palliative care philosophy are principles of *acceptance* of the individual (e.g. the patient who displays customs and habits quite unlike our own); *non-judgemental attitudes* (e.g. towards the family who will not talk about cancer and death because their religion suggests that this may take away hope); and *confidentiality* (e.g. over the life-style of the Chinese Buddhist patient, who could easily become a curiosity).

The modern hospice movement has always cherished the idea of being a community. (St Christopher's Hospice for example has, since its incep-tion, included provision for local young children to have a place through its playgroup while older people live in permanent residence in a wing of the hospice. It then provided the first home care service establishing a pattern for community-based services to develop.) It is important that the palliative care service is seen as part of the range of provision in the community and that the service is available to all the different groups/cul-tures in society irrespective of class or creed. This can only happen if the *service* is set up to give the appropriate message that *all* groups are welcome and of we as *individuals* are as comfortable as possible in working with people if differing cultural experiences and backgrounds.

Living in a society where there can be a tendency to value commonality rather than difference, palliative care workers can be faced with fears

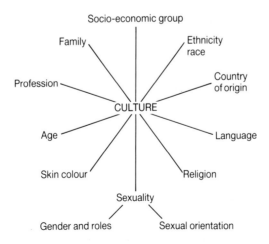

Fig. 4.2 Some determinants of culture

about people from minority groups getting preferential treatment or may be exposed to basic discomfort and prejudice. There can be real dilemmas: how much does one allow a large family to take up a constant vigil around the patient's bed with other patients in close proximity? For some staff their experience has not included relating to people who display different looks, dress, accent, preferences or humour. We have to adapt services to meet the various needs of different cultures rather than help minority groups make use of the service as provided.

Underlying all this, is a need to value diversity as giving pleasure, excitement, interest and enquiry. We are all an amalgamation of different cultural influences. We are not just referring to people who look or seem to be 'different'.

One of the challenges in working with people from various cultural backgrounds is assessing where people are in their culture, i.e. which aspects of and to what extent their cultural background is important to them. Migration to a new country, may have strengthened or diluted cultural practices and beliefs.

In the family context, there may be conflicts between members of different generations who have varying perceptions of and attachments to their own culture; people who belong to the same ethnic group and religion but from different countries may have quite differing customs. Jews born and bred in north-west London may live in quite a different style from those from Iraq or Egypt. Furthermore, 'knowledge of a country may not represent the subculture and religious denomination from which a patient comes'.[4] 'Among Asians, attitudes to death and bereavement vary with different religions, caste, and socio-economic backgrounds.'[5]

In palliative care it is vital to acknowledge the special needs of refugees or patients and families who have been subjected to persecution as a result of political, religious or racial differences. Whether the experience is recent or in the distant past, they may have experienced numerous losses and emotional trauma which are likely to be resurrected in their present situation.[6] This sense of trauma, guilt or loss will not be confined to the generation who live through it but is experienced by the next generation, as perceived in the children of holocaust survivors.[7]

Areas to be considered in ensuring multi-culturally sensitive palliative care

If you were terminally ill, which aspects of your culture would be important for you? For teaching purposes we sometimes ask students to imagine they are entering a palliative care unit in China and to identify the ten main aspects about which they would be concerned, apart from specific medical care.

In palliative care, different cultural attitudes will be held towards:

- The disease (cancer, AIDS).
- Hospice environment (food, climate, pictures/ symbols/ objects, types of staff – race, gender, status).

- Physical care (pain, analgesia, modesty).
- Talking/counselling (honesty, privacy).
- Family (who's included; roles of men/women, parents and children).
- Point of death (rituals, prayers, those present).
- Death (washing, dressing, display of body).
- Funeral (type of disposal, open/closed coffin).
- Bereavement (open expression of grief).

Access to services

Research has shown that there is unequal access to health services by black and ethnic minority and migrant workers.[8] Services are often linguistically and culturally inaccessible to people from minority ethnic groups. There is a basic lack of knowledge of services available. There is no evidence to suggest hospice services are any different.

Indeed, the indications are that people from minority cultures are less prepared to use palliative care services[9] or are under-represented. There is clearly a huge research need on the take-up of palliative care services from members of minority cultures. It is still unknown whether numbers of patients served are consistent in terms of numbers, the incidence of certain illnesses and other demographic variables with the majority population. This is, in turn, dependent on services recording the ethnic origins of those referred. In a recent survey[10] of 'Client Satisfaction with Care at the Leicestershire Hospice', the authors state: 'Perhaps the matter of greatest concern is the virtual absence of people from ethnic minority groups from the hospice. Leicester is a city with large Asian and Afro-Caribbean populations, comprising approximately a quarter of the total population, yet very few of these are admitted to the Hospice.' Similarly, in Birmingham[11] and Penarth, Wales.[4]

Part of making a service more accessible involves active reaching out to potential users and making the image of the service more acceptable to them. In order to make known the palliative care service various measures for marketing and communicating the service to minority groups will need to be considered. These include:

- *Translating* literature into the main local languages and ensuring comprehensive dissemination.
- *Making personal contact* with local leaders or providing 'open days' to discuss what is on offer. This is particularly important as minority cultures can often view palliative care services as being provided mainly by white people from the established culture or being part of a religious movement and not particularly welcoming of the minority. It is easy for people from a minority culture to be uneasy about the service and, therefore, engaging interest is crucial.
- *Addressing the image* of the service. The fact that many hospices are named 'St' and are staffed predominantly by white staff, even in very mixed areas, can, for some, reinforce the image of not being home equally for people from minority cultures. Therefore staff should

include members of local ethnic minorities. We know that patients seem to experience the service very positively once sampled, but these factors can pose barriers and create initial anxieties.

- *Targetting local general practitioners* from areas of the main minority ethnic groups.

Hospitality

Hospitality is the basis of good palliative care. It puts patients, relatives and friends at ease so that professionals and volunteers can use their skills and the person we are helping can feel safe and comfortable enough to use the help on offer.

We welcome patients, families and visitors from many cultures and religions or none, trying to communicate a deep respect for them and their customs. We want them to feel at home because their needs and wishes regarding diet, care and rituals and the whole approach to the dying person and to people during bereavement, are being met – not as an extra bonus but as their right and expectation to experience care which is in keeping with the way they have lived. They should not be made to feel 'over-special'.

Basic good practices with any patient are particularly important when dealing with the person from a different ethnic group: ensuring their names are accurately understood and recorded and also how they prefer to be called, or checking that they have understood what has been said, who is who and what plans have been agreed. Recording the patient's first language or language spoken at home can communicate care and concern.

The quality of staff is important irrespective of race but if personnel reflect the local range of ethnic groups, a powerful message is conveyed regarding the respect for difference. This does not mean that a Jewish patient should automatically have a Jewish nurse or an Asian patient an Asian nurse.

Language and Communication

'In a way I am disabled. I can see but I cannot read. I can hear but I cannot understand.' 'No agency can provide a fair or effective service to people with whom it cannot communicate.'[12]

A patient who does not speak the same language as the professional or volunteer carer (or has limited understanding) experiences a handicap and poses one for the carer. We would not try to help a patient who is deaf and has no speech without seeking assistance. Similarly, when seeing a patient where there are language difficulties, time must be taken to find and work with interpreters where possible. Otherwise we are left with a greater reliance on working assumptions, guesswork and intuition. Even people who can speak some English may forget most of it when they are ill or worried or under stress.[13]

Misinterpretation of people from ethnic groups has resulted in wrong diagnosis, e.g. the Gujerati-speaking patient from India was seen as having 'stomach pain' when he was basically indicating general 'upset'. People from some cultures nod their head to mean 'no' and shake their head to mean 'yes'.

Points to remember[13] when 'communicating across a language barrier' include:

- Speak clearly and simply and at the pace you sense is right for your patient/relative. Take care not to raise your voice as if the person were deaf! Choose words the patient is likely to know. Listen for the words the patient uses and use them yourself. If necessary, use mime and pictures to help to get the meaning across.
- Check that you have been understood and signal clearly that you are moving on to a new subject, e.g. 'Now I want to ask you about. . .'
- People who are stressed and unwell are only likely to be able to remember or absorb a very limited amount of discussion. The effort of concentrating to understand a foreign language can seriously affect the memory. You may need to write down one or two key points to which the patient and family can refer.
- Coping across a language barrier can also affect the way people behave. The person can be extra nervous knowing they cannot explain their thoughts and feelings and deal with someone in authority. The behaviour you see does not necessarily reflect the personality of your patient. Be aware of any judgements you make about the behaviour or personality of someone whose first language is not your own. Intonation is the most difficult aspect to master in a foreign language and what may sound excitable, angry or abrupt in one language, may sound perfectly acceptable in other languages. Again, beware of making judgements based on intonation or tone of voice.
- Non-verbal communication and body language is strongly culture-bound. Signals and movements which convey one thing in one culture may convey something completely different in another. For example, in English culture it is important to indicate that you are listening to someone by nodding and making eye contact and encouraging noises. In some other cultures it is not necessary to do anything special. Beware of making automatic judgements about behaviour or personality on the basis of non-verbal signals. Bear in mind too that your attempts at non-verbal communication may sometimes be misunderstood.
- Write down important instructions about how to take medications and involve relatives and friends here. Important points about drugs and treatment should be translated if possible.
- Using an interpreter is not an easy option as it involves:
  – Building up a list of appropriate interpreters.
  – Negotiating funding or input from your local interpreting service.

- Providing some preparation on the topics you are likely to cover.
- Allocating extra time for the interview.
- Debriefing time afterwards for the interpreter.

However the use of an experienced interpreter where possible has advantages. Using relatives/friends as interpreters severely limits what you can achieve as they are emotionally involved and would inevitably filter the communication you wish to have. You need to allow at least twice as much time for an interview using an interpreter. Remember, however professional, interpreters can also become very personally concerned about the painful issues often discussed in palliative care.

Family

What 'family' means to an English person may be quite different from what it may mean to someone from another culture. Our understanding of family referring to parents and children, perhaps grandparents, may to another culture include cousins, uncles, aunts, nieces, nephews and others. This will also determine who is present near the time of death and afterwards.

Expectations of how the old and the young behave within the family may be very different from our own in terms of respect, unwillingness to express anger or of younger women rather than men being the carers.

Roles, especially of women, are often different. We must be careful not to bring Western values to cultures where women's roles are very much defined in terms of motherhood and home-making. Some staff in a home care team were upset and critical of Mrs M's family, from India. With breast cancer, bony secondaries and a very oedematous arm she struggled with all the housework and shopping despite her husband and two grown-up children being at home. However, Mrs M totally accepted the expectation of her role in the family.

Cultural factors influence belief about communicating with children about death and how much children are allowed to participate in the care of family members. As professional carers, we have to be careful to work through and with the adults in the family in communicating with the children.

Stereotyping and generalizing

'She can cope with the suppositories, she's French.'
'He's a typical Greek.' 'Muslims do it like this.'

Although people may tend to categorize or generalize to 'make sense' of their experience of other cultures, it is important to avoid becoming rigid, unrealistic, denying people's individuality and increasing the assumptions about the group concerned. Every culture may have its 'tendencies' but many people are subject to several cultural influences and personal characteristics.

We have to confront prejudice and stereotypical thinking and attitudes in ourselves, our colleagues and others. There is sometimes as much difference within groups as between them. As professionals in palliative care we have never been reluctant to stand for high standards of practice. This is no less important in this area of work.

For example, we are so often exposed to images of Muslims in the media as aggressive and condemnatory of Western influences that we have to try to become aware of how one-sided images can influence our attitude towards the individual Muslim family in our care.

(There is a significant staff training implication here for any palliative care service. The most helpful publications available are those by Julia Neuberger (see Reference 16) and Jennifer Green, 'Death with dignity – meeting the spiritual needs of patients in a multi-cultural society', *Nursing Times* (1991).)

Getting to know the person

In addition to trying to understand the richness and requirements of different cultures, we need to clarify the particular preferences on certain practices of our patient or relative from a specific culture or group. We must remember that, for example, not every Jewish person keeps kosher or every Catholic wants to say the rosary.

Just because someone is categorized as Afro-Caribbean, Chinese, Hindu, etc. it does not automatically mean that they have taken on all the traditions and practices characteristic of that culture or faith. 'If we are not sensitive to this fact we may structure things in such a way that we do not allow the person to express what they are feeling in the way most appropriate to them and can sometimes actually induce guilt by implying that they *ought* to be refusing pork or lighting candles, etc.'[14]

Do not assume, either, that the patient now in front of you will match the same pattern as the previous one from the same culture. For example, the view that 'Asians are helped by having extended family support', did not apply to Nina. She continued to feel very isolated after the death of her mother. With a family business and three young children she had no space to express her grief and needed the support of the hospice bereavement service.

We cannot possibly know everything about every cultural or religious group of the person in front of us. Remember:

- Often the faith/religion given (Jew, Hindu, Muslim, Sikh) identifies the *culture* of the person rather than their religious practices or beliefs.
- Try to understand how important the culture or faith is to the individual. Not everyone from that culture automatically adheres to the conventional practices. There are many shades and variations within each cultural group from the more orthodox to the more liberal. Do not urge your understanding of *their* cultural practices – listen to what is wanted.
- Do not assume one person from a particular culture will resemble the

next person of the same culture in preferences, habits, etc.
- Many people will be 'in transition' between their family's culture and local cultural activities and practices. There may be conflict over adherence to cultural traditions between generations.
- Enquire of patient and family or friends whether there are any specific needs and requirements that you should know in respect of the particular person.[14] They are usually very happy that someone is troubling to find out their needs.

Our own attitudes

Our own culture will colour the way we assess the particular needs of people from other cultures.

It should be evident from earlier discussion that to help people from other cultures, we have to understand our own culture, race and religion or non-religion. We have to be aware of our attitudes towards people who are different from us and take care not to transfer our ideas onto the other person. 'As carers we must be aware of our own assumptions as to what is helpful or unhelpful behaviour for people in crisis.'[14]

There are potential conflicts between some palliative care principles which we hold dear and cultural influences, for example that bereaved people should express their emotions; or that ill people need not be urged by anxious relatives to keep eating or that openness and truth-telling could take away hope.[15] 'Only with a secure basis to one's own thinking can one really learn and understand other people's'.[16]

Conclusion

For each patient and family 'the journey' from life to death will be different. In palliative care, it is vital that we ensure that the journey is in accordance with the person's individual cultural values and expectations. In this way staff can find their own experience enriched and enhanced as patient and family are allowed to be themselves.

Indeed, when it comes to basics, we are talking not just about labels – Afro-Caribbean, Asian, Chinese, Hindu, Jew, Muslim, etc. but about people: people experiencing the deepest human emotions of love and pain linked to attachment and loss. In producing good palliative care, we have to listen sensitively to where the person is in their culture and give them permission to live this time using the aspects which support them most securely.

Table 4.1 Aspects of palliative care that need to be considered in making the service more multi-culturally 'user friendly'

	Issues	Practice implications
Access	Do all local ethnic, cultural groups *know* of this service? Are patients from the different cultural groups using palliative care service?	Advertising the hospice service among local ethnic and cultural groups. Targetting certain GPs/referring agents to heighten their awareness of the service. Public relations work/personal contacts with local groups. Translation of hospice information in local community languages. Should patient's ethnic group be recorded?
Hospitality	Do all groups feel welcome? What is the 'image' of the service? Could requirements be met without making person feel different/extra special?	Should there be staff from local ethnic minority groups Is the name important? What message do the symbols/ pictures communicate? Do your records identify patient/family's first language?
Language	Can the patient communicate in a language he/she finds comfortable? Should a friend/ relative be used to interpret?	Finding a reliable interpreter/ keeping register of interpreters Negotiating funding. Giving *time* for preparing and supporting interpreter.
Environment	What message would our staff mix give to someone from a minority culture? Should a patient be offered a choice of staff from same ethnic background?	Policy decisions re staffing. Staff training on the specific requirements of different cultures. Resources, e.g. books, play materials for children should have images with they can identify.
Diet	What happens when a patient requires specific food?	Arrangements for kosher/halal food, etc.
Specific requirements	Treatment – pain, method, alternative therapy. Personal care and clothing Religious practices and rituals	Operational policy on requirements related to diet, death-bed, last offices. Education and training of staff Don't make assumptions; check out with patient/relatives. Is there a place where worship can take place which a minority group would find comfortable?
Pastoral care	Do we have a Christian chaplaincy or multi-faith?	Making contacts with religious leaders of all faiths. Ensure easy access to religious leaders.
Bereavement	Does our model and assessment of bereaved people take into account the way people from other cultures express grief? Is it exclusively based on 'Western society'?	Education on different cultures' rituals and grieving patterns needed. Recruit bereavement counsellors from different ethnic groups.

Note: The above chart is a guide to thinking about different aspects of the palliative care service in meeting needs across cultures. It cannot be a prescription.

Notes and References

1. AINSWORTH-SMITH, I. In: Foreward NEUBERGER, JULIA. (ed.) *Caring for Dying People of Different Faiths*, Austen Cornish and The Lisa Sainsbury Foundation, 1987.
2. HELMAN, C. *Culture, Health and Illness*, 2nd edn, London Butterworth-Heinemann, 1990.
3. NHS Management Executive. Health Service Guidelines HSG/92/2. Meeting the Spiritual Needs of Patients and Staff. *Information Exchange, National Council for Hospice and Palliative Care Services*, No. 1, March 1992.
4. CLARKE, M., FINLAY, I. and CAMPBELL, I. 'Cultural boundaries in care,' *Palliative Medicine*, 1991, **5**, 63–5.
5. REES, D. 'Terminal Care and Bereavement.' In: McAVOY, B.R. and DONALDSON, L.J. (eds), Health Care for Asians 1990, Oxford General Practice Series 18, Oxford, Oxford University Press.
6. SCHRIEVER, S.H. 'Comparison of beliefs and practices of ethnic Viet and Lao Hmong concerning illness, healing, death and mourning: implications for hospice care with refugees in Canada,' *Journal of Palliative Care*, 1990, **6**(1), 42–9.
7. BALDER, L, and SARELL, M. 'Coping with cancer among holocaust survivors in Israel: an explanatory study,' *Journal of Human Stress*, Fall 1984, 121–7.
8. BAXTER, C. *Cancer Support and Ethnic Minority and Migrant Worker Communities*, London: Cancerlink, 1989.
9. NEUBAUER, B.J. and NEUBAUER, C.L.H. 'Racial differences in attitudes towards hospice care,' *Hospice Journal*, 1990, **6**(1), 37–48.
10. Trent Palliative Care Centre, 'Client Satisfaction with Care at the Leicestersire Hospice,' Occasional Paper No. 2, December 1991.
11. REES. W.D. 'Immigrants and the hospice,' *Health Trends*, 1986, **18**, 89–91.
12. SHACKMAN J. 'The right to be undertood.' In: London Interpreting Project (LIP) *Directory of Community Interpreting Services and Resources in the Greater London Area*, 1989.
13. HENLEY, A. *Caring in a Multiracial Society*, London, Bloomsbury Health Authority, 1987.
14. SPECK, P. 'Cultural and religious aspects of dying.' In: SHERR, L, (ed.).*Death, Dying and Bereavement*, Oxford, Blackwell, 1989.
15. ABELES, M. 'Features of Judaism for carers when looking after Jewish patients,' *Palliative Medicine*, 1991, **5**, 201–5.
16. NEUBERGER, J. *Caring for Dying People of Different Faiths*, Austen Cornish and The Lisa Sainsbury Foundation, 1987.

5

Spiritual concerns in palliation

Leonard Lunn

Pastoral care is concerned with the meaning of human experience. Its task is not to deliver answers or interpretations so much as to assist in uncovering them. A pastoral relationship thus involves a commitment to another person in his or her search for truth. This commitment is itself a witness to truth.[1]

The whole care and style of what is usually called the modern hospice movement is productive of spiritual care. The above quotation speaks of commitment to another person, i.e. a patient and his family in the context of their own search for meaning and truth. This relationship is at the heart of spiritual care of the dying, having commitment, search and probably struggle, at its heart. What gives much hospice care its essence is this 'witness to truth'. This means that spiritual care cannot be reduced to the confines of a religious or departmental concern, it is so central that it is the business of all involved in caring for the dying. Certainly just to leave it to chaplains would be negligent.

Spiritual and religious

A foundational principle of effective spiritual care is to recognize that it is much broader than religious concerns. It is as integral a component of our humanity as we feel our bodies to be.

The Christian will want to say with St Augustine, 'you have made us for Yourself, Lord, and our hearts are restless until they rest in You' and this vacuum becomes for many people much more conscious and urgent with the approach of death. That is when many non-religious dying people have their innate spiritual hunger for meaning and reconciliation surface and demand attention. This also happens to many of the bereaved.

It is helpful to distinguish spiritual from religious (See Fig. 5.1). The spiritual dimension is the deepest and is concerned with ultimate concerns, our search for meaning and values. It is often experienced in terms of relationships, possibly with God but almost certainly with others and self. Religion on the other hand is the corporate, organized and outward expression of belief systems and an attempt to describe and express faith, ordinarily in community. Doctors and nurses usually stay with the religious in clerking procedures and less formal assessments of a patient's needs because it is more easily described, less personal and far more accessible than the spiritual. If the patient or family are inarticulate about this intensely personal part of their lives it is hardly surprising that carers are tentative. The distinction is important, however, because the spiritual dimension is a common factor to us all and in the common experience of our mortality it is a liberating model after the confines of the religious. The complex shades of variables in religious faith even between members of the same denomination is bewildering and one suspects held with such deep personal investment and tenacity that we dare not tread on such holy ground. Our spirituality on the other hand, while personal and sensitive, is universally recognizable and many of the embarrassingly loaded issues raised by religion are absent.

The arrows in the diagram indicate that if the spiritual informs and shapes the religious expression then it can be perceived as humanizing the situation for all involved. This means at its simplest that any religious rituals used in the context of the sick and the dying must be adapted to the needs of the patient and family with a flexibility and sensitivity which comes from

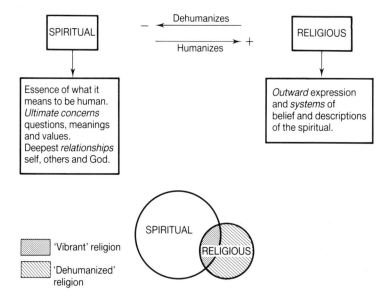

Fig. 5.1 Distinguishing the spiritual from the religious. Lunn, Leonard & Harris, Margaret. 1990. St Christopher's Hospice.

an openness to their particular needs. The reverse would be rigid religious procedures that exist for their own sake into which the patient would have to fit in on a 'take it or leave it' basis. The two circles are an estimate of the proportions that seem to exist between spiritual and religious together with the overlap. To see the spiritual as dominant is a liberating concept for most health care professionals working with the dying. It is a release from the personal religious historical baggage that many people carry around which explains the general reluctance to venture into this area of care.

Spiritual care then is about the care of persons rather than for a rigid complexity of ritual demands. This area may not be as accessible as someone's body but it is as natural a sphere for care. It also means that the whole of our work is spiritual.

But because the spiritual touches our whole being and all aspects of care it creates a discipline different from, say, medicine and nursing care. Infuriatingly for many, spiritual care cannot be translated in the style of a science or a textbook which clearly shows 'how to do it'. Spiritual care taking place in a clinical context inevitably creates a clash of cultures and often a sense of frustration that the chaplain cannot systematize spiritual care lectures to the same shape as, for example, symptom control or bowel management. So the frustration is similar to 'Why can't a woman be more like a man?' Spiritual care is a different animal.

But once this difference is acknowledged it can be used as a creative complement and there is much that can be done in response to spiritual pain.

Meaning

A major indicator of spiritual pain is a search for meaning, not often expressed in philosophical terms but as questions about what the previous seventy years have added up to, 'What is the point of my being here when I am so incapacitated and useless and will it matter to me or anyone else when I am dead this time next week?' The question of worth will be answered by the quality of care which will hopefully be an assurance but the deeper questions of meaning can only be answered by the questioner himself. As in life there are great variations of growth in dying and it is unreasonable to expect everyone to achieve great strides in their final weeks and days. Many, however, do find a place of peace because of the loving care and the space to find themselves that has been offered.

Guilt

Expressions of guilt are also major indicators of spiritual pain. There is a general guilt which affects most people when they assess their life.

> Guilt at the unfinished, the relative, the failure to develop, the talents lying fallow; guilt at a certain betrayal of oneself, one's aspirations, convictions and human vocation.[2]

This can only be addressed by acknowledging one's humanity and that there is always unfinished business. Acceptance rather than removal and some assurance of forgiveness for our weakness can be offered in an appropriate way. There are also specific areas of guilt relating to particular actions, words and decisions in the past. These can often seem trivial and sometimes hardly worthy of producing guilty feelings but they must be taken seriously and never lightly dismissed. The response will vary according to the patient's background and needs ranging from counselling, a full sacramental ritualized confession or an informal prayer following a conversation. To be listened to and to share something of another's reality or trust will be the healing agent.

Presence, being there

This is the title of Peter Speck's book[3] about the pastoral care of the sick and of itself states the simplicity and the difficulty of spiritual care. Jean Vanier, whose work with the mentally handicapped mirrors so much of palliative care, has written

> In some mysterious way
> the quality of my presence, my look
> brings to you life
> or death.[4]

The different professions may have a particular representative or symbolic presence for patients: the doctor – often authority; the nurse – competence and safety and the chaplain; God – the eternal and all the possible connotations arising from the ultimate. One patient on being introduced to the chaplain exclaimed, 'I'm not that bad yet am I?'

The patient usually needs the combined presence of a team that goes beyond their particular skills and functions. It is skill and competence with a deeply human presence that is needed. A man recently admitted to a hospice said that he felt himself to be human again, that he had returned to the human race. In explaining this he could only talk about the contrast with home when he had been left on his own for long periods. The offer of a caring presence is a major counter to the feelings of being abandoned that the terminally ill often feel.

Presence at its purest is *being* rather than *doing*, so the greatest test is whether we can just sit with people in their pain, with their suffering and unanswerable questions. Job's so-called comforters were being helpful until they started to explain the inexplicable and answer the unanswerable. The pressure to offer more than their presence proved irresistible and so they failed their friend. To what extent we can be at peace staying with unconscious patients is a good test of our spiritual care. Most of us achieve less than we care to admit. Don't just do something, be there.

Listening

What affirms people almost more than anything is a listening presence but we need to acknowledge that listening is difficult and hard work, which is why it is so little practised. So often what paralyses us in the presence of suffering and unanswerable questions like 'why is this happening to me?' is that we, having nothing to say, finding it all too easy to forget that this is the appropriate response. At the deeper level of spiritual pain the question for the carer is not 'what can I say?' but 'how can I respond?' It may be that in a listening presence we shall feel powerless and not at all in control. This again is a therapeutic response in the deeply human sense that at that point we empathize most closely with the dying whose loss of control and experience of powerlessness is total. But the professional so often needs to do something because deep down we distrust the therapeutic power of *just* listening and being present. It is in these terms that Henri Nouwen defines compassion:

> Let us not underestimate how hard it is to be compassionate. Compassion is hard because it requires the inner disposition to go with others to the place where they are weak, vulnerable, lonely and broken. But this is not our spontaneous response to suffering. What we desire most is to do away with suffering by fleeing from it or finding a quick cure for it. As busy, active, relevant ministers, we want to earn our bread by making a real contribution. This means first and foremost doing something to show that our presence makes a difference. And so we ignore our greatest gift, which is our ability to enter into solidarity with those who suffer.[5]

The most devastating description of the antithesis of this was experienced by the playwright Dennis Potter.

> One of the funniest and saddest things I saw in the hospital where I was a patient was the young chaplain, doing a swift, head-bobbing round of the infirm: an amiable fellow, with pink countenance, his nerves nevertheless stretched to the full, scurrying up and down between the beds, nodding, and grinning helplessly at each of his denomination with a 'gobble-gobble' that eventually articulated itself into 'is everything all right?' An equal panic came back from the bed. 'Yes, yes,' we would say, terrified that he might linger, and perhaps even more alarmed about the prospect of answering honestly, and thus giving too unguarded a voice to the anxiety or even despair kept for much later in the night.[6]

Other professions are capable of this 'gobble-gobble' and we can all develop defence mechanisms (hopefully more subtle) that keep us from being there. Spiritual care is something about lingering and allowing an honest answer to which we will listen and then share.

Anger and protest

One of the greatest needs in palliative care is to examine why so little anger and protest seems to be expressed by the dying and their loved ones. If we are throwing a blanket of kindness and clinical professionalism over our units and patients (albeit unconsciously) to hold down the negative responses then it is time for careful, but definite, change. This will be most effective coming from those concerned for spiritual care not least because the religious motivation and philosophy behind palliative care generally discourages anger, and in so doing not only denies therapeutic opportunities but also betrays its own roots and tradition. This is particularly true of the Judeao-Christian tradition. Abraham Heschel, a Jewish theologian writes,

> Since the day Abraham argued with God over the fate of Sodom and Gomorrah, and Jacob wrestled with and overcame the angel, many Prophets and rabbis had occasionally engaged in similar arguments. The refusal to accept the harshness of God's ways in the name of His love was an authentic form of prayer. Indeed, the ancient Prophets of Israel were not in the habit of consenting to God's harsh judgement and did not simply nod, saying, 'Thy will be done.' They often challenged Him, as if to say, 'Thy will be changed.' They had often countered and even annulled divine decrees.[7]

> One ought not to be servile even before God. Even in defeat, continued courage was essential.[8]

Some patients teach us this but usually in spite of a spiritual culture that seems to promote servility above courage.

> There are some forms of suffering that a man must accept with love and bear in silence. There are other agonies to which he must say no.[9]

If 'no' is what a patient or his family is screaming at God and life then the emotional strength and pastoral skill needs to be found for its release. The Christian patient may need to be reminded of Jesus' scream cum prayer of anguish at his own apparent abandonment in suffering and death.

> My God, my God, why hast thou forsaken me?'[10]

A legitimate question frequently felt especially by the young dying, but too rarely heard in nice hospices and hospitals.

Wilfred Owen, a deeply religious man and acknowledged to be one of the most gifted of all war poets, wrote in a preface to his 1917 poem 'Autumn for Doomed Youth':

> There is a point where prayer is indistinguishable from blasphemy. There is also a point where blasphemy is indistinguishable from prayer.[11]

But it is not that blasphemy is essential or even to be encouraged for it is frequently enough to give permission for anger and protest to God. There is power in having the idea in the bank for possible future use if things get even worse which releases the emotional and spiritual tension. Just to know that it is possible and permissible is healing and only a few need to go on to spit at a crucifix. For the religious carer the justification for this is that it is the way of reconciliation, that the shared reality of honest encounter/prayer often creates that sense of God's presence that the abandoned crave. 'God directed' wrath is an act of faith.

One of the best uses of a hospital or hospice chapel is for private prayer of this kind. It provides a legitimate target and a safe place to vent seemingly dangerous thoughts and feelings. It should also be a private place where one can be open and honest before powerful symbols that profoundly echo the spiritual distress involved in dying and loss. These symbols – the crucifix, altar, star of David, candlesticks, etc. all portable and interchangeable have enormous power even for the long-lapsed or even avowed non-believers. To be given permission and opportunity to relate honestly to what and who these symbols represent in the privacy and security of a caring environment is good palliative care. If a nurse wants to encourage a chaplain who has just visited one of her patients she will most often say something like, 'Thank you for seeing Mr Smith, he was much more peaceful after your visit.' More rarely do they evaluate spiritual care with 'Thank God you managed to help him get all that anger out'.

Mystery – having no explanation

Staying with mystery and unanswered questions is a prime function of spiritual care. This is especially difficult when all the other disciplines are very busy skilfully resolving problems about which they can be articulate and precise. The pressure to produce answers is enormous but has to be resisted. First, because many of the questions have no answers, that is why they go on being asked. Secondly, patients are not asking for an answer in the sense of explanation, most of them know that they are living with the inexplicable, and questions like the classic 'Why is this happening to me?' are there to be shared and only rarely analysed.

> Suffering is not so much a problem requiring an explanation as a mystery demanding a presence.[12]

As already said presence is our prime offer in palliative care and the Christian, of course, offers another.

At the beginning of his terrible account of his childhood in Auschwitz and Buchenwald, Elie Wiesel writes of his relationship with Moché, the Beadle in his home town in Transylvania,

> 'Why do you pray?' he asked me, after a moment.
> Why did I pray? A strange question. Why did I live? Why did I

breathe?

'I don't know why,' I said, even more disturbed and ill at ease, 'I don't know why.'

After that day I saw him often. He explained to me with great insistence that every question possessed a power that did not lie in the answer.

'Man raises himself toward God by the questions he asks Him,' he was fond of repeating. 'That is the true dialogue. Man questions God and God answers. But we don't understand His answers. We can't understand them. Because they come from the depth of the soul, and they stay there until death. You will find the true answers, Elieser, only within yourself!'

'And why do you pray, Moché?' I asked him.

'I pray to God within me that He will give me the strength to ask Him the right questions.'[13]

The dying often need the strength to address the right questions to God but though they may need assistance in the asking they often have the wisdom to know that the questions are enough. But they have to be their questions and even more their answers – not received via the ear but breathed into the heart.

Faith and hope

Faith has too often been seen as a complex effort of belief that religions have presented as hoops that can only be jumped through by spiritual and intellectual willpower. Ministering to the dying on the contrary teaches us that faith is more a reaching out with the proverbial trust of the child, a faith or trust that God accepts us as we are and that forgiveness is always offered. This reaching out can be embarrassingly simple for those used to the first definition of faith, given above, for it bypasses the lengthy instruction and preparation of the convert while disarmingly resulting in a deep and intuitive understanding of the mystery of God. We find this reaching out difficult to accept, not only for its simplicity but because it means letting go traditional expectations of the message followed by a valid or saving response. Faith as taught us by patients cuts across our need for sophistication. Jesus faced this issue in siding with the poor against the Pharisees.

A hospital chaplain's experience:

- Made him redefine evangelism.
- Made him redefine the meaning of the Church.
- Gave him a confidence to be with dying people.
- Gave him a confidence that they would come to fullness with God.
- Made him appreciate that it is not necessary to get the traditional Christian message across and obtain a traditional response.
- Led him to offer the simple but profound message of God's unconditional love.
- Led him to believe that the realization of this in a person's life is a

conversion experience.[14]

For many of us it takes courage and humility to be simple with, and for, our patients.

Hope issues from faith but not necessarily easily or in a discernable progression.

> Whenever faith develops into hope it does not make people serene and placid; it makes them restless. It does not make them patient; it makes them impatient. Instead of being reconciled to the existing reality they begin to suffer for it and to resist it.[15]

Some long-term patients who outlive their prognosis sometimes exhibit this restlessness while the impatience can be shared by equally frustrated carers. It is also not to be confused with 'pie in the sky when we die,' for genuine hope has eyes as open to present suffering as to future bliss.

> Genuine hope is not blind optimism. It is hope with open eyes, which sees the suffering and yet believes in the future.[16]

The future is often formulated in terms of heaven, which many care givers feel unsure of and are embarrassed to discuss. A sharing of uncertainties can be helpful – 'I'm not sure but I'd like to think. . .', or humour and fantasy – 'I think it will be like the Lake District' are not out of place. Hope is not so much about detail or geography but an assurance of the victory of goodness, truth and beauty; all of which are within the experience of the dying. This is made real by love added to faith and hope.

> Nothing worth doing is completed in our lifetime; therefore we must be saved by hope. Nothing true or beautiful or good makes complete sense in an individual's context of history; therefore we are saved by love. No virtuous act is quite as virtuous from the standpoint of our friend or foe as from our standpoint; therefore we must be saved by the final form of love, which is forgiveness.[17]

Traditional religious Christian care

Although this chapter is called 'Spiritual Concerns' it would be a pity if our proper emphasis on the spiritual were to exclude religious practice or imply that religion is redundant. The traditional rituals of religion have great power in the context of death and dying, separation and loss. This is true for the majority of people who are not regular participants in religious ritual at other times; it seems clear, for example, that the funeral will be the last rite of passage to be abandoned. The profoundly spiritual and cultural need for ritual is most evident in the face of death.

Different faiths and traditions have different emphases and styles of ritual that give expression to spiritual values and convictions. What follows is Christian and has a Church of England flavour because that is the author's tradition. It is also a useful model as this tradition has an inclusive tone usually making charitable assumptions about participants as well as having become intertwined into the general cultural scene, certainly in the UK.

A standard response to hospice or hospital chaplains is 'I don't go to church, vicar, but I do believe and I do say my prayers.' The way many people pray in the face of death might be seen as superstitious but is more profitably assessed as seminal or even simple faith. Some of the prayer cards that many people say that they find helpful have a sentimental and heretical flavour that health care professionals and chaplains in particular can be very snobbish and dismissive about but we need to be slow to condemn. Usually prayers with patients and families need to be short and contain some personal element, leaning toward God's love and protection rather than the problems. It is always very special to patients and their families if staff other than the chaplain pray with them. Commendatory prayers following death are a very supportive ritual to families and sometimes staff. They contain vocabulary and statements that are not only reassuring but also frank and realistic, words that might be very difficult in conversation yet help the process of letting go at a crucial point.

Baptism is sometimes asked for as part of the tidying up of loose ends that the dying often need and again it can be best seen as emerging faith and a true instinct rather than a cynical attempt at spiritual insurance. The patient must be allowed to determine whether it is administered just with the priest sitting on the bed or where family, friends and staff have gathered round in the chapel, day room or at home.

The 'laying on of hands' and anointing are very direct ways of praying for patients involving ancient and deep symbolism that speaks of healing via touch and blessing. Patients tend to understand the difference between healing and cure and it is probably staff fears of raising false expectations that inhibits a more positive ministry of healing being part of palliative care. Through touch, prayer and blessing these actions speak more deeply to the sick than we often appreciate.

Confirmations and weddings also affirm that life is primary while giving patients the opportunity to make important statements of witness to family, friends and staff. Like other rituals they should be tailored to the circumstance and preferences of the participants to allow the religious ritual to be the servant of the spiritual meaning and value that is intended by them.

Funerals are probably best conducted in the community to which the family belong but if a patient has requested that the chaplain and perhaps other staff be involved in his funeral then that may be seen as an exception. Otherwise staff should be discouraged for their own self-care and protection unless they can identify it as their own need to be present. Families often ask for the hospice or hospital chaplain because they want a continuation of the care thus far received and this may be pastorally desirable but should not be routine or done without the permission of the Parish Priest or whoever would normally be responsible. There will be an increasing number of families who will ask for a non-religious ritual and they should be advised that such is possible and perhaps desirable for them, and in some cases we may want to suggest the option. They can also be put in touch with the Humanist Association[18] who will offer sensitive advice.

For Christians of virtually all traditions the Sacrament of Holy Communion, Mass or The Eucharist is the primary healing and reconciling sacrament. This may not only be true for the committed and practising believer. Speaking directly about suffering, death and resurrection this rite with its visual, tactile symbols of a broken body and poured out life blood have immediate relevance for the dying.

Words like

> He opened wide his arms for us on the cross;
> he put an end to death by dying for us
> and revealed the resurrection by rising to new life[19]

have a resonance and a clear note of hope for the dying.

This sacrament is nothing like as exclusive in the context of sickness and dying as it is in a parish church or anywhere that does not have a focus born of pain and loss so we need not be reticent about creating an inclusive atmosphere around what is after all called a celebration.

All of these aspects of religious care and ritual should be presented in such a way that they say to patients, families and colleagues:

> God loves you, cares for you and desires your love. You are important to Him (and to us) because you are you. This service, or prayer, is for you, to help you to express your feelings and thoughts; your fears, doubts and struggle as well as your faith, hope and commitment. Be yourself, be as honest as you can. It does not matter at all if you do not understand all that this means. Relax and use this as you will, to receive something more of God's love.

Other faiths and none

There is often an apprehension about caring for those of other faiths born of the misunderstanding that a body of detailed and esoteric knowledge is needed. Added to this is the image acquired from the media that 'others' are militant and passionate about their faith, certainly in a way that is rare in the Christianised West. The propaganda which we have imbibed allows for no middle ground of gently held faith, not to mention a vast number of nominal adherents such as exist in 'Christian' countries. This fear is almost totally unfounded. We need to replace this timidity with a spiritual confidence in the spiritual power of the care patterns that are, by and large, already embedded in the tradition of palliative care. Not least this includes respect for the individual. As we listen to them they will tell us of their special spiritual, religious and cultural needs. Of course it is helpful to have a broad understanding of potential special dietary needs, post-death ritual, cultural prohibitions or modesty issues. But all of these particular requirements are likely to be communicated in the environment and relationships that are of the essence of good palliative care. In any case the response is more about sensitivity and openness than a detailed knowledge of other cultures. There will also be a variety of requirements and sensibilities within any one faith just as there is in the Christian faith so even a good general knowledge of another faith or culture will have to be checked against 'denominational' or regional variables as well as personal preferences that may confound the textbook.

The greatest problem will come with short-term patients who are unable to communicate or who die before any relationship can be established with them or their family. In such cases a list of religious leaders with telephone numbers is essential. This must also include details of whether, for example, the rabbi is Orthodox, Reformed, Liberal or ideally whether we know them well enough as people to judge whether they are likely to feel at ease with a particular patient or family.

The main question is whether the health carer can relax and treat the 'different' guest as a person, gently ask basic questions like 'Will a male doctor be acceptable?' and allow the patient and family the autonomy we offer to those from our own culture. The sad fact is that the fear that keeps peoples apart on the wider stage even infects and inhibits the most caring of individuals and teams. The result is a shyness, a nervousness and an inflated courtesy that results in a degree of separation that is destructive of what can be offered.

What a dying Jew, Muslim or Hindu needs in terms of spiritual care is precisely what is usually offered – that is, the deeply human spiritual response of acceptance, openness to his individuality, a listening respect, in a word hospitality.

> Hospitality, therefore, means primarily the creation of a free space where the stranger can enter and become a friend instead of an enemy. Hospitality is not to change people, but to offer them space where change can take place. It is not to bring men and women over to our side, but to offer freedom not disturbed by dividing lines. It is not to lead our neighbour into a corner where there are no alternatives left, but to open a wide spectrum of options for choice and commitment. It is not an educated intimidation with good books, good stories and good works, but the liberation of fearful hearts so that words can find roots and bear ample fruit. it is not a method of making our God and our way into the criteria of happiness, but the opening of an opportunity to others to find their God and their way. The paradox of hospitality is that it wants to create emptiness, not a fearful emptiness, but a friendly emptiness where strangers can enter and discover themselves as created free; free to sing their own songs, speak their own languages, dance their own dances; free also to leave and follow their own vocations. Hospitality is not a subtle invitation to adopt the life style of the host, but the gift of a chance for the guest to find his own.[20]

That is spiritual care.

Notes and References

1. RUMBOLD, B. Helplessness and Hope: Pastoral Care in Terminal Illness, SCM, 1986, p. 54.
2. TOURNIER, P. Source unknown.
3. SPECK, P. *Being There: Pastoral Care in Time of Illness*, SPCK, 1988.
4. VANIER, J. *Tears of Silence*, Darton, Longman and Todd, 1973, p. 30.
5. NOUWEN, J.M.H. *The Way of the Heart*. Darton, Longman and Todd, 1981, p. 34.
6. POTTER, D. Talk on BBC Radio 4.
7. HESCHEL, A.J. *A Passion for Truth*, Farrar, Straus, Giroux, 1986, p. 265.
8. HESCHEL, A.J. *A Passion for Truth*, Farrar, Straus, Giroux, 1986, p. 270.
9. HESCHEL, A.J. *A Passion for Truth*, Farrar, Straus, Giroux, 1986, p. 271.
10. *The Holy Bible*. Revised Standard Version, Mark 15:35.
11. Quoted in: MURSELL, G, *Out of the Deep: Prayer as Protest*, Darton, Longman and Todd, 1989, p. 154.
12. Source unknown.
13. WEISEL, E. *Night*. Penguin, 1981, pp. 14–15.
14. WOODROFFE, I. 'Towards a hospice theology,' 1989. Quoted in: *Mud and Stars. Report of a Working Party*. Sobell Publications, 1991, pp. 166–7.
15. MOLTMANN, *Experiences of God*, SCM, 1980.
16. MOLTMANN, *Experiences of God*, SCM, 1980.
17. NEIBUHR, R. *Sermon, Union Theological Seminary*, New York, 1959.
18. Humanist Association, 14 Lambs Conduit Passage, London WC1R 4RH.
19. *Alternative Service Book*, Rite A, Third Eucharistic Prayer, 1980.
20. NOUWEN, J.M.H. *Reaching Out*, Collins, 1987, pp. 68–9.

6

The Work of the Interdisciplinary Team

Tom West

Introduction

Helping people with far advanced cancer calls for more skills than any one individual can command. The interdisciplinary team approach has already been developed in disciplines such as paediatrics where the whole family needs to be involved. Nowhere is it more essential than in response to the expressed and perceived needs of patients in the terminal stages of cancer and also of their families.

The original concept of the 'total pain' of patients, with its physical, psycho-social and spiritual components has now been enlarged to include staff involvement and stress, together with all the pains that this can arouse. At the same time the importance of 'family' in the widest sense of the word, present or absent (and even alive or dead), is seen as an area to be explored and one in which there are often hidden strengths to be uncovered in otherwise impossible situations. Furthermore, working in this way does not have to be confined to independent, free-standing hospices. It can also be appropriate in caring for patients at home, in hospitals and in nursing homes, each of which has its own advantages and disadvantages.

What will now be described is based on the hospice experience of interdisciplinary functioning. It may therefore need 'translating' (rather than merely 'transplanting') if it is to be useful to teams short of time, short of staff and working in other contexts. Such crisis management will be discussed later.

Selection

The interdisciplinary team is formed from a group of individuals who will have been drawn to this work for a variety of reasons. Most caregivers have personal reasons for needing to care, and a wish to understand and be involved in the dynamics of patient and family as well as in team work is a good beginning. A successful working team must begin with careful selection. Professional competence, flexibility, a sense of humour, respect for others, the ability to support colleagues and above all an awareness of what is meant by trust will all be needed from the people composing the team.

There are as many selection procedures as there are institutions and it is hard to strike a balance between a democratic approach in which everyone has to be involved, and an autocratic appointment, which if less than a total success can be expected to bring with it much resentment. A clear idea by those interviewing, as well as by the candidate, of the common task and therefore of the accepted objectives is a good baseline for the interview. Some discussion of shared beliefs and therefore of the possibility of disagreement is important because, in spite of possessing the highest professional skills, team members may sometimes be asked to modify professional practice and the acceptability (or otherwise) of this should be explored. How 'uncertainty' can best be coped with is a further matter worth discussing with those intending to care for patients with cancer. Expediency remains one of the commonest and one of the worst reasons for making an appointment.

Following the appointment it is essential that the trial period is taken seriously and from the beginning needs to be recognized as a two-way exercise. During it there must be regular occasions for appraisal between the new team member and the team leader and both here and on into longer term team functioning there must be opportunities for growth that are not just patient centred. Although patient and family are the reason for the existence of the team and therefore for the presence of the individuals who make up the team, it is essential that team members can on occasions deal directly with each other, learning and developing in the process.

The team

In interdisciplinary work responsibility is shared. Each member of the team brings to the day's work his or her own professional skills with all the confidence that this produces. But professional traditions will also be present and may well need adjusting. The stereotype of each profession (e.g. doctor, nurse, social worker) can be almost as easily imposed as assumed. Each team member may also have to deal with personal stereotyping and work out with the team how such type-casting is best used or, if necessary, overcome.

This involves looking for and beginning to understand the professional and personal skills of other disciplines as well as one's own, recognizing the fact of professional rivalries and the temptation to compete, and learning how to share and when to hand over. It is not natural to be generous, to share the particular gifts or skills that mark one out, nor is it easy to be prepared to give up being 'the one' to complete a fine piece of work. But the symbolism and the effectiveness of professions working jointly, yet able at times to appear to abdicate roles without loss of face, is one of the major strengths of the interdisciplinary approach. The doctor who is able to step aside for the social worker and the nurse who knows when she does *not* need to call the chaplain represent effective functioning by all four of these different disciplines.

Team functions

In practice no team can afford to be leaderless. The leader makes the team. This is pre-eminently the leadership quality – the ability to organize all the forces there are in an enterprise and make them serve a common purpose.[1] If the team is to function at all decisions have to be made. Who should take the lead in reaching these decisions may vary according to the problem being addressed. In clinical decision making, for example prescribing for pain, it must be the doctor who has the final responsibility – but it would be foolish if the observations of the nursing staff were ignored. With a distraught family it is the social worker who is most likely to produce ideas on containing and resolving the situation – although someone might point out a possible role for the chaplain. In other words: 'Irrespective of position or personality, true leadership lies in the individual who knows his job, who can grasp the essentials of what needs to be done, and also the relational significance of the facts in hand.' This 'leadership of function' when recognized produces *the* leader for that specific task.[2]

In such situations the selection and affirmation of the key-worker or current 'worrier' is a task for the team leader. But it also means that every member of the team (including the leader) must have some concept of necessary personal boundaries.

Meanwhile if the work is to continue and not just rock from crisis to crisis there must be a manager to ensure day-to-day continuity. For example on a hospice or hospital ward the ward sister is the obvious manager, masterminding ward rounds in which the doctor may take a leading role, family meetings when the social worker may be the appropriate leader and coordinating such important activities as physiotherapy and occupational therapy.

But a team, as well as linking up with other professional caregivers within the institution, must also be ready to look outwards. For example, if more information about the nursing care of the patient is required it is best obtained by the team nurse from the ward nurse or district nurse who had been looking after the patient. Complicated social and family problems, perhaps involving confidentiality, will most appropriately be communicated from social worker to social worker. Details of the patient's previous investigations and medical or surgical treatments may need clarifying and here the team doctor should contact the hospital doctor or general practitioner. Such enquiries may lead to considering further more active treatment and in such situations the doctor, supported by the insight of the team, may find himself acting as the patient's advocate.

Communicating with and advising professionals outside the team is a further skill to be mastered. Discussing the pros and cons of further active therapy with an oncologist or giving advice about drugs to a general practitioner is not always straightforward. With practice, and as each side gets to know the other better, it becomes easier. Taking the trouble to meet the other person on his or her own ground and inviting them to visit the hospice or palliative care unit can transform an otherwise difficult situation.

A team must always be quick to recognize the possible importance of calling on relevant outside help. Radiotherapists, oncologists, anaesthetists and surgeons may still have something to offer even towards the end of a patient's life. Involving the available community services may enable a patient to stay at home for longer by supporting the family through a time of otherwise overwhelming stress. Clearly deciding who in the team should be responsible for making such contacts and for ensuring that things then run smoothly is part of the overall management needed if everything that ought to be done for the patient and his family is to be achieved.

To sum up: a team will need a sense of purpose and vision. The source is often hard to identify but where good management has provided a safe enough context anyone in the team may feel able to take the lead in proposing a change of plan, confident that they will be listened to with respect and then supported in their individual or collective actions. Such a team will find that it has the strength to admit mistakes and change direction without scape-goating. All this will depend on a clear but flexible organization and an acknowledgement of who, when the chips are down, has the last word.

Organization and communication

Recognizing, at any given moment, who is leading and respecting who is quietly managing is the bare bones of a system that forms the basis of good interdisciplinary work. But decisions must not only be made. In order that they are carried out they must also be communicated and recorded and even then they will still need reviewing.

Working with patients suffering from advanced disease demands not just tender loving care – there must also be skilful loving care and there will often be a need for quick decisions and quick communication. In practice it is often impossible for everyone to be informed of everything and this necessary limitation of the numbers informed calls for an exercise in trust by those who would otherwise feel excluded.

All the same this work necessitates enough time and enough staff for there to be effective day-to-day hand-overs. The time spent in good reporting from one shift to another should be treated as a priority. For example following a family meeting during the day no night staff should have to work through the night without appropriate knowledge of what went on. The next day is too late.

For less urgent matters the most economical occasion for communication is the interdisciplinary weekly team meeting. When these are well managed and well led the level of communication is amazingly high and the sources of information often surprising. It may be the physiotherapist who supplies the missing link in a problem situation. Perhaps the confidence shared with the phyiotherapist has occurred because the doctor is the doctor, nurses work in pairs and social workers do not wear uniforms. It is the one-to-one, hands-on and unhurried meeting with an obvious 'professional' that encourages the patient to talk.

At these interdisciplinary meetings as well as 'leader' and 'manager' a third skill is called for – that of 'chairman'. A flexible but real agenda, a sense of time and the ability to make the meeting feel safe enough for even the shyest or the insecure to express anxieties and make suggestions are needed. This ability to chair and then facilitate a meeting is a special skill that should be recognized and then utilized by both the organization and the team. It will pay dividends by drawing attention to anxieties, producing new ideas for the resolving of problems and prove to be the best forum of all for establishing the team's common purpose and active participation.

There are guidelines for interdisciplinary meetings that can be helpful: the right language for communication at these meetings must be learned – professional jargon even to other professionals is counter-productive; a room is needed that is comfortable enough, private enough and the right shape for easy communication; bleeps should, if possible, be left outside.

At such weekly meetings teams will slowly learn more about getting it right, as they go through match re-plays of both successes and failures, and look at the detail and the timing of personal interventions just as carefully as they plan the pharmacological ones.

Other important team activities

Ward rounds should be fixed points in the week's programme. (In home-care teams the regular review of patients fulfils the same function.) It is useful if an interdisciplinary discussion can take place before the patients are visited. Here the manager – usually the senior nurse – can bring the other disciplines up to date with patients and their families; fore-warned can be fore-armed. Possible changes in treatment can then be discussed and provisional plans of action proposed.

Who visits the bedside depends on both availability and appropriateness. Three or four people are usually the maximum that can sit round a bed without it feeling oppressive. Here it is usual for the doctor to be leader while the senior nurse or the social worker may well be cast in the role of patient's advocate. During discussion it is important that while any two are engaged in conversation the others are observing reactions on both sides and picking up clues as to what is really being asked or understood. People round the bed can be drawn into the conversation to help prevent any feeling of an unequal duel between patient and doctor and it is particularly satisfactory if the patient (or sometimes a family member) ends up by taking a leading part in the discussion.

When the ward round is completed team members must take time to go over what has occurred and what they observed. Plans of action can now be confirmed or altered. Decisions will then be recorded and appropriate people (for example, the patient and family) will need to be informed.

Of course it is also important that team members do rounds alone, giving the patient the opportunity for a more private interview or a thorough physical examination. But it is essential that such solo visits are immediately and fully reported back to the staff responsible for the ongoing management of the ward.

Home visits may often have to be carried out by a single member of the team. Again as much knowledge as possible should be gathered beforehand from those already involved. It is useful if a check list of the current problems has been drawn up so that these can be checked out and proposals for dealing with them formulated. The visit itself takes place on the patient's territory and it is worth remembering that good manners are as important here as they are at the hospital bedside. Recording and reporting are vital if continuity of care from one visit to the next is to be maintained by the team and links with the wider multidisciplinary community services are to be forged and strengthened.

Family meetings are sometimes anticipated with a degree of fear by team members. Doctors in particular have often had little experience of facing an angry family except perhaps when protected by a white coat or a large desk. A brief team-meeting beforehand is essential. The strengths as well as the weaknesses of the family should be rehearsed. The objectives of the meeting can be decided on and a provisional agenda and seating plan proposed. If the family concern is primarily medical the doctor will take the initiative. At other times it will be the social worker or the team member closest to the family who starts off as leader. But often a family member rapidly takes over as the spokesperson for the whole group and not infrequently it is the youngest person present who asks the question no one else has the courage to voice.

Perhaps at no other time is the interdisciplinary team approach more obviously appropriate. The family will see the team's wide-ranging concern for their needs while, at the same time, they experience a model of different people trying to work together in ways that can often be usefully applied to their own situation. Recording such meetings while respecting confidentiality can be difficult, but again it is important that team members not present are informed of matters that have arisen and are relevant to their ongoing care of the family.

Assessment visits are a special skill. Those carrying them out must have real experience of the possible course and problems of the disease. They also need to be aware of the current strengths and weaknesses both of the team and of the institution they represent. It is irresponsible to take on a patient or family that the team, for whatever reason, is not able to care for appropriately.

Building and maintaining the team

From all that has been said it is clear that teams do not function just because they exist.[3] A team begins as a group of people with a common purpose learning to work together. Its strength is in the diversity of talent which it brings to the task; its vulnerability lies in its necessity for coordination and the time this takes.[4] A concise statement of the attitudes, values and beliefs about issues that are considered important will provide a sense of direction and common ground from which to work. The selection of new members for the team, along the lines already described, should take place in the context of this clear (but not rigid) philosophy of care. Teams, like buildings, require regular maintenance. This will involve periodic discussion of the common goals and opportunity for the team to evaluate their achievements and if necessary to redefine their aims. Team members need to be encouraged to discuss their individual roles in such a way that people feel supported rather than criticized. The interdisciplinary team meeting (see above) is one good place for such communication to take place. But an interdisciplinary team is made up not just of different individuals but also of different professions. There is a proper place of *uni*disciplinary appraisal, discussion and support groups, though here again there will need to be trust and relevant interdisciplinary communication.

Building a good team and then ensuring that it is properly maintained will result in that most important morale factor of all – job satisfaction.

Other matters

Reporting and confidentiality

If the interdisciplinary team is to function reasonably smoothly then reports, recording and handovers have to be conducted efficiently. It is not always easy to distinguish what is relevant and important from what is routine trivia. Yet the ability to distinguish what is currently of prime importance from what is an optional extra or merely (like 'the bowels' or 'religion') of traditional importance is what distinguishes a useful handover from one that is both unmemorable and an expensive waste of time.

When matters of confidentiality are involved it must be explained and then accepted that not everyone has to know everything. Indeed no one needs to know more than will enable them to fulfil their own role in caring for the patient. If a patient chooses to unburden personal matters to a member of the team it can be very helpful to say something like: 'Thank you for sharing such an important and difficult thing with me. Would you mind if in turn I shared it with other members of the team?' Almost always the person, pleased to be the centre of such real concern, will agree.

Teaching

An important function of the interdisciplinary team should be to teach. Sometimes this may feel like an unwanted and heavy load but in fact it can be both stimulating and a first-class antidote to battle fatigue. Teaching other people what is on offer and how best to use the team and its individual members obviously makes good sense. Experience will then help to show them when the team's skills really should be called on, when team involvement is quite unnecessary or when all that is needed is back-up from the team.

Teaching non-team members appropriate skills in hospice and palliative care will only succeed if they are also given sufficient confidence in their ability to take on these rather wider roles. Nothing succeeds better in building confidence than giving appropriate praise. Nothing is more destructive than public criticism.

Further questions

There will always be further questions for a team to address if it wishes to continue to develop:

- How can the team cope with the problem of the 'team splitter'? This can be caused by either a patient/family member or a team member. Perhaps the patient most likely to split the team is a longer term or very dependent person. Such a patient can easily give rise to differing aims and expectations particularly among the nursing team and, as an expression of helplessness, at the same time become difficult and manipulative. Often a member of the team from another discipline will have a clearer insight into the root of the problem.

  Team nursing will reduce the numbers of people involved and there-fore the amount of potential conflict. Meeting to acknowledge the problem and to agree on a fairly strict plan of care will re-establish the common objectives and therefore the trust between team members. A firm statement of intent to the patient (and probably to the family) will then help to put the situation back on the rails.

  Dealing with the team member who is a problem is not easy. (This may especially be the case if they are the only representative of their profession on the team.) The individual's manager should be approached and the situation explained. Confrontation should be handled firmly and communication needs to be clear. Problems need to be dealt with one at a time and as far as possible without putting down the individual concerned. If honest communication across the whole group has been established there is a good chance that conflict can be resolved and trust and competence restored.[5]

- What makes people tired? Genuine pressure of work, ill-health, personal problems, battles with administration, communication problems, inadequate resources, unrealistic expectations are some of the factors that a tired team (or a team with a tired team-member) would be wise to explore.
- How does a team take on a new member? Marriages may be made in heaven, but they certainly have to be worked at on earth. Taking the trouble to make space for the newcomer can help turn what feels in the first place an intruder into a valued addition to the team.
- How does the appraisal system fit in? It will of course help leaders, managers and staff members to monitor their personal progress. But in working as a multidisciplinary group it is important that the appraiser takes the trouble to find out how well the appraisee is fitting into the multidisciplinary scene. Ideally each person should feel satisfied (though not complacent) with their own professional performance and at the same time consider that they are a fully paid-up member of the interdisciplinary team.
- How does a team cope when it is short staffed, short of time and there is still a mountain of work that has to be done? It is extraordinarily difficult to lower standards or to cut corners, though the real choice may end up between leaving work undone or, for the emergency, to work faster. Yet most teams know from experience that it is at times like these that ethical issues or personality clashes seem to emerge. Rather than allowing pockets of discontent to accumulate the team leader should call a full team meeting to address the problem. Such 'crisis management' will enable a good team to achieve an acceptable resolution within the day and, because of their involvement, the team members will now have a personal investment in once again getting it right.

Summary

The interdisciplinary team has to look outside itself and recognize and learn how and when it is appropriate to incorporate different disciplines. Occupational therapy, physiotherapy and the other important therapies, volunteers, the administrative staff all have vital roles to play. Too often lip service is paid to their supportive membership of the team, when in practice not enough care has been taken in first carefully defining their special function and then appropriately including them in.

The interdisciplinary team approach is an exercise in learning, caring, working together, teaching and appraisal. It cannot succeed without enough individual professional skill and enough trust and understanding between the professions to give each member the courage to follow his own judgement when that is what seems appropriate. Taking such considered risks is often only possible with the knowledge that the team is providing a solid enough stage for actions that may lead to a positive approach and real creativity in otherwise overwhelming problems.

Team work is often more untidy than tidy – so is the rest of life. But honest reviewing by the team of the work as it proceeds will usually result in a sense of job satisfaction rather than one of despondency. And just because it is not possible to take on new commitments when there is too much unfinished business still in hand, the occasions taken by a team to affirm achievements and to acknowledge the ending of successive pieces of work is good use of their time.

Finally, it is difficult to overrate the importance of appropriate praise and a respect for such phrases as 'Good morning', 'Thank you' and occasionally, 'I was wrong, I'm sorry'. Good manners can enable a team to get through times of misunderstanding and also to cash in successfully on crisis situations when, just by *not* playing it safe, often the impossible is achieved.

Notes and References

1.   GRAHAM, P. *Integrative Management*, Oxford, Basil Blackwell, 1991, p. 120.
2.   GRAHAM, P. *Integrative Management*, 1991, p. 136.
3.   JACKSON, L. 'Team building.' In: SAUNDERS, C. (ed.), *Hospice and Palliative Care*, London, Edward Arnold, 1990, pp. 14–25.
4.   ZIMMERMAN, J.M. *Hospice. Complete Care for the Terminally Ill*, Baltimore: Urban and Schwarzenberg, 1981, pp. 97–125.
5.   CHANNON, H. 'The Team Splitter.' In: SAUNDERS, C. (ed.), *Hospice and Palliative Care*, London, Edward Arnold, 1990, pp. 60–4.

Further reading

HANDY, C.B. *Understanding Organisations*, 3rd edn, Harmondsworth, Penguin, 1985.

7

The Cost to the Professional Carer

Barbara Monroe

Palliative care makes difficult and personal demands on those who provide it. Working closely with the pain and loss of others makes professionals acutely aware of their own losses, both those already experienced and those feared in the future. It also makes them more aware of their own death and its implications. Palliative care workers can enrich their work from their personal experiences of loss, but the commonality between these losses and those of patients and families can present a problem which requires help. It is important that all palliative care professionals have adequate support systems, both within their work places and personally.

When considering the shape of such support systems perhaps one of the most important requirements is a sense of perspective and proportion. In the literature on palliative care much has been made of the concept of 'burn-out'. For a time it was suggested that there was probably a 'shelf-life' for those working in the field, a point beyond which negative self-concepts, job attitudes and a loss of concern for patients were inevitable. This is not so. Palliative care is not a uniquely stressful profession. Many of its pressures are to be found in other environments and require similar solutions. What is needed is professional attention to staff support which includes issues of recruitment, orientation, training, appraisal, communication and team-building.

It is interesting that numerous surveys,[1] including Vachon's[2] seminal study of occupational stress in the care of the dying and bereaved, have reported that care givers feel that far more of their stressors emerge from their work environment and occupational role than from their direct work with dying patients and their families. None the less, it is also clear that professionals need to feel comfortable with themselves and their own losses in order to listen attentively to those of others. Professionals must accept their own needs for support and care and a proper support system will include both personal and organizational mechanisms.

Sources of stress

Institutional

Dr West's chapter in this book has highlighted the value of a team approach to palliative care. However, poorly managed teams are themselves a source of stress. Team communication problems, role ambiguity, interdisciplinary conflict, uncertain or unrealistic objectives and a lack of clear leadership can all contribute to a negative view of the workplace. These difficulties may be exacerbated by poor managerial and administrative practices in the institution as a whole. Problems in teams may simply result from exhaustion, a failure to match workload to resources. Teams, like individuals, need to find a balance between giving and receiving. Most damaging of all is an organizational failure to set clear goals and to give all staff regular recognition for their achievements and regular opportunities to develop new skills against known gaps and deficiencies.

Patient and family

Professionals find it hard to assess the results of their work when their patients die. They receive much of the fear and anger carried by patients and their families and often feel that they are being asked to solve the insoluble. In this atmosphere, unexpected behaviour in patients and families can upset the team; relatives who refuse to visit, those who arrive drunk, those who will not communicate. Patients sometimes resolutely resist dying the way the professionals want them to, leaving the team with a sense of failure and disappointment. The appropriateness of strategies to manage difficult situations, such as sedating a distressed and confused patient, can become a source of conflict if not openly discussed.

The attitudes of the professional

Stress can be a stimulus, it can also disable. Many of the professionals attracted to palliative care disable themselves with an unrealistic set of attitudes and objectives. They expect themselves to be thoroughly competent in every situation they meet, to be able to respond to every demand, to feel warmth towards every patient and family and to be loved and appreciated by all their colleagues and clients. Such 'supermen' confuse helping with rescuing. They tend to become over-involved with patients, feeling indispensable and working extremely long hours. Their actions not only diminish the patient and family, they also disable the rest of the team. Apparent infallibility is very daunting.

The personal life of the professional

The patients and families with whom professionals most readily identify, perhaps because of age or life situation, can trigger off powerful reactions in them. They can raise unexpected and sometimes unresolved personal issues relating to loss and bereavement. The home life of the professional can be supportive but may also be stress intensifying if it includes concurrent emotional demands such as a difficult teenager, illness and marital difficulties. Everyone needs someone to talk to about their work and its problems, but partners and friends may become resentful if they represent the sole source of off-loading or analytical response available to the professional carer.

Signs of stress

Organizations with a high level of employee stress will be characterized by power struggles and rivalry, hostility towards team leaders, unrecognized conflict displaced onto convenient scapegoats, rapid staff turnover, high sickness rates and a general lack of enthusiasm, particularly for new initiatives. The individual may exhibit stress through irritability, depression, loss of self-esteem, over-involvement in work, sleep disturbance, weight loss or gain, tension, headache and other minor illnesses, rigidity, cynicism, apathy and a general sense of feeling overwhelmed.

Clearly palliative care organizations will wish to avoid these consequences. They will do so through a mixture of routine measures available universally and a sensitive and flexible response to particular individuals for whom work and personal pressures have coincided. For example, bereavement in a staff member needs a personally adjusted amount of time off, timed to the needs of the individual. Some may find that they need it two or three months after the death rather than immediately when work colleagues and routines may represent an important source of support. For others the opposite will be true. Many professionals will welcome a brief recognition of their difficulties by a colleague where more detailed probing would be resented or the exposure of explanation become an additional pressure.

Supporting staff

The institution

It is important to devote time to team-building both formally and informally. Opportunities must be created for colleagues to share expertise and beliefs, to exchange opinions, to develop a team philosophy with shared objectives and to review work undertaken. Ward rounds will need to be supplemented by full interdisciplinary meetings in which all staff can stand back and examine the effect that patients and families are having on them, as individuals and as a team, as well as planning for their care. In these, contentious issues can be debated and it is safe to share vulnerabilities, to admit to not knowing what to do, or to not liking a certain patient. Working with loss often seems to cause a loss of professional confidence with individual staff members feeling that only they stand speechless in front of the patient who declares 'Talking can't help, can it?' or that only they retreat in relief from a potentially difficult conversation because the patient has his friends with him or appears to be asleep. Shared, such fears are a source of cohesion and increased understanding, held in isolation, they paralyse.

Talking to colleagues is likely to remain one of the major sources of support for many professionals, both in formal settings but also the hug or cup of coffee following a difficult meeting. Professional review, the process of acknowledging what went well and what went badly, must be accompanied by personal exchange and the time to get to know colleagues as individuals. Opportunities need to be found to develop a certain level of intimacy so that in a crisis staff feel safe enough with one another to take short cuts. Examples would be going out for meals together or joint writing or teaching projects. Teaching and writing are important counter-balancing activities to work with dying patients. They are essentially creative and allow an overview and some sense of control. In a professional area where so much unfinished business is inevitable it is vital to find activities that have a beginning, a middle and an end. Developing a supportive team culture also helps, with common expectations about time-keeping, taking time off in lieu, going off site for team 'away days' and so on. In addition everyone in the organization should know clearly the boundaries of their own responsibility and have the opportunity to participate appropriately in decision making. An active policy of delegation is a benchmark of a healthy organization.

Organizations engaged in palliative care also need to employ strategies more directly aimed at staff support. A regular, formal 'supervision' session between a professional and their manager can provide time for reflection and direct skill development. Appraisal allows monitoring of achievements and difficulties and suggests requirements for personal development and training.

All staff will need a safe institutional framework within which to express their grief and learn how to let go. It may help to have a regular slot in ward meetings to remember the dead, beds might be left empty for 24 hours after a death and permission given for staff to attend funerals. For most professionals some deaths will become particularly significant and attending such a patient's funeral will permit grieving for many other deaths at the same time, providing a useful release valve in addition to being much appreciated by families. Equally, staff members not directly engaged in bereavement care need some reassurance that vulnerable families will continue to be cared for, even if not by themselves. Thought should be given to ways of helping them to express their own concern appropriately, for instance via anniversary cards or presence at institutional memorial services.

For many professionals such strategies will be sufficient. Not everyone wishes to share on a more personal level within the workplace. Some, however, will welcome specific support groups, facilitated by an outsider and usually more successful if requested by the group itself around a particular issue. Many organizations also offer individual counselling to staff members. Such help should be provided on a confidential basis and limited to two or three meetings aimed primarily at examining options and, if necessary, identifying an appropriate external agency to provide additional help. Long-term individual counselling should not be offered to staff within the workplace, particularly in the field of palliative care where personal and institutional objectives are all too likely to be confused.

Personal coping mechanisms

All professionals will have different strategies for looking after themselves and will need to respect this variety. However, some factors are common to all; the need to recognize personal limitations, that resources are not inexhaustible and to learn how to say 'no' sometimes, to forgive mistakes in self and others and to ask for help. Perhaps even more difficult for most people is the task of remembering what they are good at and sharing it. A sense of pace is important, starting the day with an already packed diary and trying to squeeze in several more impossibilities is a certain recipe for stress.

Everyone needs to keep a regular check on their own emotional bank balance. Is it in credit or overdrawn? It varies and if things are badly awry the individual should be prepared to commit himself to one specific and realistic change to alter the balance. This may involve examining commitments at work and at home, setting priorities and taking action such as planning a holiday, a training course, or leaving the telephone off the hook for once.

Individual professionals also need to be alive to ways of strengthening personal resources and finding renewal. These might include:

- Developing a particular area of work as a personal specialism in which satisfaction can be taken even when compromises have to be made elsewhere.
- Treats; a meal with friends, a cream cake, a hairdo.
- Physical activity; gardening, golf, swimming, squash.
- Creativity; painting, cooking, DIY.
- Relaxation; reading, music, yoga, prayer, a bubble bath.
- Doing something different on a structured basis. Just flopping is not always the answer; learning German, hang-gliding or lace-making may help with a sense of achievement.
- Cultivating a sense of humour and the occasional act of delinquency. An ice cream in the park with a colleague after a difficult home visit, before the return to work, can make a lot of difference.

Managing endings

Palliative care professionals are in the business of endings. They need to take them seriously, not just for patients and families but for themselves. The way professionals finish with a family can sometimes help to model a different and perhaps more satisfactory ending than that of the death of the patient. In crisis families need someone external to hold a sense of security when their world has become unreliable, to convey optimism where they are hopeless. But they do need to separate. The professional is not offering friendship and families need his confirmation of their strength and independence. Professionals are also a scarce resource and will not be able to help new patients and their families if they are full of 'loose ends'.

Pauses

Pauses are important. A pause to let go of what has just been done and to focus on what is to come. The professional cannot really listen if his head is full of the last interview. The gaps between meetings matter. It is vital to remember that people change and work in the spaces between seeing professionals. It is arrogant and patronizing for the professional to expect to find people where he left them. Similarly, silences in an interview often represent the patient's thinking and feeling time. If the professional interrupts too readily by guessing, 'Are you feeling angry?', he puts the patient where he thinks he is, when what is important is to know where the patient thinks he is, 'You've been thinking for quite a while now – would it help you to share your thoughts?'

Review and rehearsal

These help people to close a session or series of sessions. 'Where were we, where are we, what more needs to be done?' In bereavement counselling for example it may help to plan how the bereaved person will tackle a specific future task on his own. Coping skills and achievements must be identified and confirmed.

Respect the relationship

When ending a contact the professional should offer patients and families some feedback on what the relationship has meant to him. Such an acknowledgement of personal involvement helps to return the meeting to the level of two independent adults rather than helper and helped. At the end of a single meeting the question 'How will it help you most to go from here?' will serve a similar function, returning responsibility and control to the patient or family.

Mark the ending

Marking the ending in some way, by ritual or touch, may help; a prayer, a last visit to the grave, shaking hands, a hug.

De-role

It is important for the professional to be clear at the end of the working day about what has been stirred up in him. What belongs to the patients and families and what feelings are properly his own. Time must be taken to separate the two or the professional's own family may suffer. Again a ritual may help, particularly in creating a buffer zone between work and home; loud music in the car, sitting in the car for two minutes on arrival home, consciously taking the doctor role off and putting husband and father on. Good written recording helps in leaving things behind, as does asserting the right to five minutes of a colleague's time to de-brief following a particularly stressful interview. The professional must also develop the ability to trust colleagues to carry on in his absence.

Conclusion

All professionals in palliative care need good personal, social and institutional support systems if they are to function effectively. It also helps to be realistic; the major goal of the palliative care team is to support patients and their families, not to be endlessly sensitive to the personal needs of team members. Professionals must also avoid letting their vision of 'total pain', their desire to treat the 'whole person', trip them into thinking that they must treat every problem. Most people are seeking support not protection, someone willing to listen to their problems rather than someone who can achieve a miracle. Probably the most important element in maintaining personal and institutional morale is a sense of job satisfaction and competence in the work role. This requires affirmation from the organization, and a personal acceptance that 'good enough' care linked to a knowledge that things are better than they would have been without the team's intervention, often represent enormous achievements.

References

1. ALEXANDER, D. and MACLEOD, M. Stress among palliative care matrons. *Palliative Medicine* 1992, 6(2), 111–124.
2. VACHON, M. *Occupational stress in the care of the critically ill, the dying and the bereaved.* Washington: Hemisphere, 1987.

Additional recommended reading

GARDENER, D.R. *Stress Management*. Birmingham: Pepar Publications Ltd, 1990.
VANIER, J. *The broken body*. London: Darton, Longman & Todd, 1988.

8

Interpretation of Palliative care in Different Settings

The primary health care team

Bruce Cleminson

Terminally ill cancer patients usually wish to die at home[1] and, even when death occurs elsewhere, the majority of these patients are at home for most of their terminal illness.[2] Recent work has shown that symptom control at home can be as good as in hospital. Indeed, when physical, emotional and social parameters are considered, skilled care in the patient's own home is seen to be the more effective.[3]

In Britain, the care of the terminally ill patient in his own home will be, largely, carried out by the relatives, helped by the primary health care team (PHCT).

The family doctor

The family doctor is particularly well placed to help in these circumstances. He has a long-term view of the patient, his family and the family's health experiences. He may also have been involved in the original diagnosis of cancer or even before that discussed related subjects in a health promotion role.

He can usefully act as the patient's advocate, e.g. in ensuring that adequate information is transmitted by the hospital and understood by the patient. He can press specialists for treatment when opportune, and liaise between patient and specialist to stop inopportune treatment, coordinating services to obtain as far as possible the type and place of care the patient wishes to receive.

He is readily available both in the surgery and by home visits to meet the needs of the patient. He does not have to wait to be called to make contact, indeed, patients value highly 'spontaneous visits' where the family doctor elects to visit without being called – this means that the patient's problems can be picked up sooner and distressing symptoms minimized.

He can ensure continuity of care, mobilizing the different disciplines of the PHCT and even extending it to meet the individual patient's needs.

The PHCT

The PHCT looks after people in the community, seeing them either in the health centre (or surgery), or in their own homes.

The PHCT will be made up of several members, usually including the family doctor, district nurses, health visitors, community physiotherapist and community psychiatric nurse, social worker and occupational therapist. Not all these will be involved in every case but those particularly involved will liaise so that optimal care is given.

When the PHCT is involved in the care of a dying patient and his family, the basic care will usually be given by the family doctor and district nurse, and others will be brought in as need arises, especially the social worker (for finances and for family distress), the occupational therapist (for aids and adaptations), the physiotherapist and home help.

In unusual cases the team might be widened to include the health visitor for the elderly, the stoma nurses and the continence advisor. Hospital specialists doing domiciliary visits can also be a useful extension to the team.

Where physical care is proving too much, hospice type home care teams and Marie Curie night nurses can be incorporated to make the PHCT more effective and help sustain the patient at home.

In Australia, twenty-four hour nursing in the patient's own home has been used and found to be no more expensive than hospital care.[4] In this era of the internal market and fund holding, such care, presently virtually unknown in Britain, may become more common.

It has been reported that terminally ill patients consume five times the average amount of PHCT time,[5] but this input varies, depending on how far before death it is measured, and is probably an underestimate.[6]

In order to do this work the PHCT member needs to be skilled in the work to be done.

The doctor must be competent in the area of symptom control, being able to come to understand the mechanism of symptoms, with a minimum of tests, relying mainly on clinical skills. He also needs to be aware of the variety of treatment options available so that he can use medicines appropriately and also involve other normal members of the PHCT, and wider team members, such as medical specialists, at the correct time. The family doctor also needs to be aware of the value of a syringe driver when patients are vomiting or no longer able to take medicines orally. (Should the practice not have one, it may be borrowed from a local hospice, or hired from Help the Hospices.)[7] He therefore needs a certain amount of training, as well as the ability to discuss the options with other members of the PHCT and specialists where appropriate.

The nurses likewise need to be excellent at their work. The required skills are possibly best learnt by a hospice attachment, or by having an experienced hospice nurse, e.g. a Macmillan nurse, working alongside as a resource.

Both doctors and nurses need to be highly skilled at communicating with the terminally ill patient and his family, listening carefully, not only to what they say, but what they mean. Though this can be taught to some degree, it also has to be practised.

Support for the team

Because of the intensive nature of this work there is a considerable emotional cost to PHCT members – mainly to the district nurses because of their much longer time commitment than any other PHCT member. This emotional strain can only really be dealt with by the team members talking to each other, saying how they feel and gaining help from each other. This may be a formal support group, or as part of the weekly PHCT meeting or informally with the affected members of the team seeking out other members for a coffee and a chat. A formal group input could usefully include a psychiatrist, psychologist, psychiatric nurse or other members of the caring professions such as a clergyman if they have appropriate skills, time and willingness, and the PHCT feels confident in them.

For the family, home care can be exhausting and emotionally draining. Adequate time must be spent with the family so that they can verbalize their feelings. These may be fears, such as being unsupported at the time of the patient's death, or that the death will be terrible. They may just become exhausted by the continued hard work, specially if the person is very dependent. The use of 'sitters' or, if necessary, respite care can allow time for physical recovery.

Communication

In order to function effectively, especially when the team is extended, communication between team members is of vital importance.

The basic PHCT probably already has a formal meeting weekly, or more often, to discuss a variety of patients and their problems. In the early stage of terminal illness this forum may prove adequate.

However, later on, when there are PHCT members going in to the patient's home daily or more often, a weekly meeting is clearly inadequate. At that stage the members mainly involved are the family doctors and district nurses, and these will probably meet frequently or communicate by telephone especially when something happens that requires the other to visit, or alters the other's treatments.

In a large practice it may be helpful to have one family doctor nominated as coordinator for the medical services to prevent confusion.

Where doctor and nurse rotas for night cover mean that a variety of them cover different nights, those responsible in the day must communicate with those covering at night. A telephone call may be enough, but notes may need to be left in the patient's home if there is more than one practice involved in the rota, or especially if the deputizing service is being used.

The likely problems that will befall the terminally ill cancer patient should be anticipated. Before the patient is bed bound, the commodes, bottles or bedpans should be delivered, and before the patient stops swallowing, a syringe driver should be set up to deliver essential medicines, such as hyoscine and opiates, and oral medications discontinued. In hospital or hospice, such needed equipment may be only yards away. In general practice it may be miles away, making this area much more important.

In a small rural practice it is not usually necessary to leave any special drugs for injection in the patient's house as these will be available at the surgery, if not already in the doctor's suitcase. However, in a large urban practice where there are a number of doctors and nurses involved, especially for out of hours calls, it may be valuable to leave hyoscine, opiates and sedatives at the house for use if needed. There may be local rules relating to the nursing staff with drug treatment charts or it may be less formalized. The doctors must, however, communicate with each other and the nurses so that all know what drugs are to be used in which situations, including dosage and route, and whether the doctor needs to be contacted before they are given or not.

Conclusion

In the care of the dying, the PHCT is particularly well placed to give quality care to the dying patient and his family, because as well as being readily available, the members both know and are known by the patient and family, and they are already trusted.

With the skilled assistance of the hospice, hospital and Macmillan team, there is little that can be done institutionally that cannot be done at home.

References

1. BOWLING, A. 'The Hospitalisation of death: should more people die at home?' *Journal of Medical Ethics*, 1983, **9**, 158–61.
2. DOYCE, D. 'Introduction', *Domiciliary Terminal Care*, Edinburgh, Churchill Livingstone, 1987, p. VII.
3. VENTAFRIDDA, V. 'Comparison of home and hospital care of advanced cancer patients', *Tumori*, 1989, **75**, 619–25.

4. GRAY, D. 'A comparative cost analysis of terminal cancer care in home hospice patients and controls,' *Journal of Chronic Disease*, 1987, **40**(8), 801–10.
5. URQUHART, A.S. 'Care of malignant disease in an urban practice,' *Journal of the Royal College of General Practitioners*, 1986, **36**, 326–8.
6. CLEMINSON, F.B. Audit of terminal care of cancer patients in General Practice for Shetland Health Board, March 1992.
7. Help the Hospices, 34–44 Britannia Street, London, WC1X 9JG, Telephone: 071–278 5668.

The complementary home care team——

Penny Smith

Specialist home care teams transferring the principles of hospice care into the community began in the late 1960s, and have mushroomed at a great rate so that today about 360 teams exist in the UK.[1]

In a study looking at the structure and function of twelve urban hospice based home care teams Boyd showed how two separate working models have arisen. The more traditional approach was where the home care team had direct involvement with patients and families in conjunction with the primary health care team. The second model was of an advisory service with the home care team acting as a specialist resource to the primary health care team. Initial assessments would be undertaken by an appropriate member of the home care team but further patient and family contact would be at the instigation of the primary care team.[2]

The majority of home care teams have a role that is advisory and supportive to the primary health care team, thus enabling the general practitioner (GP) and district nurse to remain in the front line of care. Specialist home care teams should be a resource for the primary health care team, patient and family, in order to augment care given and not replace it.

Over the past thirty years the proportion of patients who die at home has fallen from 50 per cent to 25 per cent. With the reduced number of patients dying at home and advances in care of the dying this may lead to a loss of confidence by the GP in managing the terminally ill at home. GPs with a case load of 2500 patients would only expect to look after six terminally ill patients each year with two or three dying of advanced malignant disease. In a study by Copperman (1986)[3] of GPs in North West London 63 per cent of 196 GPs frequently expressed difficulties in patient management and 50 per cent indicated that they had problems frequently or always in coping with the emotional distress of patients or relatives.

This section sets out to describe the role of the home care team and how it complements care given by the primary health care team and the family. In order to achieve this objective the home care team needs to be confident in its skills, specialist knowledge and professionalism and therefore can enable other health professionals to care for the dying.

Structure and role of the home care team

The focus of hospice care is multidisciplinary where each person's views and skills are valued as an integral part. The home care team needs to have the disciplines of nurse, doctor and social worker with secretarial support. Other disciplines such as phsyiotherapist, chaplain, occupational therapist and pharmacist could also be part of the team. The teams need an appointed and not assumed leader/coordinator. It should have identified aims and objectives with a philosophy of its values and beliefs. The operational policy stating its way of working needs disseminating to those health professionals who are likely to use the service. A leaflet for patients and families explaining the service and how to use it is helpful and may avoid the confusion of roles.

Such policies and structures are formed in order to provide and maintain a high standard of care and teams should think carefully before altering their agreed policies. It is right that from time to time this is done but it is almost never without consequences, and will need careful review. It is helpful to have a written referral completed by the GP or hospital doctor with full medical and social details. This enables its appropriateness to be assessed and the needs prioritized. Where the primary health care team are able to meet the needs of the dying, referral to a home care team may not be necessary. For a number of others the role of the home care team will be solely to give telephone advice to the GP and/or district nurse. However, others will require more intensive input. Permission to make a visit should be sought from the GP if the referral has come from a hospital doctor.

Having been accepted by the home care team for an assessment visit the team must decide who will go. It is usually appropriate that first visits are made by the nurse. If it is known that patients and families have identified psycho-social issues or are requesting specific help, for example, how to talk with their children about the illness, it may be helpful for the social worker to join the nurse on the first visit.

If a district nurse is known to be involved contact should be made with her prior to the visit. She will already know the family and add to the information given. The home care nurse can also ascertain any anxieties that the district nurse has in caring for this patient. In some cases it will be possible for the district nurse to join the home care nurse on the assessment visit. If there is likely to be a delay in visiting the GP should be contacted and informed thus enabling him to talk through any problems that he is having in controlling the symptoms of the illness.

The role of the home care team will only be complementary to others if it is functioning well. It is therefore important that the roles of different disciplines are understood by other team members. The nurses are clinical nurse specialists, experienced practitioners skilled in palliative care and with a knowledge of the working of health care professionals in the community. They are usually best suited to making initial professional contact with patients and their families. They will also be the coordinator of care in the home care team, making an ongoing assessment and evaluation of patients' and families' needs. This will be by face-to-face contact and by telephone. Visits need to be planned carefully with other members of the primary health care team in order to work together and not to overwhelm a family. It will be the nurse who has the main contact with the primary health care team relaying suggestions of management of care previously discussed by the multidisciplinary team. However there will be times when the team doctor is the most appropriate person to liaise with the GP, particularly when there are complicated medical problems that need discussion.

The major role of the doctor in the team is consultative, advising on symptom control and patient management. Where a further medical assessment is needed the doctor may see patients and families in an out patient clinic or make a home visit. Part of their role is to teach and affirm the nurse in her role.

The role of the social worker on the team is less easily defined but just as vital. The social worker helps the team keep the focus of care family orientated, helping the team to plan the management and appropriate level of family care needed. A significant part of this role is to pass on skills to other team members. The social worker should be available to occasionally make joint visits with either the nurse or doctor. A joint approach can be very useful in the home enabling two individuals to be seen separately and then brought together. Two disciplines working together can model an approach to care that helps the patient and family feel safe. It helps them to recognize that the two disciplines are working together for the good of them and their family. The social worker will also provide more in-depth counselling for some patients and their families. Working with children and adolescents facing bereavement is often part of their role. Some teams will have a welfare worker who helps patients and families with their financial and practical problems but in other teams this role is also undertaken by the social worker.

Home care teams need a leader in order to function well. The leader is responsible for monitoring standards of patient care and clinical practice. On a small team it is important that the leader remains clinically involved. A major focus of the role is the well-being and smooth running of the team paying particular attention to managing areas of conflict and maintaining staff morale. On a regular basis the team will need to review how they are functioning and what the objectives are for the coming year. The team leader is a key person in helping to foster an atmosphere where each individual's contribution is valued, honest discussion can take place and conflicts worked through.

A team cannot develop mutual trust and supportive working relationships unless they meet together. Ideally this means time each day set aside for the team to discuss problems encountered the day or night before and to look together at the needs of new patients seen. It is helpful to have a review system where on a regular basis care is evaluated and future patient and family management planned.

It can be useful to have a time each month to look in depth at one or two patients and families who are causing particular concerns. The primary health care team members involved could be invited to participate, thus emphasizing collaborative working and mutual support. Other issues facing the teams involved could also be discussed at this time.

Most team support happens informally between team members and in the structured daily meeting. However, all members will also need to be seen formally probably monthly by their manager with a yearly appraisal undertaken. On occasions teams will need some extra supportive sessions. An outsider to the team could be helpful to facilitate these. From time to time the team will need to review their past achievements and failures, setting new goals together.

Relationships with the primary health care team

Communication with the primary health care team is the most essential ingredient if the home care team is to be complementary. The role is generally highly valued by patients and particularly carers.[4] It has probably enabled patients to spend a larger proportion of their illness at home or to die there.[4] District nurses and other health professionals generally value this service.[5]

Potential pitfalls lie in de-skilling the primary health care team and a tendency to encourage dependency upon the specialist team, thus displacing the GPs and district nurse from their key position and preventing the family from developing their own strengths and resources. The home care team's role is in affirming the skills of the primary health care team and negotiating a joint approach to care. This will have the consequence of helping the patient and family feel secure in their own home with a competent wider team caring for them. Drugs should not be prescribed or changed without the GP's agreement and he should remain the first line of contact for the patient and family. Regular discussion with the GP and district nurse regarding the management of patients is essential. Although telephone contact is often the chosen mode of communication, for any more difficult situations face-to-face contact should be strived for. With the more complicated patients and their families the health care professionals may find it helpful to meet together for a case discussion. Also in such situations it can be helpful to have a meeting, after the patient's death, of the professionals involved. This enables care to be reviewed acknowledging success and failure and learning lessons for future working. It can be a time for professionals to take down their masks and acknowledge their own vulnerabilities. Sharing thoughts and feelings in this way can lead to professional growth. The

GP may ask the home care nurse to convene the meeting at the GP's surgery or health centre.

Home care teams can offer support to their community colleagues by being a resource for information and by teaching. The educational remit of home care teams should be a significant part of their role, sharing their up-to-date knowledge in their specialist field and responding to the agenda of the primary health care team. Sessions at individual health centres can be an effective way of teaching both for unidisciplinary and multidisciplinary groups. Nurses on home care teams should see their role as directly supporting the district nurses by one-to-one communication and by facilitating group support sessions, particularly where district nurses are carrying a heavy case load of dying patients.

Inviting district nurses to spend time with the home care team can help facilitate good working relationships. It is important that a member of the home care team is available to respond to the needs of GPs and district nurses. This means that one member of the team should carry a bleep in order to be easily contacted to give advice regarding patient care. It is debatable whether or not home care teams should provide an on-call service out of hours. My own feeling is that an on-call advisory service should be available with a visiting service according to local need. Home care teams must not see themselves as indispensable.

It can be helpful to patients, families and district nurses for home care teams to have easy access to equipment which may take the local authority longer to acquire. In some circumstances, where a patient's condition has deteriorated quickly and their pharmacological needs have not been anticipated, it can be supportive to all involved for the home care team to access medications needed, prescribed by the team doctor with the permission of the GP and delivered to the patient.

The home care team working in collaboration with the primary health care team are also in a position to pursue different avenues of possible treatment, for example, nerve blocks, radiotherapy, chemotherapy needed to palliate the symptoms. They are also in an ideal position to liaise with the local hospice in patient unit and explore day care facilities for the patient.

Conclusion

Like other modes of health care the future of the care of the dying will lie increasingly in the community. As the public becomes better informed about services available and society continues its increasing openness about the taboo issues surrounding death and dying, greater numbers of people will choose to die at home. The role of the home care team must continue to develop to meet the needs of other health care professionals. Home care teams are therefore likely to become less involved in direct patient care and more educationally involved in enabling and em- powering others. The challenge for the specialist home care team is to facilitate this change in direction, becoming an even greater resource to the primary health care team.

Notes and References

1. 1992 Directory of Hospice Services produced by St Christopher's Hospice information 51–59 Lawrie Park Road, Sydenham, SE26 6DZ.
2. BOYD, K. 'The working patterns of hospice based home care teams,' *Palliative Medicine* 1992, **6**, 131–9.
3. COPPERMAN, H. 'Domiciliary hospice care – a survey of general practitioners,' *Journal of the Royal College of Practitioners*, 1988, **38**, 411–3.
4. PARKES, C.M. 'Evaluation of an advisory domiciliary service at St Christopher's Hospice', *Postgraduate Medical Journal* 1980, **S6**, 685–9.
5. KINDEN, M. 'The role of hospice home care nurse as perceived by Macmillan nurses, district nurses and health visitors,' MPhil thesis, unpublished, University of Edinburgh/RCN Steinberg collection.

The palliative care team

Jo Hockley

Introduction

The fact that hospice practice is not just a building but a philosophy of care means it can be adapted to several locations. The palliative care team is the medium whereby hospice can be introduced to the hospital environment. Palliative care teams form what might be seen as the 'second generation' of the hospice movement. They have become the means by which the hospice movement has come full circle back into the acute setting.

There are a number of reasons why such teams have been set up. First, the majority of cancer deaths occur in hospital. Secondly, the unpredictability of the terminal phase of non-malignant disease make it difficult for hospices to accommodate more than just a small proportion of those patients dying from diseases other than cancer. Thirdly, hospice education has often only been able to attract those professionals already interested in the care of the dying. It is important that the philosophy of hospice care be seen as standard care for the dying rather than the exception, i.e. just for those privileged to receive it within the hospice setting. There is a need to bring such education to the place where not only a majority of people die but where health care professionals are exposed to it while in training.

The history of palliative care teams

In the early 1970s a nationwide study on the care of the dying[1] stressed the importance that the expertise developed in hospices should be more widely disseminated in geriatric departments and acute ward situations, so that *all* dying patients could benefit. At the same time an interest in the idea of a 'roving' hospice team, working within the acute hospital, was emerging at St Luke's Hospital, New York and in operation by 1974. T. Bates[2] established the first palliative care team in Britain in 1977 at St Thomas' Hospital, London, after which other teams evolved. Such teams have risen from differing specialties of care, e.g. community medicine, radiotherapy, anaesthetics, chest medicine and oncology. There are five major aspects (see Table 8.1) concerning the role of a palliative care team which form part of its everyday function.

There are now around 140 such teams in Britain varying from a fully operational, multi-disciplinary team with hospital/community/day-centre facilities, to teams composed of nurse specialists. It is important that teams evolve according to the circumstances around them. Where it is important to have a multidisciplinary representation such as in a teaching hospital, a team consisting of a doctor, nurse specialists, social worker and secretary would be the minimum requirement. Unfortunately, some teams have failed to become established[4] especially when administrative, medical and nursing co-operation is not achieved. However, once established their effect, although difficult to measure and quantify, can be significant. In the case of one team, complaints from relatives dissatisfied with the terminal care given were reduced from 8.6 per cent of all complaints to under 1 per cent over a four-year period.[5]

Why people die in hospital

Where people die is often unfortunately an outcome of chance rather than choice. Cartwright *et al.*'s (1973) study concluded that those most likely to die in hospital were the unmarried, wives rather than husbands, those that had been ill for less than two years, people aged under forty-five

Table 8.1   Aims of palliative care team

- To assist in the relief of distressing symptoms and to give emotional, social and spiritual support to patients who have a terminal illness.
- To provide counselling and support to relatives and the bereaved.
- To provide support and advice to the staff caring for their patients.
- To take part in education programmes on a multi-professional basis (where at all possible) with both students in training as well as those already trained. This includes both formal and informal meetings.
- To research areas of interest within symptom control and issues surrounding the emotional impact of dying.

Source: adapted from Dunlop and Hockley[3]

years and those without children (particularly daughters) to care for them. Fifteen years later a study looking at why patients referred to a palliative care team died in hospital, found that 33 per cent of patients were still receiving radiotherapy/chemotherapy, or were being investigated for first presentation of advanced cancer; 28 per cent had made no other choice – generally no contingency plan had been made, either because of denial of disease, or because the patient and family had such close links with the ward that it was appropriate that the patient should die on the ward; 24 per cent wanted transfer home or to a hospice but by the time arrangements were made the patient was too ill to travel – a further 12 per cent were too ill to consider any other option than stay in hospital and 3 per cent died suddenly.[6]

Advantages of palliative care teams

One of the main advantages of palliative care teams is the bringing of hospice expertise to those who do not want hospice transfer or for whom a non-malignant disease precludes transfer to a hospice facility. Such a team is a resource for other professionals, making hospice relevant to all terminally ill patients and their families and not just to cancer patients. Good symptom control is easily the most applicable area of hospice care within the acute setting. One of the main reasons for setting up the team at St Thomas' Hospital was to help with the symptom control of terminally ill patients and thereby enable such patients to be at home for longer periods and even to be able to die in their own home. Symptom control and appropriate care can therefore be maximized from an earlier point in the disease process without necessarily waiting until the end stage of an illness.

It is unusual for palliative care teams to be involved with all the dying. In many situations it seems to be between 40–50 per cent. More time is then utilized for those patients and families who have complex problems that the ward team find perplexing. A good rapport can be built up between the various medical and surgical teams as long as the respect for who is responsible for the patients' care is adhered to. When advising on care the team have the opportunity of suggesting relevant expertise from other professionals who might not already be involved. Being involved at a much earlier point in the disease process provides an opportunity to try to plan ahead for appropriate care rather than be faced with a crisis situation during the dying phase.

The palliative care team represents a visible standard of care. It is more difficult for a sub-optimal practice of care for the dying to be practised if ward staff are being reminded and supported by a specialist team. There is the opportunity of revitalizing the care of the dying within the clinical setting where often ward teams have been subject to an upward spiral of pressure. Palliative care teams can enable ward teams to take the time and have the satisfaction not only of thinking through basic problems, but of seeing how much work can be done with a dying patient. Such teams provide continuity of care for patients and their families amidst a changing hospital scene of staff rotation. The palliative care team is the ideal medium whereby knowledge and skill of symptom control and the psycho-social aspects of care for both patient and the family can be shared and passed on, not only via the medical and nursing school curriculum but also via a 'role-model' method of teaching. It is difficult to teach the psycho-social skills of the dying didactically. However, with a multidisciplinary team of specialists who have already been trained within a hospice environment these skills can be passed on within the very real and natural setting of the ward. This 'role-model' of teaching does require good organization ensuring that the relevant health professional is available to share in the session with the team member.

A palliative care team is reasonably inexpensive to run as it operates within the existing hospital structure. Expenses can often be shared throughout a number of specialties as most areas of care within a hospital use such a team and experience difficulties associated with dying patients. However with the new NHS 'purchaser and provider' aspect of care, the team, unless it makes significant help in patient care and even in reducing patient stay in hospital, might be seen as a luxury even though quality of care for the patient is meant to be the present NHS emphasis. Some hospital trust documents envisage a palliative care team within the oncology structure as being a most important asset to have, especially when competing with other oncology services that may be without such a facility.

In many ways the palliative care team acts as a bridge to a hospice home care service or hospice unit. Its role too as 'ambassador' for the local hospice unit can be a benefit to both hospital and hospice service; keeping each up-to-date with the most recent change in technologies and techniques. It is important that no facility thinks it is more important than another. All are promoting expert, compassionate care and advice for the dying within their appropriate situation. Having examined the advantages of palliative care teams it is important to detail some of the difficulties that such teams face.

Difficulties facing a palliative care team

Bates stresses that the presence of a palliative care team can cause potential confusion over responsibility of care. However involved a team member is with a patient, the responsibility of care rests firmly with the consultant in charge of the patient unless for one reason or another they have given over the care completely. In some cases this happens but most palliative care teams have no authority to admit patients, so continued written communication in the notes is vital to keep the referring team as involved as possible.

There is a danger that a team which was meant to improve the standard of care for the dying in hospital becomes an agent for doing the work itself, so that the ward team then has an excuse not to be so involved. This does not happen where there is a true desire within a ward to care for the dying, but it can easily happen (and not just in hospital) where the incentive to care is taken away because the patient relates to the specialist team instead of the primary team. Team members must act as a role-model rather than take over the care. If due attention is not taken to involve ward staff with patient and family interviews, there is a danger that any inclination towards the dying will be dismissed, and de-skilling of ward staff will occur.

One of the difficulties of working on a palliative care team is the compromise that is sometimes necessary. Although the specialist team is there in the hospital to represent hospice principles, nevertheless, there are times when one cannot carry out the care one would be able to within the uniformity of the hospice setting. Sometimes appropriate compromise is an important issue for future referrals rather than 'holding out' on an issue just for the sake of it.

A palliative care team within the hospital may experience a lower number of deaths compared to colleagues within other aspects of hospice care. However, the work is no less demanding. The fact of not having total management over patients, a different philosophy over truth-telling, or having to wait for the ward team to carry out suggestions, can all cause considerable tension. It may seem easier to do the task oneself, and, of course, there are some situations where it is appropriate to; but this should not become the 'norm' otherwise the team's potential will be diminished.

Within the hospital environment the palliative care team is working in an atmosphere that is highly charged. The checking of the appropriateness of further active treatment, understanding the patient's wish and knowing whether to challenge a decision made by the referring team, can give the sensation of 'swimming against the tide' of normal hospital practice. The very atmosphere of working in the acute situation can heighten anxiety and therefore at times diminish effectiveness with patients and their families. In hospital there is considerable overt pressure on beds and a member of a palliative care team can often feel pressurized to transfer a patient inappropriately, or face the difficult situation of knowing a patient needs re-admission without an available bed.

Any palliative care team runs the potential risk of conflict not only as it interfaces on the ward but also within the team. Respecting that ward staff have their own expertise which may not be in palliative care is important especially in preventing antagonism. Team members should be wary of confronting conflict against them on the ward, but within the team it must be resolved. The difficult and challenging situation of a hospital often attracts strong personalities onto a palliative care team. To a certain degree it is important for team personnel to be able to stand on their own, but this should be through skill and expertise rather than a overly strong ego.

In many ways the roles of team members are less well defined than the normal roles of health care workers within the hospital or indeed hospice situation. The nurse specialists' role is perhaps the most blurred with its extension into both the doctors' and social work role, through symptom control and counselling advice respectively. However, the physician's role within a team is specific to backing up the symptom control advice of nurse specialists, debating the merit of further treatments and highlighting the importance of both teaching and research. The social worker's role is channelled towards the more difficult psycho-social and emotional issues, especially where children are involved, and to anticipatory and post-death grief work.

Conclusion

The appropriateness of the palliative care team has been described along with its evolution from within the hospice movement. Although these teams can vary considerably in personnel, a skill mix of disciplines is most appropriate. There are a number of advantages but also difficulties working on such a team, but good symptom control, psycho-social care and family interviewing, and support of ward staff and teaching are the main channels whereby the ideals and philosophy of hospice care can be brought to those patients who might otherwise not benefit.

Notes and references

1. CARTWRIGHT, A., HOCKEY, L. and ANDERSON, J.L. *Life Before death*, London, Routledge and Kegan Paul, 1973.
2. BATES, T.D., HOY, A.M., CLARKE, D.G. and LAIRD, P.P. 'The St Thomas' Hospital terminal care support team – a new concept of hospice care', *Lancet*, 1981, i, 1201–3.
3. DUNLOP, R.J. and HOCKLEY, J.M. 'Setting about meeting the need.' In: DUNLOP, R.J. and HOCKLEY, J.M. (eds), *Terminal Care Support Teams – The Hospital/Hospice Interface*, Oxford, Oxford University Press, 1990, pp. 13–27.
4. HERXHEIMER, A., BEGENT, R., MacLEAN, D., PHILLIPS, L., SOUTHCOTT, B. and WALTON I. 'Short life of a terminal care support team: experience at Charing Cross Hospital', *British Medical Journal*, 1985, **290**, 1877–9.
5. HOCKLEY, J.M. DUNLOP, R. and DAVIES, R.J. 'Survey of distressing symptoms in dying patients and their families in hospital and the response to a symptom control team', *British Medical Journal*, 1988, **296**, 1715–17.
6. DUNLOP, R.J., HOCKLEY, J.M. and DAVIES, R.J. 'Preferred versus actual place of death – a hospital terminal care support team experience', *Palliative Medicine*, 1989, **3**, 197–201.

How the acute team can provide palliation

Carol Haigh

Nursing today seems to be composed of 'specialists', specialists in stoma care, diabetic care, mastectomy care and specialists in palliative care. Such specialists are an asset to the nursing profession, providing expert knowledge for others to utilize. However, it must also be acknowledged that even in today's nursing environment the generalized acute care setting is often in the front line of palliative and terminal care.

Since this is the case, it is important for the acute clinical area to set the highest standards it can for the provision of palliative care. The most important of the various factors that are required to achieve this is the recognition, by the whole of the ward team, of the importance of good palliative care and a commitment to its delivery.

It may be difficult, at first, to see how these factors can be assimilated by the average acute care ward. Whether consciously or unconsciously the main expectation of both staff and patients in acute care settings is that the patient will eventually recover. If we begin to suggest that the provision of good palliative care is a ward priority, are we not also acknowledging that there are some patients within the acute care setting that will die? The answer, of course, is yes we are, and by acknowledging that we are reflecting reality. How then can the acute ward team provide palliation? Perhaps there are two elements which together can help to create a palliative care environment within the acute clinical setting, namely:

- A ward philosophy of care.
- A commitment to the provision of comfort.

Let us examine both of these in more detail.

Ward philosophy

A ward philosophy is simply a statement that outlines, for the benefit of all concerned, the beliefs, values and attitudes of the ward team. It is important to stress that a ward philosophy is not a statement of intent or a standard of care but highlights the qualitative concepts that the ward team are striving to achieve.

The important aspect to remember when formulating a ward philosophy is that all members of the ward team should be involved. Everyone, from the ward manager to the nursing assistants, should be given the opportunity to participate. This will ensure that not only will the philosophy be understood by all of the team, it also will be owned by them. We have already stated that the one important factor in the delivery of good palliative care is the commitment of *all* ward staff to that ideal. A ward philosophy can help to generate this commitment, it is, 'the rock upon which all else is built' (Wright, 1986).

Careful crafting of a ward philosophy will ensure that all the staff are standing in the same place, looking in the same direction and using the same values when making judgements. This can be of paramount importance when providing palliative care.

Areas that are of concern within a clinical area can be explored, rationalized, justified and incorporated into a ward philosophy. This can be demonstrated by examining some elements of a ward philosophy which was developed in an acute care area.

The staff were concerned that patients were not being fully informed of their prognosis, thereby compromising the trusting relationship between nurses and patient. This was discussed at the philosophy meetings that the ward held and was incorporated into the finished philosophy and expressed as follows: 'Every patient has the right to be kept informed of their diagnosis, prognosis and progress.'

Every member of the ward team had agreed that if a patient had the courage to ask if they were going to die, they had the right to the truth. This gave the ward team a solidarity that it had not known before when dealing with the dying patient and their relatives. This solidarity was generated because the whole of the ward team had acknowledged a need to improve and had discussed strategies for doing just that in continuing and sensitive relationships.

Furthermore, the ward had previously experienced difficulty in obtaining expensive equipment to complement their palliative care techniques. By creating an element in the ward philosophy that stated: 'Every patient has the right to the best possible nursing care we can provide' the team had provided themselves with an argument to back up further such requests.

Patients requiring palliation were enabled to participate in their own care or to 'opt out' of the routine if they felt so inclined. Relatives were also acknowledged within the philosophy by an element which stated: 'Relatives/carers should be given the maximum opportunity to participate in the care of their loved ones.' This reassured relatives that they were welcome to participate in providing palliative care for their loved ones, as partners and with the support of the entire ward team (Haigh, 1990).

This illustrates how the provision of palliation in the acute clinical area can be facilitated by the generation of a ward philosophy. Once a specific set of beliefs and values have been identified by the ward team this aspect can become a foundation of a ward's stated attitude to care. Being included in the generation of a ward philosophy and the planning of palliative care can be beneficial to each member of the ward team but it is important to stress that the whole team will require the trust and strong support of the ward manager if good palliative care is to be achieved.

The ward philosophy that forms our example was actually generated for use in the area of acute orthopaedic trauma but because palliative care had been identified as a ward priority many of the elements within the finished article were highly relevant to that subject also. This illustrates how, if a secure ward philosophy exists it will permeate any care and philosophy that the team will provide.

Once a ward philosophy of care has been formulated it can be used to support and justify the second of our identified components of acute care palliation.

Providing Comfort

Raphael (1984) notes that the giving and receiving of comfort is one of the most basic human responses to distress. However, it must be recognized that very often, within the acute care setting, comfort is sacrificed to care.

The distinction between comfort and care is a most important one. When speaking of 'care' one can identify all of the skills that the acute ward can provide. This includes medical and nursing intervention in acute physiological crisis, physiological observations, and general rehabilitation. Every single one of these concepts is important within its own right, is given acceptable priority when planning care in the acute setting and implementation is generally subject to quality measurement in the form of standards which are often quantitative in nature.

However, these concepts can be dangerous to the acute ward team who are providing palliation, since they can form a satisfying check list for patient care. They provide grounds for nurses to believe that they are providing good care simply because they have supplied all of the acute care requisites that were identified for that particular patient. The provision of patient comfort, although closely allied to patient care in many instances does however, differ in certain important ways.

The provision of patient comfort requires that the nursing staff acknowledge that the patient is entitled to whatever they want, whenever they want it. Good palliative care is patient centred. If the patient wants to 'opt out' of the ward routine, if they want to be visited on the ward by their pet dog, wear their own clothes or eat special foods provided by their relatives, no obstacle should be placed in their way. Equally, if they do not wish to participate in unpleasant and often useless investigations or procedures, no pressure should be brought to bear to try to make the patient conform.

Obviously, a ward must have a routine if it is to run efficiently, and it can be difficult for the staff if that routine is disrupted. However, it can be argued that acute care wards rarely contain enough palliative care patients to make the provision of these simple comforts an impossible proposition, and indeed from the perspective of routine the acute setting can be more flexible than the specialist area.

For the purpose of this work, we can define care as a physical concept, for example effective symptom control with medication, of sufficient strength, at the right time for the patient. Within the same context comfort may be defined as more empathetic in nature, for example allowing the patient the certain knowledge that the medication will always be provided at the right time regardless of who is in charge of the ward and that its effects will be carefully discussed and assessed.

These examples demonstrate very clearly the difference between the two concepts. Care can be perceived to be the 'doing' of nursing, whilst comfort can be perceived to be 'doing' (or in certain circumstances *not* doing) coupled with the demonstration of total commitment to another individual's well-being. It is possible to care without necessarily comforting but it is not possible to comfort without caring.

Within the concept of palliative care this commitment to well-being should be demonstrated even if the benefit of an activity is not immediately apparent to the health professionals within the ward team. For example, many hospitals now enforce a 'no smoking' policy. All health care professionals understand the dangers of smoking. However, if a patient who is dying expresses a desire for a cigarette it may be an act of comfort if the ward manager is prepared to bend hospital rules for the well-being of that patient.

In that circumstance we could argue that true patient care would be to provide health education for the patient on the hazards of smoking. However patient comfort would provide the cigarette and a place to smoke it. This is not to suggest that nurses should disregard the dangers of smoking but to highlight that the application of this knowledge is not always appropriate.

Hospital regulations, like ward routine are a necessary evil. There have to be recognized rules that lay down acceptable standards of behaviour in any large institution or anarchy will reign. However a ward team that are committed to providing good palliative comfort will be prepared, using their professional discretion and accountability, to 'bend' certain rules in the interests of their terminally ill patients.

Various areas can be improved by this provision of palliative comfort rule bending. If a patient feels better in the mornings than in the evenings, a ward team committed to comfort will encourage their relatives/carers to visit before lunch time regardless of any effect on the ward routine. If a patient is close to death and relatives are reluctant to leave the ward it is an act of comfort to provide food for them in any way feasible. By the same token, if relatives want to stay overnight with a very ill patient, bedclothes and a pillow will at least ensure they will be comfortable in a chair by the side of the patient's bed.

One of the most important comfort strategies is to ensure that someone is with a dying patient at all times. If relatives cannot attend then the nursing staff can perform this service. No-one should have to die alone and if ensuring that means altering the ward routine in some way, so be it.

It can therefore be seen that the provision of comfort in the acute care setting can be extended to include the whole of the patient's support network. This can be seen to be holistic nursing in its truest sense, in providing comfort for those our patients care about we are acknowledging their importance to the patient. The provision of comfort for patients' carers/relatives can be achieved by the extension of the empathy, hospitality and friendship of the ward team and an inclusion in any relevant 'comfort rule bending' that may be required. It is important to note that during the course of a hospitalization there will be times when comforting activities will be focused as much upon the relatives/carers as on the patient.

We have argued that if an acute care ward is to provide good palliation there must be a recognized team commitment. It has been shown that this commitment can be incorporated into the ward philosophy of care. That ward philosophy can further be used to support, justify and defend rule bending, comfort providing strategies.

Such strategies appear simplistic and self-evident when written down but the provision of patient comfort is very often neglected in an environment that is primarily concerned with the provision of acute nursing care.

References

1. WRIGHT, S.G. *Building and Using a Model of Nursing*, London, Edward Arnold, 1986.
2. HAIGH, C.A. 'Adopting the hospice ethic,' *Nursing Times*, 1990, **86**(41), October, 10–17.
3. RAPHAEL, B. *The Anatomy of Bereavement. A Handbook for the Caring Professions*, London, Unwin Hyman, 1984.

The day hospice

Anne Gibson

This chapter describes the philosophy of care which underlies the programme of activities provided at St Christopher's Hospice Day Centre. It is based on the experiences of commissioning and then managing the day to day service provided to both in-patients and out-patients.

The expansion of hospice services into day hospices has led to the development of a wide variety of models. Some are set up as socially led centres. These bring people away from the loneliness of their four walls, give them time out from their illness, offer companionship and support together with a programme of diversional activities. Other centres provide an intense service following a medical model where all physical, social and spiritual needs are addressed within one building.

At St Christopher's the day hospice complements the work of the in-patient services and the home-care team. With the support of a caring professional team the patient has greater autonomy in choosing whether to remain at home as opposed to an early admission. We have found that attendance can provide the first link with the hospice services often easing the way for a future admission. Out-patients can become in-patients and vice versa. The service may also assist in the transition period from curative to palliative care.

Whilst focusing on maximizing the present quality of life within the limitations of the disease, the individual patient is assisted with the help of a key worker to remain as independent as possible and to attain an improved level of physical and mental well-being. Needs are assessed, choices are identified and attainable goals set. Thus by helping them to be in control, dignity and self-respect are maintained. Moreover, a better understanding of themselves and their position can take place within a time of inner healing.

The belief is that good symptom control is not the only objective. Having achieved control, one can go forward and assist the individual to have a better quality of life and continue *living* within a nurturing environment. With this as our aim, we have a planned programme of activities, covering self-care, occupational needs, leisure activities, emotional needs and carer's needs.

Self-Care and physical needs

Here, the emphasis is on a comfortable environment. There are areas set aside for activity, for companionship and for quiet withdrawal. The well-equipped, professionally staffed hairdressing salon, bathing facilities, and a treatment room are all important provisions. There is access to an adjoining physiotherapy department which also plays an important role. Gentle exercising to music and relaxation sessions are regular features of our programme. It encourages an optimum level of mobility and independence. The use of gentle massage is considered to be helpful for it eases communication, and lifts the mood. It ultimately leads to a reduction in levels of anxiety and stress and to an improved body image. 'For patients who create barriers to communication touch through massage can be a means of bridging gaps without offence or invasion of personal space.'[1]

Occupational needs

A regular and structured programme of activities is offered. In this way patients may choose to attend the centre on the day of the week that suits their interests. Consideration is also given to the existing membership of a group and whether the individual will benefit from the companionship offered by attending on one particular day over another. The use of creative activities are more than just diversionary as they are seen to stimulate and enrich life and encourage self-expression. This above all results in a sense of achievement and a sense of being valued. Wherever possible we introduce crafts and set projects which can be completed in a short space of time. More often than not these crafts are new to the individual so that there is no sense of failure from a comparison with previous achievements.

Nor need they be restricted to the individual for much can be done to redress the feelings of loneliness with a group, for instance, sitting around a large table working on a joint project such as making a patchwork quilt. We have noticed that by encouraging participation in purposeful activity the new interest has led not only to greater productivity but also to an increase in levels of energy and feelings of well-being. Conversely, passivity increases dependency and a slide into the sick role – a receiver only.

The sense of achievement gained from the creation of an object enables the individual to give a tangible reminder of themselves to their family and friends. This tangible memento can also be derived from the creation of a poem, the writing of a diary, a short essay or a piece of reminiscence writing. The need by some to be able to give something back to the community is also fulfilled for they can contribute to fund raising activities and other charitable trusts. For example, teddy bears were knitted and sent to children in refugee camps throughout the world.

Socializing and leisure activities

For many, the socializing aspects available at the day hospice are of the most value. Reminiscence group work, talks by visiting speakers, demonstrations, entertainers, musicians, and outings all allow time out from their illness and a day to look forward to. 'Recalling of past accomplishments and good feelings . . . is frequently seen in social interaction among hospice staff, patients, and care givers. This positive reminiscence assists in the adaptation to multiple losses and the maintenance of self esteem.'[2]

Friendships made, experiences shared, laughter and joy have all assisted in restoring levels of self-esteem and self-confidence thus benefiting relationships within the family and with carers.

Emotional and spiritual needs

Patients need to be supported in their search for some meaning in their personal lives. We have found that the use of art, music and writing in a trusting relationship can open lines of communication with previously isolated and withdrawn patients. 'Certain patients get stuck in the surface level of their experience and need help with the process of healing by being able to move from the surface to the deep level.'[3]

Support can also be given within the more formalized setting of a patient's discussion group facilitated by members of staff. Members of the Chaplaincy Department help with regular visits to the department. They lead a useful session for staff and patients entitled 'Remembering Friends' where time is set aside for reflection, for coping with loss, for feelings of sadness, and for a celebration of those who have died, focusing on their special contributions to the centre.

Carer's day off

This is an important side benefit of the day hospice in that it gives support and respite to the carers. We can share with them the burden, ease the pressure on community support systems, and reduce the tensions at home enabling the carer to have a day off even if that only means catching up on sleep or managing to complete household chores.

Carers can also be invited to join the outings and attend social events at the centre. This indeed often leads to memories of recently shared happier times together when they had thought that these would not be possible to achieve anymore.

Conclusion

At St Christopher's we have set our aims beyond that of just the control of symptoms. With a well-researched and structured programme of activities we have enabled patients to continue to participate in life and achieve the possible. As the focus of a developing health service moves forward into community based care, the Day Hospice is well placed to respond to the needs of the palliative care team for the benefit of the individual patient.

Notes and References

1. BYASS, R. Soothing body and soul, *Nursing Times*, 1988, **84**, 40.
2. WHOLIHAN, D. *American Journal of Hospice and Palliative Care*, 1992, 33–34.
3. KEARNEY, M. 'Palliative Medicine – just another speciality?' *Palliative Medicine*, 1992, **6**, 45.

Suggested reading

4. TIGGES, K.N. 'Independence through Occupational Performance,' paper presented to UK National Society for Cancer Relief, Addington, December 1980.
5. CONNELL, C. 'Art therapy as part of a palliative care programme,' *Palliative Medicine*, 1992, **6**.
6. CORR, C. and CORR, D. 'Adult hospice day care,' *Death Studies*, 1992.

Overview of spread of palliation: starting a new service outside Europe and North America———————

Avril Jackson

'Hospice brings together people who would not normally meet.'[1] This statement was a central theme in a paper on bridging the racial gulf in hospice care given by Christine Dare at St Christopher's Sixth International Conference in May 1991. The conference, attended by doctors, nurses, social workers, chaplains, administrators, physiotherapists and volunteers from thirty-eight countries was truly representative of the worldwide hospice community that has developed in recent years. Hospice now spans six continents and is already established or planned in almost sixty countries. Palliative care is a recognized specialty in the UK, Canada and Australia where academic posts have been established and the launching of national coordinating organizations in both the UK and Australia should lead to greater government recognition. However, in other continents, and particularly in developing countries, the spread of palliative care has been more gradual. Yet it is in the developing countries, where more than 90 per cent of people who develop cancer will die from it, where the need is greatest. This chapter, written from the perspective of the Hospice Information Service, presents a glimpse of worldwide development.

The Hospice Information Service, part of St Christopher's Hospice since 1977, is an international link and resource for those involved in hospice or palliative care. Rooted in a teaching and research centre of international reputation we receive a privileged global view. Our small office is often a meeting point for visitors from many lands anxious to share news of their hospice or to obtain publications relevant to the planning or management of a new service. The literature from St Christopher's Librarian or from our series of Fact Sheets (including accounts of how some UK hospices have initiated a home care service, a day centre, or an in-patient unit) can be a useful starter for an overseas group. But the inspiration for a hospice starts far earlier. Sometimes it is a traumatic personal experience which may provide inspiration or occasionally the chance reading of an article or attendance at a lecture on the hospice movement which has impelled an individual to pursue a better way of caring. More often the impetus evolves from a desperate need to change existing health care for the terminally ill. The inspiration for the Nairobi Hospice (established in 1990) grew out of the recognition by cancer nurses that 'many patients of all ethnic backgrounds and socio-economic groups were dying of advanced cancer, some alone, and almost all dying in pain with no medical and psychological help and support.'[2]

Sadly, there are many barriers to the implementation of a palliative care programme often in the very countries where the need is greatest: lack of pain relieving drugs and the problems of legislation enabling their use, lack of education for both health care workers and the public and lack of finance for research and development. Sometimes, too, there is an underlying current of fear: fear of creating a 'death house' and the health care professional's fear of losing the management of their patients. Thus the information and experience we share with our overseas colleagues must be adaptable to local needs and take account of cultural differences. The big, impressive hospice building may be unlikely: indeed for many patients the noise and closeness of the family home would be infinitely preferable to a hospice in-patient unit. The World Health Organization recommends as wide a coverage as possible by the provision of home care services and certainly most overseas hospices have begun by initiating a home care or patient outreach service.

The first steps

For many, the first step towards setting up a hospice service may be through attendance at an international conference on hospice care. Some delegates who attended St Christopher's Sixth International were asked to submit a report six months after the conference explaining how attendance had influenced their present work. Some had been inspired by individual workshops or plenary lectures; all emphasized the importance of sharing experiences and ideas, the knowledge and understanding gained, the encouragement to continue, and the confirmation that they were 'on the right track'. A strength of international meetings is the chance to forge personal links with others involved in similar work although the opportunity for a fruitful exchange of ideas and experiences may arise just as easily from a chance meeting in the coffee queue as from the formal meeting. Certainly the idea for a European Hospice Clergy Conference (held in Poland in autumn 1992) stemmed from informal discussion amongst three chaplains from Germany, Poland and England whilst at an international conference in London. Interestingly, the Polish chaplain spoke not a word of English and the English chaplain not a word of Polish. But hospice has a way of building bridges!

In Nigeria there is at present no national programme of palliative care. In Lagos, Mrs O.K. Fatunmbi is chief nurse of the Ajuwa Clinic, (part of the Kelu Specialist Hospital) an eight-bedded clinic providing medical care for cancer patients. By the end of the conference Mrs Fatunmbi had written to the Federal Minister of Health for Nigeria urging him to consider the need for a hospice, preferably a home care service, in their country. In her report to St Christopher's she described how her attendance had provoked changes in care:

> We have tried with a measure of success the palliative care on patients with involvement of their relatives. A case in point was a 67 year old patient with advanced cancer of the prostate

gland. He had been bed-ridden for the past 6 months because of secondaries in the spine and femurs. We have been able to maintain a tolerably clean environment at his residence through counselling, general nursing care and regular changing of his indwelling urethral catheter. The home visits by doctors and nurses gave him a lot of encouragement as this type of visit is rare in this part of the world.

The task ahead is enormous: general recession coupled with Nigeria's transition from military to civilian rule are not the most welcoming background to a new concept. But already Mrs Fatunmbi has awakened interest in hospice care amongst her professional colleagues and, in her most recent letter to us, says that she has 'made up her mind to start singlehandedly, if need be in a shed, a free counselling service as soon as possible'. Hospice is not simply bricks and mortar. It is a blend of skills, principles and attitudes which are capable of being transposed to suit the needs of different environments.

In Southern Africa hospice has developed considerably during the past decade responding to the needs of different racial, language and cultural groups. In South Africa, where there are presently about 22 hospice services, St Luke's Hospice in Cape Town first demonstrated that hospice could cross the bridge of racial prejudice. In her paper, Christine Dare described the need to respect the different cultures and attitudes of both patients and staff, to listen to and learn from each other, and recalled the words of an Afrikaans visitor: 'Coming to St Luke's was like a window opening. . . so many people could work together in harmony and peace.'[1]

In Swaziland, one of the smallest countries in southern Africa with a population of just over 700 000, a small hospice home care team has been caring for patients with advanced cancer since 1990. Swaziland Hospice at Home, was initiated by a former UK hospice nurse who was shocked to discover on her arrival in Swaziland a complete lack of terminal care facilities and neither were there radiotherapy or chemotherapy units or a cancer specialist. Encouraged by friends and local residents the founder, Stephanie Wyer, 'started a hospice from scratch' assembling a band of willing helpers and a few donations. The project was 'blessed' – but not funded – by the Ministry of Health. Contact with the Hospice Information Service was first made in July 1990 when Stephanie wrote to us requesting literature to support a course she had been asked to organize for industrial nurses. Attached to her first letter were the aims of the hospice group: to train volunteers, raise funds, establish a library for learning materials and equipment, to achieve acceptable pain and symptom control (at the invitation of the patient's doctor), to offer bereavement counselling, to provide a meeting place, to train and employ a Swazi nurse and to do home visits.

Now, in autumn 1992, the team has grown to four nurses and a programme administrator whose base is a caravan donated by the British High Commission. Over thirty-five patients have been cared for by the team and, like other overseas hospices, the long-term goal includes provision of service for other areas of the country, a day care centre and on-going educational programmes for both health care workers and volunteers. A vision becomes reality.

Although the above example may be regarded as a fairly typical beginning for a hospice service, other services have stemmed from a more traditional medical background. In India with its teeming population of 900 million, one in eight people will get cancer and 80 per cent will seek treatment when it is too late and palliative care becomes the only humane option. At St Christopher's First International Conference in 1980 L.J. de Souza, chief of the gastro-intestinal service of the Tata Memorial Hospital, Bombay, spoke movingly of the problems specific to developing countries: hunger and poverty as well as physical pain. 'It is bad enough to be old and feeble. But to be old, sick with advanced cancer and poor and hungry with nobody to care for you is often the height of human suffering.'[3] He put forward his imaginative plans for a purpose-built hospice to be established in Bombay with the capacity for extra beds to be added later and described how he had waited until a religious order of trained nurses, the Sisters of the Holy Cross, had agreed to undertake the work. In November 1986, after much fund-raising abroad and sufficient funds invested to cover running costs, the Shanti Avedna Ashram, the first hospice in India, opened with one ward of ten beds. Now, in 1992, the hospice has 50 beds, each with a sea view, and cares for 400–500 patients annually. Families are encouraged to help and both wards have facilities for families to stay if they wish. A sister hospice has been opened in Goa, plans are proceeding for a further unit in Delhi and the Shanti Avedna Ashram celebrated its fifth birthday by hosting the first international hospice conference in India in November 1991. The conference entitled 'Sharing Hospice Concepts – East Meets West', was attended by members of the World Health Organisation and by almost 300 hospice personnel from India and other Asian countries as well as from Australia, Brazil and several European countries. Although oral morphine has been legally available only since 1988 (only six states out of twenty-two are legalized to use it) palliative care is spreading and further services are now developing in Manipal, Kerala and Madras.

Education and training

The emphasis on education is a hallmark of palliative care no matter where in the world: increasing professional and public awareness, training staff, volunteers and patients and carers alike. In La Plata, Argentina, the ten-strong multidisciplinary team at the Fundacion Mainetti Palliative Care Unit combine patient care with a teaching role at La Plata University Medical School and in a school of nursing. In Singapore, where hospice care has been provided since 1985 by several charitable organizations, Cynthia Goh, a leading specialist in palliative care, would like to see nationwide coverage with input from the government. As a first step, the Hospice Resource Committee, of which she is a member, has been set up by the Ministry of Health to formulate standards and guidelines for hospice and will also recommend directions for future development. A free-standing hospice is now planned with the promise from the government of substantial funds towards building and running costs.

Where on-the-spot training is not available, many overseas staff will avail themselves of training and work experience programmes offered by other countries.

The International School for Cancer Care is a British-based charity providing advice and assistance for people from overseas for whom education and training in palliative cancer care is not readily available in their own countries. The School offers both short and long-term fellowships at palliative care centres in the UK and will also provide teaching support for workshops and seminars overseas. In the first two years since its inception the School helped to run seminars in Singapore, Kenya, Poland, Colombia and Brazil.

Gilly Burn has made several visits to India[1] in the course of her work as a peripatetic nurse tutor with Marie Curie Cancer Care, the first visit in response to a call for teachers from the World Health Organisation. She has now set up an organization, Cancer Relief India, to raise money for equipment and education of medical and paramedical staff working in palliative care. Recent fundraising initiatives in the UK have enabled the purchase of syringe pumps, training and translation into Hindi of the WHO publication: 'Cancer pain relief and palliative care'. Numerous other UK hospice workers are frequently invited to participate in overseas training programmes, sometimes taking time out from an overseas holiday to visit the local hospice service! Earlier this year a group of palliative care doctors and nurses from the UK took part in a conference in Romania to launch the establishment of a small hospice ward in Brasov. The conference carried a strong message; first, that hospice will flourish only if it is truly indigenous and appropriate to the social, economic and human situation of that country and secondly that many problems encountered in caring for the dying are common to all cultures. In a subsequent report of the conference Dr Mary Baines, physician to St Christopher's and a member of the conference team, remarked:

> The Brasov Conference created a great deal of interest among local doctors because it attempted to address important questions which are rarely tackled in conventional medical training – neither in Romania nor elsewhere. And yet these topics arise daily in a cancer ward: how to control pain and other distressing symptoms, what to say to patients and their relatives, the best place for someone to die.[4]

Access to literature on palliative care and general advice are also highly valued by overseas colleagues and certainly the mail order service offered by St Christopher's book shop and the Hospice Information Service is extremely well used. Catherine Krings, project director of the newly established Patient Outreach Service in the Philippines, refers to the literature purchased during her recent training in the UK as 'my great helpers in doing the work'. Much literature on palliative care available from St Christopher's bookshop has now been translated into other languages including French, German and Japanese. The two WHO publications which address cancer pain relief, *Cancer Pain Relief*[5] and *Cancer Pain Relief and Palliative Care*[6] have been translated into a number of languages. '*Cancer pain relief*' has already been translated into more than seventeen languages and the Bulgarian and Bahasa Malaysian and Indonesian versions are in preparation. The more recent '*Cancer pain relief and palliative care*' has been translated into four languages and Chinese, Japanese and Spanish editions are in preparation.

But as hospice reaches out across the world there can be heartbreak too. The Omega Foundation, established in Bogota in 1987 by Isa de Jaramillo, had been caring for patients at home and in hospital for just one year when the building which was to be the eventual location of the team's in-patient and day unit was severely vandalized. The house, which had been purchased from donations and a bank loan, was destroyed by members of the local community who feared the arrival of patients with AIDS. Undaunted, however, the work goes on and the Omega Foundation still intends to open its inpatient unit.[1]

Determination, faith and courage are common characteristics throughout the worldwide hospice community.

Acknowledgements

I would like to record my deep personal gratitude to the following for making available to me unpublished material: Stephanie Wyers and Stuart Craig, Swaziland Hospice at Home, Mrs O K Fatunmbi, Adjuwa Hospital, Nigeria. Dr Catherine Krings, Patient Outreach Service, Philippines and to my colleague Ann Eve, who helps me to run the Hospice Information Service.

Notes and References

1. Recorded proceedings of the Sixth International Conference of St Christopher's Hospice, Hospice: building bridges. *Bridging the racial gulf*, Dr C. Dare; *A Window on the Hospice World*, London Gilly Burn; Dr P. Bejarano (Colombia).
2. 'Out of Africa – a hospice in Kenya', *The Hospice Bulletin*, No. 11, January 1991, London, The Hospice Information Service.
3. SAUNDERS, C., SUMMERS, D. and TELLER, N. (eds.) *Hospice: the Living Idea*, London, Edward Arnold, 1981.
4. 'A Hospice for Brasov', *The Hospice Bulletin*, No. 16, July 1992, London, The Hospice Information Service.
5. World Health Organization, *Cancer Pain Relief*, Geneva: WHO 1986.
6. World Health Organization, *Cancer Pain Relief and Palliative Care*, Geneva, WHO 1990.

9

Ethical and legal considerations

Ethical considerations

Peter Byrne

General

Terminal care is defined in this study as the treatment of patients who have an irreversible, fatal condition, where death is expected relatively soon and the focus has shifted from treating the primary disease to easing of the patient's symptoms and support of him and his family. Such care is bound to be surrounded by ethical considerations. It is committed to goals and ideas which are partly ethical in character, relating to the idea of a good death. It assumes relations with patients which take members of the caring team into the details of personal and family life and presuppose a degree of intimacy between patient and carer. This section explores some of the ethical issues surrounding terminal care in greater detail.

Wisdom in dealing with the moral problems which arise out of terminal care will grow out of the thoughtful practice of those involved in giving and receiving it. Practitioners should be particularly wary of the thought that only by listening to or reading moral philosophers can they come to an understanding of these problems. Such a conclusion may be suggested by the notion that the ethics of medicine is governed by a range of general principles (such as those of justice, autonomy, beneficence and non-maleficence adumbrated by Beauchamp and Childress[1]) which require philosophical competence in order to be understood properly.

General principles may quickly prove of limited value once the messy world of practice is confronted. Moreover, concentration upon them may take attention away from the unique needs of particular patients and the demands that relationships with them place upon doctors, nurses and others. A sound ethics for terminal care will more properly focus on the demands of right relationship between patient and carers and the problems these demands give rise to. Some of these problems can be illustrated by reference to truth-telling and truthfulness.

There has been a welcome shift toward telling terminally ill patients the truth about their condition within the last two decades.[2] Both the internal demands of the doctor-patient relationship and the goals doctors bring to the practice of good terminal care appear to place a premium on honest disclosure of diagnosis and prognosis to the terminally ill. The necessary kinds of contact between carer and patient require the latter to have trust in the former. This is always likely to be destroyed if members of the team are involved in weaving a web of deceit around the patient. Relations between carers, patient and family will likewise be more difficult to manage if carers use a different standard of disclosure to patient on the one hand and to relatives on the other. Good terminal care is also likely to aim at goals for the patient which, leaving behind attempts to cure his primary condition, focus on general life enhancement and well-being in his final months. This may well give carers a direct interest in getting the patient to attend to needs, such as those of family reconciliation, which entail in turn facing up in some measure to the realities of his dying. Above all deceit represents a direct violation of what is owing to another encountered as a person in moral relationship.

However, despite all that may be said in favour of truth-telling toward the terminally ill, the uniqueness of each patient and of the demands of each doctor–patient relationship necessitate the abandonment of any inflexible policy of disclosure. Fidelity to the patient and the specific relationship with him dictate concentration upon his needs and capacities. This may reveal in the individual case a positive desire not to know, or a desire to have truth hinted at rather than openly acknowledged. Dialogue and communication are implied in a relationship with the patient that embodies a true respect for him but such dialogue may reveal that respect for *this* individual involves withholding or masking the truth. This is not deceit: it need entail no lying. The patient must be allowed to ask questions but not all questions are requests for information; some are requests for reassurance. Fidelity implies truthfulness but may rule out the spelling out of truth regardless of the patient's desire and capacity to know.[3,4]

The governing model of an ethics of respect for persons-in-relationship should exclude our thinking of the issues surrounding truthfulness in terms of a clash between principles such as autonomy and beneficence, still less in terms of a conflict between the interests of patient (in 'self-determination') and doctor (in 'paternalism' and 'benevolence').

Euthanasia

The licitness of euthanasia is an inevitable question when discussing the treatment of the terminally ill. Since the patients concerned are relatively close to death, decisions about their care may have implications about the time of their end. Good terminal care focuses on the palliation of distressing symptoms and on improving the quality of the patient's remaining days, and typically eschews the use of aggressive measures to eke them out. Given these points advocates of euthanasia will want to know how a consistent medical ethics for the terminally ill can rule out euthanasia.

There is no way these questions can be pursued profitably unless a sharp definition of 'euthanasia' is employed. Clarity of thought forbids using the term to refer generally to 'easing or assisting dying'. Such phrases denote no precise act whose morality we can debate or about which we may have a view.

What is in question here is medical killing and whether there are circumstances in normal medical practice in which doctors may kill. Objections that 'killing' is too emotive a word to allow the case for euthanasia to be heard are crass. We are familiar with the notion of justified homicide in ethics and law. Those who wish to change ethics and law in relation to euthanasia want the idea of justified homicide extended to include a range of acts that doctors may perform for the terminally ill (or the handicapped – but that is another discussion).

Used with precision 'euthanasia' denotes an act-type with three main features: first, its *intention* or *objective* is to bring about death, hence it is a member of the species homicide; secondly, its *motive* is typically to avoid further harm (in the way of suffering or degradation) to its victim. I assume here that the best case for euthanasia will concentrate on the good it brings to its victim and not on the harm to others it may prevent (as in avoiding a 'waste' of resources); thirdly, its *circumstances*, which are presumed by its apologists in the most favourable case to be ones where the only means of avoiding the gross forms of harm specified in its typical motive are those of using medical skill to kill. Thus euthanasia as an option for medical carers is a form of homicide presumed to be justified in certain circumstances by an extension of the same motives of benevolence which drive other, licit acts of medical care.

So defined, euthanasia for the terminally ill is open to easy objection. Most people believe that killing is in itself a drastic form of action. If it is so, then it can be argued that it cannot be warranted by the motives and circumstances found in good terminal care. Two reasons may be offered for this conclusion. First, there are usually much less drastic means of securing the ends good terminal care seeks, namely by offering patients the best kind of symptom control and palliative care.[5,2] Secondly, even if there are at present a small minority of patients whose symptoms even the best available care cannot fully mitigate, killing is so drastic a step that it is not to be contemplated. This second point can be strengthened by reference to arguments appealing to the long-term consequences of an open practice of euthanasia. Euthanasia, it may be urged, is liable to generate bad results for the practice of terminal medicine. An established practice of this sort will promote distrust between doctor and patient, will make the dying fearful of the wishes of relatives and generally increase their sense of being a burden on the living, rather than being persons who matter. It is much better to adopt a social policy of investment in the development of palliative medicine to whittle away at those cases where euthanasia appears to be the only or best option for care.

These stock arguments against euthanasia as an option in terminal care are cogent only to the extent that we regard killing as a serious harm which requires strenuous justification in any circumstances. Contemporary defenders of euthanasia are able to circumvent arguments of the form outlined above by appealing to a voluntaristic ethic of homicide and of the value of life. Thus they will sharply distinguish voluntary euthanasia (with the patient's consent or at his express wish) from involuntary euthanasia (against the patient's wishes) and nonvoluntary euthanasia (upon a patient who has lost the capacity to express a wish about continued living). Voluntary euthanasia is then defended as the last, and most important, right of self-determination any human subject can enjoy. Its refusal is allegedly a fundamental denial of autonomy or an interference with privacy.[6] The value of a life is made conditional on its possessor having a reflective desire to continue to live.[7] No harm is then done if a person is killed at his express wish. Medical killing done with consent does not represent a drastic response to the problems of the terminally ill to which alternatives should always be sought.

This voluntaristic ethic is at the heart of defences of the established practice of voluntary euthanasia in the Netherlands.[6] It represents an extension into the ethics of homicide of the stress on the importance of autonomy and privacy characteristic of many contemporary philosophical and social developments. Because of the ramifications of its underpinnings no attempt can be made here to discuss it thoroughly. Enough, however, can be said to indicate how those involved in terminal care can take their bearings with respect to it.

First, we should note that at a deeper level such views must lead to the licensing of non-voluntary euthanasia. If the underlying view is that a person's life is of value to the extent that he has a reflective desire to live, then those who through lack of competence or self-consciousness can no longer form such a desire have lives which are of no value. Thorough philosophical defences of the voluntaristic ethic agree in predicating the distinctive value of human life in the possession of the ability to form autonomous choices, continued living being valuable if a choice for life is present.[8,9] Accepting the voluntaristic ethic will have, and is designed to have, major consequences for the treatment of the demented, the handicapped and the newborn as a result. These consequences should make us pause before accepting it.

Those who are involved in terminal care will have reason to question the reliability of appeals to patients' expressed desires as the measure of life's value. Terminal illness is frequently characterized by feelings of dependence which may turn into fears of being a burden on others. Expressed desires to be killed may have a complex and confused motivational background. The 'right to die' cannot be a simple privacy right if it entails a duty on others to kill. What is claimed is not mere non-interference of others in a private process: as a plea for euthanasia it requests the performance by others of a public act, concerning which their consciences are necessarily engaged. There is no way in which appealing to the patient's autonomy can easily triumph in any conflict between his wishes and others' perception of their duties (not least, because *their* autonomy is equally in question).

A voluntaristic ethics can also be seen to be in conflict with much else in medical practice. Consider a surgeon's decision to amputate a patient's limb. The patient's wishes are certainly relevant here. Without consent the act will be a gross violation of the latter's bodily integrity. Some grounds for amputation may be affected by judgements of the patient's wishes. But there is no way in which the mere desire of a patient to have a limb cut off constitutes a convincing reason in itself for mutilating his body. This is normally thought of as a serious harm, to be justified not because the patient desires it, but because medical necessity dictates it. That is, if it is justified it is the only means of warding off even greater harm (such as death). Granted that medical necessity is the prime justification, then of course it can be performed in an emergency *without* consent. The doctor cannot fail in such a case to form a view about the harms involved in undertaking drastic acts to ward off great evils. Patient's wishes, where known, are relevant to forming such a view, but they can never dictate it. If tests of medical necessity must be applied to proposed acts of euthanasia, we would once more find that voluntary euthanasia is licit only if non-voluntary euthanasia is sometimes licit.

On a whole range of acts, law and social policy in the UK and the Common Law countries support the anti-voluntaristic stance of much medical decision making. It is no defence against a charge of serious assault on another that your victim desired it (hence the need for the surgeon to plead necessity to justify his invasion of the body). Still less is consent of the victim a successful plea in defence of a charge of murder. Social policy, for good or ill, recognizes a wide range of alleged harms that are too serious to be visited upon a victim merely because he desires it. Killing another is a paramount example of one of these harms. Very large parts of medical practice are predicated on this aspect of social policy. Defenders of euthanasia, in my view, have not begun to take seriously the changes that their voluntaristic ethic would require in medicine and social life in general if it were consistently accepted.

A soundly based practice of terminal care will take requests for euthanasia by patients very seriously. The beliefs and motives behind them will need to be explored carefully; the anxieties that prompt them dealt with. Such requests may constitute important crises in the relationship between patient and his carers. If euthanasia were openly approved and practised, then such requests would take on an entirely new meaning. For the reasons indicated above, it is arguable that if the doctor were seen as the potential supplier of death on request his relationship with the terminally ill patient would be radically altered.

That killing someone is a serious harm does not entail that there are no circumstances where it can be justified. Our notion of justified homicide allows us to suppose that the harm of taking life can in some cases be outweighed by other goods and harms. It is surely possible to imagine cases (as, classically, on the battlefield) where the only, and the right, thing to do for a dying, suffering person is to kill him. In cases where normal medical care is not available or has broken down, such acts of mercy may become licit even on a traditional understanding of the value of life. The question for terminal care is how far expected, real-life cases in the practice of normal care for the dying can come close to such instances of justified killing. The assumption of this section, and presumably of this whole study, is that, if sufficient resources are made available, they need not.

A final issue in consistently distinguishing good terminal care from euthanasia relates to how we may separate the foregoing of aggressive measures to prolong life as long as is physically possible from deliberate acts of euthanasia. The traditional answer is in terms of double effect. In euthanasia the hastened death of the patient is not merely foreseen as a possibility but intended. In non-aggressive terminal care which focuses on life enhancement, hastened death may or may not be foreseen, but it is never intended. Therefore, good terminal care is not tantamount to killing, regardless of whether or not it actually foregoes opportunities to prolong life. *If* not prolonging life to the greatest possible extent *is* an effect of the best terminal care, it is merely a side effect.

There is now a considerable literature on double effect and whether it can be used to draw distinctions between those medical acts which kill and those which do not. Much of it is sceptical of the distinction.[10] In my view this scepticism betrays a failure to analyse properly the notion of intention. Lacking a proper understanding of the import of saying that death is 'intended' in a true act of killing, sceptics about double effect conclude that the distinctions it gives rise to are trivial. Let it be noted that in good terminal care death is not pursued as an object of acts or policies. If a patient's death were the real object of a doctor's actions then they would constitute an endeavour to kill him. They would have to be adapted to achieving this result as changing circumstances demanded. They would exclude the performance of other acts which might have effects opposite to the one intended, so would rule out doing anything that might prolong life. Finally, yet other plans (such as for further admissions) would be predicated on the successful pursuit of this objective.[11,12]

There may well be borderline cases where distinctions between euthanasia and non-aggressive management of the dying are hard to draw. This is to be expected. Their existence need not devalue the reality and usefulness of a general distinction between euthanasia and other ways of avoiding burdens upon the dying. In this brief discussion I have tried to argue for the conclusion that a policy and practice of euthanasia would damage the peculiar relation between patient and carers that is at the heart of both good terminal care and of the ethics of such care.

Notes and References

1. BEAUCHAMP, T.I. and CHILDRESS, J.F. *Principles of Biomedial Ethics*, New York, Oxford University Press, 1989.
2. SAUNDERS, C. and BAINES, M. *Living with Dying*, Oxford, Oxford University Press, 1989.
3. BYRNE, P. 'Hospice Care: weighing the issues,' *Palliative Medicine*, 1991, **5**, 195–200.
4. BYRNE, P. 'Comments on an obstructed death,' *Journal of Medical Ethics*. 1990, **6**, 88–9.

5. British Medical Association, *Euthanasia*, London, British Medical Association, 1988.
6. LEENEN, H.J. 'Euthanasia in the Netherlands.' In: Byrne, P. (ed.), *Medicine, Medical Ethics and the Value of Life*, Chichester, John Wiley, 1989, pp. 1–14.
7. HEYD, D. 'The meaning of life and voluntary euthanasia.' In: Carni, A. (ed.), *Euthanasia*, Berlin, Springer, 1984, pp. 155–65.
8. GLOVER, J. *Causing Death and Saving Lives*, Harmondsworth, Penguin, 1977.
9. HARRIS, J. *The Value of Life*, London, Routledge, 1985.
10. KUHSE H. *The Sanctity of Life Doctrine in Medicine*, Oxford, Clarendon Press, 1987.
11. BYRNE, P. 'Homicide, medical ethics and the principle of double effect.' In: Byrne, P. (ed.) *Ethics and Law in Health Care and Research*, Chichester, John Wiley, 1990, pp. 131–60.
12. BYRNE, P. *The Philosophical and Theological Foundations of Ethics*, London, Macmillan, 1992.

Legal considerations

A McCall-Smith

The legal implications of the treatment of the terminally ill have become of increasing concern in view of the greater involvement of the courts in the practice of medicine. This involvement is reflected in a variety of contexts, most notably in the considerable increase in the incidence of medical litigation, with patients being apparently readier to press claims against negligent doctors. Then there has been a small, but significant group of cases in which the guidance of the courts has been sought as to the appropriate parameters to treatment of vulnerable patients (mainly handicapped or terminally ill infants).[1] And, finally, there has been a series of highly publicized prosecutions brought against doctors for negligent manslaughter.[2] All of these factors have combined to make it increasingly important for doctors to be guided not only by their sense as to what is ethically right in a particular case, but also to be aware of the legal restraints on their freedom of clinical action.

Not everyone welcomes this development. The harrowing and inappropriate spectacle of the 'judge at the bedside' with the courts monitoring the care of unconscious and gravely ill patients in the face of family determination that life supporting measures should be stopped, has distorted terminal care in the United States to a considerable extent and led to the emergence of a 'natural death' movement.[3] This is very far removed from the ethic of the hospice movement, for example, but even if the United

Kingdom has been spared this distressing development there are none the less legal considerations to be borne in mind by doctors involved in terminal care. The law in the United Kingdom is not interventionist in this area of medicine, but it does set limits to what is permissible. These are fairly wide and allow the individual doctor considerable room for the exercise of discretion.

The legal bedrock principle: human life is sacrosanct

The starting point of any discussion of the legal implications of terminal care is the well-established legal principle that the deliberate taking of human life amounts to homicide and punishable by the criminal law. The deliberate killing of another is murder (or, in certain circumstances, at least manslaughter) whatever the motive of the person who takes life. This means that euthanasia is a serious criminal offence even if the deceased had a short time to live and is saved from unendurable suffering. Nor is the consent of the patient a defence in such a case. One who kills another at that other's request is not relieved of criminal liability by virtue of the consent, a principle which is applied even to cases of serious assault, where the consent of the victim is irrelevant to the question of criminal guilt.

There have been persistent efforts to change the law of homicide to permit medically regulated voluntary euthanasia, but these moves have met with no success. The introduction of a lesser offence of 'mercy killing' has been raised as a possibility by law reformers, but this has not attracted official support. We are left, therefore, with a situation where the only prospect of mitigating the criminal guilt of one who carries out an act of euthanasia is the raising of a plea of diminished responsibility, the effect of which is to reduce murder to the lesser offence of manslaughter. This tactic might recommend itself in cases where the patient's life is taken by a relative who, say, suffered psychologically from the strain of the terminal illness, but it is obviously unlikely to apply in the medical context. Consequently, no doctor should be unaware of the fact that euthanasia involves a possible conviction for murder, followed by a mandatory life sentence for murder.

The severity of the law in this area has caused considerable misgivings. Yet such is the level of legal opposition to euthanasia that there is only one Western jurisdiction which has openly sanctioned euthanasia. In the Netherlands, euthanasia practised under certain conditions is no longer prosecuted, and its incidence has apparently become remarkably high.[4] For many, this is a disturbing development which is unlikely to be followed elsewhere. Yet it does represent a significant precedent.

Assisting others to die

Rather different from the takings of steps directed towards killing one who wishes to die is the provision to such a person of the means of ending his own life. Suicide is no longer a crime in English law, and has never been a crime in modern Scots criminal law. Yet under the terms of the Suicide Act 1961, the legislation which decriminalized suicide itself in England and Wales, the crime of aiding and abetting another to take his own life is preserved. This means that it is an offence under this statute to provide for another the means to kill himself, as long as one knows of his intention, and as long as there is a reasonably immediate link between the provision of the means and the attempted suicide. In the case of *Attorney General* v. *Able*[5] it was held that the provision of advice, as opposed to material assistance, could amount to a breach of this provision, and this decision served to inhibit for many years the publication of guides to what the pro-euthanasia societies term 'self deliverance'.

In Scotland, and in other countries where there is no statutory prohibition directed against aiding and abetting suicide, the same result might be achieved through the application of common law principles. A person who gives another the means of committing suicide may be considered to have caused the death, and this may amount to homicide. Alternatively, the person who gives the means of suicide to one who intends to take his own life may be said to act recklessly, and could be prosecuted for a homicide offence on these grounds.

Even if it is criminal to assist another to take his own life, this is not of everyday relevance to those who are professionally involved in the treatment of the terminally ill. More pressing to them is the question as to the limits of the obligation to prolong life and the identification of the point at which medical efforts can be directed towards either hastening death or ensuring the comfort of the patient rather than his or her continued survival.

The fundamental obligation to the patient and the provision of care

In assuming responsibility for a patient, a doctor undertakes to provide an acceptable degree of care. The definition of what is acceptable depends on a variety of factors, including the availability of resources and the patient's condition. There is no duty to provide everything that medical science can offer; material limitations will prevent this, apart from anything else, and there are other reasons, too, why it might be inappropriate to resort to certain treatments. In essence, only productive treatment need be offered; treatment which is medically unproductive, in that it exacerbates or prolongs the patient's suffering and provides no real hope for the future need not be adopted.

How does the law distinguish between a failure to discharge basic obligations on the one hand and, on the other, a reasonable medical choice not to pursue a treatment which is considered productive? This distinction is difficult ethically as well as legally, and a hard and fast answer is likely to prove elusive. It is possible, though, to identify the broad contours of the legal approach to this issue, accepting that every case is likely to depend on a variety of individual factors.

The most basic obligation to the terminally ill, as to any other patient, is the duty to provide physical care. It might be thought that this is uncomplicated, and yet there lurks here at least one difficult issue – that of the duty to provide nutrition and hydration by artificial means.[6] There is no doubt but that a doctor or any other person caring for a dependent ill person must provide food and water for that person as well as undertaking basic nursing tasks. Medical staff cannot decide to stop feeding a person who is still capable of taking food and who appears not to reject such care. It may be that stopping food and water is judged to be the most convenient way of ending a patient's suffering, but to do so amounts to an omission to perform an important basic obligation and is punishable under the criminal law. There are many cases which support this view, the majority of them involving the failure by relatives to look after elderly people in their charge, but at least one, the *Arthur* case,[7] involving a nursing care only instruction given by a paediatrician in respect of an uncomplicated Down's Syndrome infant whose parents did not wish it to survive. The fact that a criminal prosecution was brought against Leonard Arthur surprised many doctors, and yet it demonstrates the clear boundaries which the law imposes in this area.

Yet even if the law is clear in relation to the obligation to provide this basic care, does the obligation extend to a duty to resort to the provision of nutrition and hydration by naso-gastric tube? This precise point arose in *Airedale National Health Service Trust* v. *Bland*,[8] a case in which the court was asked to consider the plight of a young man who had spent three years in a persistent vegetative state and who was sustained by these means. The court was clear in its view that feeding by naso-gastric tube amounted to medical treatment and that there was no obligation to provide treatment in those cases where this would merely prolong the life of an insensate patient with no hope of recovery. Discontinuance of treatment in such circumstances was held to be in the patient's best interests, as the court could not imagine what possible benefit the patient could derive from his continued existence in the persistent vegetative state.

In *Re J (a minor)*[9] the Court of Appeal considered another invasive procedure, artificial ventilation, and concluded that such treatment was not necessarily required in the case of a grossly handicapped baby. This constitutes a further recognition of the limits to which medical efforts should go, and emphasises the pointlessness of prolonging suffering when the prognosis for the patient is unambiguously bleak.

The extent of the duty to treat?

Basic care, as we have seen, is always required, no matter how limited the patient's prospects may be. But what does the doctor have to do beyond that? Does the law expect him to provide whatever treatment is available, as long as it holds out some prospect of prolonging the life of the patient?

Neither morality nor the law require that a doctor should take active steps to prolong a life when the general quality of that life is so unacceptable that prolongation will merely lead to further suffering. In the past, legal discussion of this topic tended to stress the distinction between 'ordinary' and 'extraordinary' treatment, the former being legally required and the latter not. This terminology is potentially misleading, as the crucial factor to be taken into account is whether the treatment was required for that particular patient, given the patient's particular circumstances. An antibiotic may be the ordinary treatment for a chest infection in the case of an otherwise healthy young adult, but this does not mean that it should be considered ordinary treatment for the elderly patient with advanced malignant disease and a very poor quality of life. A more appropriate distinction is between 'productive' and 'unproductive' treatment, a distinction which allows for consideration to be given to the treatment's implications for that particular patient.

Decisions as to which treatments are productive and which are unproductive will clearly be delicate ones of clinical judgement, and the law provides only the broadest guidelines as to the legal limits in this context. The standard against which such decisions would be measured legally – if the law were to be involved – would be the standard of the reasonable doctor. A failure to provide treatment in circumstances which any reasonable doctor would provide might amount to culpable neglect, and therefore constitute manslaughter, but this would probably be so only in an extreme case. It is true that recently there have been more frequent prosecutions of doctors for negligent homicide, but none of these has involved the withholding of treatment. A decision not to treat terminal illness aggressively does not amount to euthanasia, and would be unlikely to be regarded as such by the criminal law.

The administration of pain-killing drugs which may have the incidental effect of shortening life is also legally proper, provided that the motive for which the drugs are administered is the control of pain. A substantial dose of morphine, which may have the effect of suppressing respiration and hastening death, will not amount in the eyes of the law to a deliberate taking of life, provided that the predominant intention behind the administration of the drug is the legitimate one of helping the patient through pain.

It is apparent, then, that the law in the United Kingdom does not intervene in terminal care decisions to anything like the extent it does in the United States. The excessive prolongation of life out of fear as to legal consequences does not occur here, and this is to be welcomed. At the same time, the courts have set the outer limits of medical discretion

– almost entirely in those cases concerned with the treatment of handicapped infants – and these limits should not prove unduly hampering to doctors.

Patient autonomy and the law

In spite of the general absence of antagonism between doctors, family and patients in matters of terminal care, there is a growing awareness in the public mind of the extent to which medical technology can sustain human life beyond the point of what might be termed 'natural death'. Concern is felt by some that it may be difficult to avoid the undue prolongation of life in the face of medical assumptions that a lengthy survival rate amounts to therapeutic success. To this end there is growing interest in 'advance declarations' or 'living wills', documents which purport to instruct doctors that certain treatments should not be pursued in the event of incapacity.[10] Once again, this is primarily a North American development, but the use of English and Scottish equivalents appears to be becoming more common, even if there is little evidence that medical practice here justifies such fears.

The typical advance declaration states that should the grantor become incapable of expressing a view as to medical treatment, and should his or her condition be deemed to be terminal, then certain treatments should not be undertaken. For example, the declaration circulated by the Voluntary Euthanasia Society of Scotland, states that in the event of the development of a listed condition (including severe and lasting brain damage, advanced disseminated malignant disease, and dementia) life should not be sustained by 'artificial means' such as life support systems or intravenous fluids and drugs.

The legal effect of these declarations has yet to be tested in the United Kingdom. In principle, it is difficult to see why they should not be given legal effect, subject to certain safeguards, as they amount to a clear withholding of consent to treatment on the part of the patient. If the law requires, as it does, that any treatment should in normal circumstances be consented to by the patient, then there is no reason why this consent should be excluded in advance. Against this view it can be argued that a decision of this nature simply cannot be given in advance. It is one thing to say that one would not wish to be treated in a particular way in the event of a particular condition being developed, but how is one to be certain of one's view as to treatment when faced with imminent death? It is quite possible that the patient will undergo a change of mind and want to continue living. The possibility of such a change of mind has been taken in some quarters as grounds for refusing to recognize the validity of an advance declaration.

Another argument against the laying of too much store by the advance declaration is that to do so unduly hampers the doctor in the exercise of judgement at the time when treatment decisions have to be made.[11] It might be said that the person who is most likely to understand what a patient wants, or indeed wanted in the final weeks or days of life, is the doctor or the nursing staff. To tie the doctor's hands by requiring the cessation of treatment could constitute an interference in a delicate and subtle professional relationship.

The arguments against giving legal effect to advance declarations are powerful ones. Yet it is clear that many of those who go to the trouble of filling in advance declarations have strong feelings on the subject of their mode of death, and they see control of the means of dying as being an important part of their autonomy. To override this is a serious step, and it might be one which the law will avoid taking, should the issue come before the courts. There is, of course, a compromise position, which would treat the advance declaration as an important piece of evidence of the incapable patient's wishes at an earlier stage, but to treat these wishes as being a significant factor to be taken into account by the doctor in the making of any decision. This gives some recognition to the principle of patient autonomy while at the same time taking into account the significance of the doctor's own views.

Conclusion

A survey of legal developments in this area over the last decade reveals comparatively little change and certainly should give rise to little concern on the part of doctors that medical practice in this area is becoming unduly invaded by legal considerations. In pronouncing on the treatment of terminally ill or seriously ill children, the courts have effectively left the decision as to when to draw the line and refrain from further treatment initiatives in the hands of the doctors. The active ending of life has been declared to be legally unacceptable, but this really represents no change from the traditional legal interdiction of homicide and there is no evidence that organized medical opinion wants this changed. Life remains sacrosanct in the eyes of the law, although its undue prolongation is clearly not a legal duty. The law therefore continues to mirror closely the professional and ethical consensus, a position which still appears to afford a satisfactory degree of protection of the interests of the terminally ill. Ultimately the real protection of the vulnerable ill lies not so much in a highly vigilant legal system (which cannot possibly police every case) but in the ethical sense of those who provide medical care.

Notes and References

1. For example, *Re B (a minor)* [1981] 1 WLR 1421; *C (a minor)* [1989] 2 All ER 782; *Re J (a minor)* [1990] 3 All ER 930.
2. DYER, C. 'Doctors convicted of manslaughter,' *British Medical Journal*, 1990, **303**, 1156.
3. For general discussion of American developments, see Mason, J.K. and McCall Smith, R.A., *Law and Medical Ethics*, 3rd edn, London, Butterworths,

1991, 338–43.

4. WACHTER, M.A.M. 'Euthanasia in the Netherlands,' *British Medical Journal, 1990,* **300**, 1093.

5. [1984] 1 All ER 277.

6. For discussion of this issue see Dresser, R.S. and Boisaubin, E.V. 'Ethics, Law and Nutritional Support,' *Archives of Internal Medicine* 1985, **145**, 122.

7. *The Times*, 6 November 1981; Brahams, D. 'Putting Dr Arthur's Case in Perspective,' *Criminal Law Review*, **387**–389.

8. [1990] 3 All ER 930.

9. *The Times*, December 10, 1992.

10. For discussion of advance declarations and their possible effect, see Age Concern, Institute of Gerontology and the Centre of Medical Law and Ethics, King's College, London, *The Living Will*, London, 1988.

11. This consideration clearly weighed heavily with the Scottish Law Commission in their discussion paper, 'Mentally Disabled Adults,' Edinburgh, Scottish Law Commission, 1991.

Wider applications of palliative care

Robert Dunlop

Introduction

The hospice movement has established new standards of care for patients with incurable cancer. This new movement has captured the hearts and minds of the lay community. Hundreds of hospice programmes have been set up throughout the United Kingdom and the rest of the world; many of them are largely or wholly community funded, with volunteers playing a major role in the provision of care.

Why has the hospice movement had such an impact? Because it has reestablished the art of medicine in an age where high technology investigations and treatments focus predominantly on the science. This chapter examines the exciting prospect that the principles of cancer palliation developed by the hospice movement, can be the leaven for a whole new dimension of care for people who suffer from progressive non-malignant disorders.

What are the principles of cancer palliation?

The principles of cancer palliation have been examined in detail elsewhere in this book. There are three basic tenets which are relevant to this chapter:

1. *Symptoms from a disease should be treated, even if the cause cannot be corrected*: In the past, doctors who were faced with a cancer patient for whom there was no curative treatment would tell the patient that nothing more could be done. The patient and family were left to confront the worst part of the illness with little or no prospect of relief from the relentless effects of the disease. The hospice movement cast aside this pessimism by using the scientific method to understand

the mechanisms which produce symptoms. As a result, creative and constructive strategies are now available which can provide relief from all manner of problems.

2. *The patient is far more than just a physical illness*:   Medicine teaches how cancer affects the physical body but hospice considers the person as a highly individual, complex interwoven pattern of physical, psychological, social, and spiritual dimensions.

3. *The person and their family must be considered the unit of care*:   Any illness, but more particularly any incurable illness, affects more than just the patient. The impact on the family extends even beyond the death of the patient, sometimes dominating their lives for many years.

It is the attention to detail and yet the recognition of the whole which explains the revolutionary effect of the hospice movement.

Are the principles of cancer palliation relevant to other conditions?

The answer to this question is definitely yes. This conclusion is supported by a review of the needs of patients with chronic progressive conditions and their families.

Needs of Patients

Physical needs

There have now been several studies of people with non-malignant conditions who are terminally ill (Hockley, 1988; Hinton, 1963; Cartwright 1973). These studies have revealed that patients are just as likely to have symptoms and many patients have multiple symptoms. The relative frequency of these symptoms is a little different from the hospice experience with cancer patients. Pain, breathlessness, anorexia and weakness are very prevalent but patients with non-malignant conditions are less likely than cancer patients to have their symptoms relieved.

Psychological and Spiritual needs

Many patients describe themselves as feeling depressed, particularly if they are suffering from unremitting and distressing symptoms. The prospect of a slowly progressive condition such as chronic obstructive respiratory disease can cause patients to become severely depressed.

Anxiety is also common, particularly if the patient is breathless, has young dependents or a 'tepid' religious faith (Hinton, 1963). The complex technologies required for treatment and diagnosis increase anxiety, as does any prolonged wait for the results of tests or treatments.

Surprisingly, anger is relatively uncommon. Those patients who do get angry often direct their frustrations and anger onto the relatives, which adds to their burden of care.

Any progressive illness will cause people to confront deeper spiritual issues. Even though non-malignant diagnoses may not evoke the same immediate realization of impending death as cancer, feelings of helplessness, guilt, and self-deprecation can emerge as the patient's condition deteriorates and may cause profound anguish.

Needs of relatives

Physical symptoms

Given the chronicity of many progressive diseases, it is not surprising that relatives frequently become fatigued (Wilkes, 1984). It is more surprising that only 20 per cent of relatives actually develop a physical illness from the stress of trying to care for their loved ones. It is important not to underestimate the physical cost on the carers.

Psychological needs

Depression and anxiety are also common with relatives who are trying to cope with the impending loss of the patient. They have great difficulty coping when the patient indicates that he or she is going to die. They try to be optimistic but feel depressed at the breakdown in their previously trusting relationship.

If the patient is experiencing distressing symptoms, relatives feel helpless and fearful. Fear is made worse when there is a perceived lack of general practitioner support. Many relatives are afraid that the patient will fall or die suddenly at home.

If the patient is admitted to hospital, relatives often feel guilty that they have let the patient down (Hockley, et al. 1988). Relatives also have difficulty obtaining accurate information about the patient's condition and prognosis. They often receive conflicting statements from doctors and nurses which reflects the greater degree of medical uncertainty about non-malignant conditions. Very often, they do not get information because they do not want to disturb the routine of the doctors and nurses.

Social needs

A progressive debilitating illness can have very profound effects on the structure and integrity of the family. There may be loss of earning power, particularly if the patient is younger. The long-term financial consequences can be devastating despite the presence of a number of benefits. A re-distribution of roles is often required which further compounds feelings of depression and anxiety. The patient and spouse often find themselves becoming socially isolated. The impact of changes in the patient's sexuality will often go unrecognized by health professionals.

Why are patients with non-malignant diseases and their families less likely to have symptoms controlled and other needs met?

The evidence clearly shows that major problems impact on the lives of these patients and their families. In contrast to the management of terminal cancer, it is disturbing that there has been little change since Hinton highlighted the problems with his study in 1963. If changes are to be made, we must understand the reasons for this inertia. Some of the issues include the following.

Doctors have difficulty coping with fatal illnesses

Doctors are trained to recognize and treat illnesses which can be cured. For example, Grand Round presentations often focus on dramatic success stories, and other doctors' mistakes which might have caused the death of a patient are frequently quoted in ward rounds. Consequently, doctors have difficulty in coping with illnesses which cannot be cured or which get worse despite treatment. Doctors also have difficulty relating to terminally ill patients because they are reminded of their own mortality.

Doctors have difficulty recognizing when patients are terminally ill

Very few doctors have ever seen patients die other than from a cardiac arrest, and they often fail to recognize when someone is entering the terminal phase of a progressive condition. Junior doctors, who have the least experience, are often responsible for the care of these patients while the concern of the consultant and registrar is focused on the 'acute' cases. It is little wonder that patients and families often receive conflicting information.

Doctors can experience the feeling that 'nothing more can be done' for some non-malignant conditions

There is an increasing range of medications available which treat the abnormal physiology of many non-malignant conditions, such as diuretics and vasodilators for heart failure. When this is not the case, as with motor neurone disease, patients and families are more likely to find themselves cut adrift from medical follow-up. However, the recent review of St

Christopher's Hospice experience with motor neurone disease (O'Brien *et al.*, 1992) confirmed that good control of symptoms can be achieved by applying the principles of palliation for cancer. Whereas most patients had symptoms on admission to the Hospice, over 90 per cent of the 124 patients were peaceful and settled when they were dying.

Discrepancies can arise between the aims of the doctors and the patients

Paradoxically, the availability of medications to treat the condition may not benefit the patient. Doctors will often feel that they can make the patient 'better': examples include reducing the oedema of congestive heart failure with diuretics, and using a higher dose of corticosteriods and bronchodilators for chronic obstructive respiratory disease. In patients with end-stage disease, treatments may improve some objective manifestations of the illness but fail to improve the patient's overall physical capacity and quality of life.

Doctors are unlikely to ask about symptoms which are not specifically related to the illness

The medical model emphasizes that certain symptoms are associated with particular diagnoses, e.g. paroxysmal nocturnal dyspnoea, orthopnoea, and breathlessness on exertion are all features of congestive heart failure. Doctors routinely ask about these symptoms, whereas other symptoms such as nausea from gut congestion and pain from liver congestion will be overlooked. Any symptom which distresses the patient, should be considered important, whether it is caused by the disease or is unrelated.

Patients and families are less likely to be distressed by the diagnosis

The very word 'cancer' can trigger extreme distress in many patients and families thereby precipitating referral to hospice services. Patients and families are less likely to be aware of the prognosis of non-malignant conditions, particularly when doctors feel they have beneficial treatments.

When patients have an inherited condition such as Huntington's Chorea, they will be very aware of the outcome if other family members have been affected.

Patients and families often accept symptoms as inevitable and do not complain

This situation is common to both cancer and non-malignant conditions. Many people still have a low expectation about what can be achieved on their behalf; rarely some people believe they deserve to suffer. Patients minimize their symptoms when questioned by their doctor, much like a child trying to avoid displeasing a parent. Nurses frequently relate how patients will tell the doctor 'I'm feeling fine, thank you', having just told the nurse about their pain. In home care, general practitioners should always confirm a negative response with the family.

A slowly progressive disorder can make some patients and families complain more bitterly and frequently because they cannot see any end to their suffering. These patients are often labelled as 'difficult' and are then ignored.

Health professionals fail to recognize less obvious symptoms

Symptoms such as vomiting and diahorrea are very obvious. However, symptoms such as nausea, pain and constipation are not readily apparent and tend to go unrecognized.

Inadequate doses of medications are prescribed for controlling symptoms

This is particularly the case with morphine. Although many of the fears and myths about morphine for cancer pain have been exploded by the experience of hospices, there is still considerable fear about using morphine for non-cancer pain or breathlessness. The effectiveness and safety of morphine have been clearly established for patients with motor neurone disease, not only for treating pain but also dyspnoea and insomnia (O'Brien *et al.*, 1992).

Health professionals may feel that the patient has 'deserved' the illness

When patients are considered culpable for their illness, they are likely to receive less attention. Some examples are: AIDS, smoking related diseases such as emphysema, heart disease due to obesity, and alcoholic cirrhosis.

How can professional carers become more responsive to the needs of these patients and families?

Palliative care is already having an impact on the management of patients with non-malignant conditions. This can be attributed in part to the practical examples provided by hospice. Hospital and domicillary nursing staff have become more aware of the positive difference that cancer patients experience under the care of hospice. Even when staff do not directly observe this difference, hospices do have an indirect effect which encourages staff to become more proficient at controlling pain for example (Parkes, 1985). Some hospital staff with an interest in cancer patients have begun translating the principles of cancer care to their other patients. Palliative care teams are having a much greater influence in hospital settings. Lay people are becoming much more aware of the positive influence of hospice and it is not uncommon for families to express anger at the paucity of services for non-cancer patients compared with cancer patients.

There are three main ways in which this impetus for change can be accelerated: by teaching, practical example, and support. The training programmes for doctors and nurses should contain more information about the management of distressing physical symptoms, particularly pain and breathlessness. Hospital staff also need to be taught how to recognize and manage psychosocial issues. The teaching content must be tailored to the requirements of the staff, for example first year student nurses have different requirements from senior staff nurses.

Didactic teaching methods are useful but must be supplemented with practical experience. Undergraduate medical students, nursing staff and other health professionals should be encouraged to visit and study at hospices whenever possible. One or two senior nurses from a ward or rest home can undertake post-graduate study and then become resource persons. Palliative care teams are in an excellent position to provide practical teaching within hospitals. Team members have to be familiar with the strategies to effect change in medical and nursing practices (Dunlop and Hockley, 1990).

Palliative care teams and other people working in an advisory capacity can indirectly improve patient and family care by providing emotional support for staff. The staff are then able to deal with personal issues that otherwise cloud difficult clinical decisions. Nurses are more receptive to emotional support; they bear the greater burden of care for the patients and families.

What are the problems which hospices experience when managing non-malignant conditions?

Very few patients, usually less than 10 per cent with non-malignant conditions are referred to hospice services; they usually die in hospitals. Some of the reasons for the lower rate of referrals have been reviewed previously in this chapter. But there are also a number of problems for hospices who manage patients with non-malignant conditions and new hospice programmes need to be aware of these:

- The uncertain trajectory of some illnesses such as chronic obstructive airways disease can require a long-term commitment to the care of the patient, longer than the twelve months criterion used by many hospices. When a chronic illness is punctuated with frequent episodes of deterioration followed by recovery, greater demands are placed on staff who are used to caring for patients who deteriorate steadily.

- Hospice staff may be unfamiliar with medications for the treatment of non-malignant conditions. Hospice training usually focuses on cancer patients. Because staff have much less exposure to non-malignant conditions, they may feel uncomfortable managing these patients. Palliative care team members who have trained in hospices can become very stressed in the hospital setting where patients are more likely to receive 'active' treatments which the team are not familiar with. The post-graduate palliative care training programme for physicians will help overcome these problems.
- Some doctors think of hospice as a 'dumping ground' for patients and families with difficult psychosocial problems, especially when the patient requires long-term placement. Patients with progressive non-malignant conditions are often hospitalized in acute medical beds when the family reach crisis point. Doctors quickly recognize the problem is not a medical one and they become angry with the thought of 'being used' by the general practitioner. The anger is translated into pressure for early discharge or transfer, and hospice in-patient beds will be considered if there is a long wait for long-term placement beds.

  Home care teams can be asked to provide home nursing care on a daily or more frequent basis because the relatives have become exhausted by the constant physical care. Hospice home care usually involves empowering the relatives to perform the cares. Few teams have the personnel resources to sustain a high level of input for more than a few days or weeks. This can be overcome by maintaining a good liaison with other community services, such as district nurses, who frequently provide a high level of support for non-terminally ill patients extending over months and years.
- In the current climate of decreasing central funding for health care, there is increasing pressure from patients and families to use hospice services which do not charge.
- Although hospice programmes are very familiar with the use of opioids for cancer patients, there can be significant concern and uncertainty about their use for patients with non-malignant conditions, especially the fear of causing addiction if the patient has an indeterminate prognosis. Even when hospice staff feel comfortable, there can be concern about adverse comment from other health professionals which would be detrimental to service growth.

What are the principles guiding the use of opioids in patients with non-malignant conditions?

There is no doubt that opioids can relieve some of the distressing symptoms, particularly pain and breathlessness, experienced by patients with progressive non-malignant conditions. However, doctors are more concerned about opioids causing addiction. For example, what about the emphysema patient who initially appears to be dying of an acute infection, is helped by oral morphine but then survives the chest infection and returns to a stable but symptomatic plateau – will the patient have to take morphine thereafter? Physical dependence will develop after 10–20 days but this can be overcome by reducing the dose gradually. There is no clear evidence that opioids cause addiction in patients with chronic non-malignant pain, and experts such as Melzack (1990) and Portenoy (1990) feel that opioids should not be withheld from these patients if these are the only option for relieving the pain. Our experience is that dyspnoeic patients can reduce their morphine dosage if breathlessness improves.

Given that the issue of addiction should not determine whether opioids can be used, the first principle is to make sure that opioids are appropriate for the patient's symptom. In particular, any decision to prescribe opioids for a patient with a chronic pain problem should be taken in consultation with a multidisciplinary pain clinic (Schug *et al.*, 1991).

When treating pain, it is important to make full use of other analgesic options. Morphine should not be considered as the panacea for all pain. The step-ladder method of pain control, starting with simple analgesics progressing through weak opioids to strong opioids, is very useful in many patients with non-malignant pain.

Non-malignant conditions often produce intermittent symptoms, for example angina chest pain with heart failure and breathlessness with emphysema. Continuous morphine therapy can cause more side effects, especially drowsiness, because the symptoms are not continuous; it is more appropriate to give shorter-acting opioids before any incident which will produce symptoms.

Several non-malignant conditions are associated with liver and renal dysfunction from direct involvement by cirrhosis or chronic renal failure for example, or as an indirect effect of an illness such as severe heart failure. In these patients, the dose and frequency of administration should be modified to avoid toxicity from the delayed metabolism and clearance of morphine.

It is easier to initiate morphine therapy in a hospice in-patient unit because the staff are all familiar with its use. Difficulties are likely to arise when patient care is shared with non-hospice health professionals. Hospice home care teams and hospital-based palliative care teams are frequently confronted by the need to persuade other doctors to start morphine. If the patient has a non-malignant diagnosis, the medical practitioner will need more reassurance and support than usual.

Summary

Patients with progressive non-malignant conditions are just as distressed by the physical and mental effects of their illness as cancer patients are. The families of these patients are also subject to considerable anguish. The principles of hospice care are very relevant to these patients and families. The challenge that faces the hospice movement is to make other health professionals more aware of the needs and the options which are available to meet these needs. Although the magnitude of the challenge is considerable, the objective of more compassionate and humane health care has to be worth the effort.

References

CARTWRIGHT, A., HOCKEY, L. and ANDERSON, I.L. *Life Before Death*, London, Routledge and Kegan Paul, 1973.

DUNLOP, R.J. and HOCKLEY, J.M. (eds). *Terminal Care Support Teams: the Hospital–Hospice Interface*, Oxford, Oxford University Press, 1990.

HINTON, J. 'The physical and mental distress of the Dying,' *Quarterly Journal of Medicine*, 1963, **32**, 1–21.

HOCKLEY, J.M., DUNLOP, R.J. and DAVIES, R.J. Survey of distressing symptoms in dying patients and their families in hospital and the response to a symptom control team, *British Medical Journal*, 1988, **296**, 1715–17.

MELZACK, R. 'The tragedy of needless pain,' *Scientific American*, 1990, **162**, 19–25.

O'BRIEN, T., KELLY, M. and SAUNDERS, C. 'Motor neurone disease: a hospice perspective,' *British Medical Journal*, 1992, **304**, 471–3.

PARKES, C.M. 'Terminal care: home, hospital, or hospice?' *Lancet*, 1985, i, 155–7.

PORTENOY, R.K. 'Chronic opioid therapy in nonmalignant pain,' *Journal of Pain and Symptom Management*, 1990, **5**, S46–62.

SCHUG, S.A., MERRY, A.F. and ACLAND, R.H. 'Treatment principles for the use of opioids in pain of nonmalignant origin,' *Drugs*, 1991, **42**, 228–39.

WILKES, E. 'Dying now', *Lancet*, 1984, i, 950–2.

Index